COACHING SCIENCE

COACHING SCIENCE
THEORY INTO PRACTICE

Terry McMorris and Tudor Hale
University of Chichester

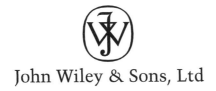

John Wiley & Sons, Ltd

Other Wiley Editorial Offices

John Wiley & Sons Inc., 111 River Street, Hoboken, NJ 07030, USA

Jossey-Bass, 989 Market Street, San Francisco, CA 94103-1741, USA

Wiley-VCH Verlag GmbH, Boschstr. 12, D-69469 Weinheim, Germany

John Wiley & Sons Australia Ltd, 42 McDougall Street, Milton, Queensland 4064, Australia

John Wiley & Sons (Asia) Pte Ltd, 2 Clementi Loop #02-01, Jin Xing Distripark, Singapore 129809

John Wiley & Sons Canada Ltd, 6045 Freemont Blvd, Mississauga, ONT, L5R 4J3

Wiley also publishes its books in a variety of electronic formats. Some content that appears in print may not
be available in electronic books.

Library of Congress Cataloging-in-Publication Data

applied for

British Library Cataloguing in Publication Data

A catalogue record for this book is available from the British Library

ISBN – 13 978 0-470-01097-6 (HB) ISBN – 13 978 0-470-01098-3 (PB)
ISBN – 10 0-470-01097-5 (HB) ISBN – 10 0-470-01098-3 (PB)

Typeset in 11/14pt Sabon by Thomson Digital
Printed and bound in Great Britain by Antony Rowe Ltd., Chippenham, Wiltshire
This book is printed on acid-free paper responsibly manufactured from sustainable forestry in which at least two
trees are planted for each one used for paper production.

Contents

Series Preface

One of the most astonishing cultural phenomena of the twentieth century has been the exponential growth in our knowledge and understanding of the importance of sport and exercise to human kind. At the beginning of that century, sport was principally a force for moral development, whilst strenuous exercise, though necessary to ensure military personnel were fit to engage in combat, was medically proscribed. The academic study of sport – what there was of it – was restricted largely to the history of the Olympic Games and philosophical arguments for the moral case for team games. A hundred years later, the picture is very different. 400 million people turn on their television sets to watch the Opening Ceremony of the Olympic Games and soccer's World Cup Final; millions of people jog, go to the gym, or work out in front of the television; and the academic study of sport embraces physics, chemistry, biology, biomechanics, physiology, psychology, politics, sociology, social anthropology, and business studies as well as history and philosophy. Over the last twenty years the number of degree courses in the academic study of sport and exercise has grown phenomenally, attracting students from a wide range of backgrounds. It is against this background that the new series *Wiley SportTexts* was conceived.

This new series provides a collection of textbooks in Sport and Exercise Science that is rooted in the student's practical experience of sport. Each book covers the theoretical foundations of the contributing disciplines from the natural, human, behavioural, and social sciences, and provides the theoretical, practical and conceptual tools needed for the rigorous academic study of sport. Individual texts focus on a specific learning stage from the various levels of under-graduate to post-graduate study.

The series adopts a student-centred, interactive, problem-solving approach to key issues, and encourages the student to develop autonomous learning strategies through self-assessment exercises. Each chapter begins with clear learning objectives and a concise summary of the key concepts covered. A glossary of important terms and symbols familiarises students with the language and conventions of the various academic communities studying sport. Worked examples and solutions to exercises together with a variety of formative and summative self-assessment tasks are also included, supported by key references in book, journal and electronic forms. A website is planned for the series, containing specific information on individual titles, supplementary information for lecturers, important developments in the academic study of sport, and links to other sites of interest.

Eventually, it is intended that the series provides a complete coverage of the mainstream elements of under- and post-graduate degrees in the study of sport.

Tudor Hale
Jim Parry
Roger Bartlett

Preface

When we began coaching we had little knowledge of the underlying scientific theories involved. We soon became aware that, unless we spent some time finding out about them, we were always going to be limited as coaches. Studying theory and then applying it in practice was not as simple as we imagined. Sometimes it was difficult to see where and how what the scientists had to say was relevant to us as coaches. The more we studied and coached, however, the more we became able to see the relevance of coaching theory. Sometimes things worked in reverse. Coaching practice led us to explore areas of science other than those recommended in the literature. We could see that a practice worked but had to find out how and why. This leads us to the purpose of this book. We are writing it in the hope that we can help you to shortcut many of the processes through which we had to go. We hope, however, that you will not simply accept our explanations and applications of science but develop your own.

In our journeys through the theory and practice of coaching, both of us have received a great deal of help from many individuals and we are very grateful to them. We do not intend to try to name them as we are sure that we will miss someone out. What we would like to say to you is that you must talk to other coaches and to sports scientists and listen to what they have to say. It won't always be correct but you can still learn a great deal. We have learned a lot from watching other coaches; coaches from all different types of sport, and from talking to sports scientists. We have been able to use other people's ideas in our coaching. It is one area in which 'plagiarism' is acceptable.

The book is primarily aimed at first and second level students working towards coaching science/studies and physical education degrees. It should, however, be useful to practising coaches and those studying for national governing body awards. We hope that it is also of use to anyone interested in coaching. The chapters in Parts I–IV are divided into a theoretical and research based first part followed by a section on practical implications. We have also tried to include as much sports-specific applied work as possible even in the theoretical aspects of the book. Part V deals totally with application and draws on all of the theory covered earlier.

The book is divided into five parts. The first part covers some of the socio-psychological factors affecting coaching. There is an abundance of sports psychology texts that examine these factors from the point of view of the sports psychologist, but in this book, we have tried to examine these issues from the coach's perspective. Part II looks at the psychology of skill acquisition. Again we have examined it from a coaching point of view. Moreover, we have tried to avoid the inclusion of research and theory based on many of the esoteric, laboratory based experiments often used in motor learning texts. It is not possible to completely avoid these, however. This highlights the fact that the link between theory and practice is still comparatively in its infancy and we hope that this book inspires some of you to carry out research in this area using ecologically valid research designs. This part of the book, and Parts IV and V, are written by Terry McMorris, who has a wealth of coaching experience in many sports, especially football, which he coached at every level from school-boy to full-time professional. Terry is Professor of Motor Behaviour at the University of Chichester.

Part III examines what the exercise physiologist has to say to the coach. What are the factors that limit performance? How do we get athletes fit? This part of the book was written by Tudor Hale, Professor Emeritus at the University of Chichester. Tudor has a wide range of coaching experience and was responsible for setting up the Sport UK Sports Science Support Programmes for the British Olympic boxing, cycling and sailing teams. These have been among the most successful of the British Sports Science Support Programmes over the years, with many gold, silver and bronze medals among them.

In Part IV, we look at some of the developmental factors affecting coaching. The emphasis is on coaching young people but we have not forgotten older athletes. As older people become fitter they are continuing to play sport for much longer than previous generations. Part V is a very practical based examination of how to integrate physical, technical, tactical and psychological training and practice. Much of it is based on Terry's experiences of having to coach a variety of sports with limited time and facilities. This is the reality for most coaches. However, our experiences, even when we have had more than adequate facilities and plenty of time, have led us to believe that there is a need to develop more and more integrated practices. After all, when you compete you do so as a complete individual. Your physical, motor and mental components interact with one another; therefore, why not practise like that?

In line with the other books in the Wiley SportText series, this book is written in a 'user friendly' way. It does not follow the conventions of academic texts. We have only used citations of authors' names when absolutely necessary. In most cases we have resorted to the phrase 'research has shown'. Those of you studying for degrees in physical education, sports coaching and sports science and/or studies will probably be expected to use a formal academic style of writing when completing assignments. You will need to be aware of your university's rules and regulations. It is normal practice to actually cite the names of the authors who have carried out the research. While academically this is correct, it can be 'off-putting' when reading a book and often spoils the flow. The editors of the Wiley series believe that, for beginners, a more friendly approach is necessary.

Also within the text we have introduced a number of tasks for you to complete. These vary greatly from the practical to actually just sitting down and thinking. They can be used by individuals but can also form the basis of discussions either formally, in a seminar, or informally among friends. You can go down the pub for a discussion and tell your tutors or parents that you are studying. In fact, you would be as long as you kept the alcohol consumption in check.

There are many people whom we would like to thank for their help in writing this book, in particular Celia Carden from Wiley. Both of us are more than grateful to Celia for her help, encouragement and patience. We would also like to thank colleagues in the School of Sport, Exercise and Health Sciences and the School of Physical Education at the University of Chichester, in particular Steve Fitzsimons for information about basketball and also for his photography skills; Paul Robinson for help and advice on hockey; Neal Smith and Mike Lauder for their comments on the biomechanical aspects of the book and John Kelly for help with photography. Thanks to the students who acted as models for the photographs. Finally, thanks to the many people whom we have coached over the years and the coaches whose ideas and practices we have 'stolen'. Without them we could never have written this book.

Terry McMorris
Tudor Hale

I

Socio-Psychological Factors

Introduction

This part of the book is concerned with some of the major socio-psychological factors that affect coaching. I have not, by any means, covered all of the factors. My aim is to highlight the major areas of concern to coaches. In the chapter on motivation, we examine not only athletes' motivations but also the motivation of coaches. The interaction between the athletes' motivation and the coach's in terms of intensity and direction may be very important in developing coach–athlete relations. Coach–athlete and athlete–athlete relationships are examined in Chapter 2. The importance of team cohesion is discussed in that chapter.

Chapter 3 examines the effect of anxiety on athlete performance. In particular, we look at how the coach can help the performer to overcome problems of anxiety. I have approached this problem from a coach's point of view rather than one of a sports psychologist. The inter-relationship between a coach and a sports psychologist is also discussed. While coaches' leadership styles are examined in Chapter 2, in Chapter 4 we look at the interaction between coaching and learning styles. I have seen few attempts to examine this interaction but I feel that it is an important one. In particular, we discuss whether or not it is possible for coaches to change their styles in order to accommodate the athletes.

Additional reading

Carron, A. V. and Hausenblas, H. A. (1998). *Group dynamics in sport*, 2nd edn. Fitness Information Technology: Morgantown, WV.

Weinberg, R. S. and Gould, D. (2003). *Foundations of sport and exercise psychology*, 3rd edn. Human Kinetics: Champaign, IL.

1

Motivation

Learning objectives

At the end of this chapter, you should

- know the difference between intrinsic and extrinsic motivation
- understand achievement motivation theory
- understand achievement goal theory
- know how coaches can develop their athletes' motivation.

Before discussing motivation, we need to provide a working definition. It is generally accepted that motivation describes the *direction, intensity and persistence of behaviour*. Direction refers to the types of activity that we choose to undertake. Intensity describes how hard we are willing to work at these activities or how much effort we are willing to put in. The length of time that we are willing to work at the task is termed persistence. Although intensity and persistence are related they do not refer to exactly the same process. Some individuals will work very intensely at a task but lack persistence – if things start to go badly they will give in, while others will continue to practise tasks for long periods of time but the intensity of the practice may be limited. Obviously the ideal to is to have both intensity and persistence. Examples of this abound in the world of sport. One of the best examples is Sir Steve

Coaching Science Terry McMorris and Tudor Hale
© 2006 John Wiley & Sons, Ltd

Redgrave, who put himself through an extremely gruelling training regime (intensity) for *four* Olympics (persistence).

Task 1 Assess your own intensity and persistence in your main sport. Try to be honest. Ask friends or family to assess you also. You can use a 1–5 scale with 1 as 'very little' and 5 as 'obsessed'.

Research has shown that motivation can be sub-divided into *intrinsic* and *extrinsic*. Intrinsic motivation refers to a desire to perform the activity for its own sake. Intrinsic motivation is thought to be related to our inherent need to demonstrate self-competence or self-efficacy. We enjoy performing the activity because, through it, we can demonstrate our self-worth. Extrinsic motivation, on the other hand, refers to the need for social recognition. We wish to compare ourselves to other performers. It is related to status. Extrinsically motivated people are interested in winning medals and other accolades.

Research examining the effect of the different types of motivation on performance and participation has tended to suggest that intrinsic motivation leads to greater intensity and persistence, especially when things do not go well. However, we are motivated *both* intrinsically and extrinsically. Winning competitions and receiving extrinsic rewards is very pleasant, even if one's motivation is primarily intrinsic. There is also an interaction between the two. One professional football player told me that he had enjoyed playing as a schoolboy and as a junior professional much more than he did as a senior professional. The need to win and the money involved had taken away some of the enjoyment that he had experienced when younger. The extrinsic motivation that is inherent in being a professional had affected his intrinsic motivation. Similar effects have been demonstrated in American football, where varsity footballers stated that they were less intrinsically motivated than they had been at high school. On the other hand, extrinsic motivation can lead to intrinsic motivation. Individuals who take up activities because they feel that they might win something or do so to impress a friend often find themselves becoming intrinsically motivated. The ability to get extrinsically motivated individuals to become intrinsically motivated is one that youth coaches need to possess.

Task 2 To what extent are you intrinsically and extrinsically motivated? What is the evidence for your claims?

Motivational theories

In this section, I outline some of the major theories related to motivation. These are by no means exhaustive. I have ignored theories, such as Zuckerman's sensation seeking theory, which are more concerned with direction than intensity and persistence. As we are studying coaching, we are more interested in intensity and persistence than direction. We assume that the athlete has chosen this sport for the right reasons. I accept that, with young children pressed into taking part in an activity by parents or peers, direction may be an issue. This is more of a topic for social psychology and physical education texts.

Achievement motivation theory

The achievement motivation theory of McClelland and Atkinson (see McClelland *et al.*, 1953) is built on the assumption that we have a *need to achieve (nAch)*. The intensity of one's nAch will depend on the interaction between a number of factors. The two most important are our *motive to succeed (Ms)* and *motive to avoid failure (Maf)*. The difference between Ms and Maf is further affected by the *probability of success (Ps)* that any situation brings. A person high in Ms and low in Maf will wish to undertake tasks that are difficult. There is no reward for these people in doing simple things. There has to be a challenge. An individual high in Ms and comparatively high in Maf, however, will choose moderately difficult tasks. They will keep away from the very difficult because Ps is too low, thus exposing them to the possibility of failure. They prefer moderately difficult tasks to easy ones because success in easy tasks will not satiate their Ms. Those individuals low in Ms and high in Maf will tend towards easy tasks because Ps is great, therefore little chance of failure.

Although this may appear to be concerned with direction of motivation it does affect intensity and persistence. Where Maf is high there is always the possibility that athletes will stay in low level competitions. They will not wish to take on greater challenges. I have seen this in amateur and semi-professional sports. Some players who are good in lower level competition will not move up to the next level even when they do well. It is also very prevalent in children's sport and it is here that coaches must try to get the children to reappraise their motivation. Those high in Maf are that way for some reason. As coaches, we need to find out what that reason is. It may be a personality factor or can be the effect of significant others, e.g. 'pushy' parents or peer pressure.

Another factor highlighted by McClelland and Atkinson is the fear of succeeding or *motive to fail (Mf)*. Mf occurs when, for some reason, the athlete is afraid to be successful. The person wishes to fail because that way they can remain in the background and so not look to differ from their peers. It is not as uncommon as one might think and is particularly prominent among adolescent girls. To many girls winning at sport is unfeminine and so it may help them to remain popular with their group of friends if they fail. Although I personally have not experienced this as a coach, I have seen it many times when I was a schoolteacher. I have even seen it with girls who were close to international standard. These girls withdrew from competition and even deliberately under-performed in class activities.

Task 3 *How would you evaluate your Ms and Maf? Do you know anyone who shows signs of Mf?*

Achievement goal theory

This theory has been developed for sport and particularly for children's participation in sport. It is derived from Nicholl's (1978) perceived ability theory, which was aimed at explaining motivation in education. To me, the theory is good at explaining behaviour in athletes of all ages and is particularly helpful to coaches when devising their strategies for training and competition. According to achievement goal theory, individuals are *task oriented* and *ego oriented*. Task orientated individuals are said to possess *mastery* motivation. These people are concerned with how well they perform a task. They wish to perform well for the sake of performing well. They do not compare themselves to others but to standards they set for themselves. This is intrinsic in nature. Ego oriented individuals are said to possess *competition* motivation. These people compare themselves to other people. Positions in leagues and rankings are very important. This is extrinsic.

At first glance it would appear that to be mastery motivated would be the better. However, closer observation shows that there are some problems with this kind of motivation. Mastery motivated individuals will demonstrate greater persistence and, to some extent, greater intensity but the latter is not always certain. They set their own standards and it does not follow that these standards are all that high. If they lose but are satisfied that they have achieved their own criteria, they will not see the need to increase effort and practice. On the other hand, the competition motivated individuals are more likely to 'drop out' if they cannot achieve a high position in the rankings. Defeat can have a negative effect. However, if they feel that extra practice will lead to winning next time, they may well demonstrate intensity of motivation. This will only last for a while, however. Further defeats will highlight their weak persistence. It should be remembered that we possess *both* mastery and competition motivation. The energies of those high in mastery and above average in competition motivation can be harnessed so that the person works hard at their skills and develops into an outstanding performer.

Task 4 To what extent are you mastery and competition motivated? How does this affect your behaviour?

Summary

Achievement motivation theory is based on the premise that we have a need to achieve and/or a need to avoid failure. This is not unlike one of the theories that we have not so far mentioned, namely Albert Bandura's (1977) *self-efficacy theory*. According to Bandura, we are motivated to demonstrate competence in one or more activities. We will take part in sports if we perceive ourselves as being competent in them. Experiencing success leads to the desire to continue working at a sport in order to achieve even more success. It is termed self-efficacy because people see the success as being due to their own efforts. This is not dissimilar to Robin Vealey's (1986) theory of *sport confidence*. Vealey believes that we possess an enduring trait called the *sport confidence-trait* (SC-trait). Those high in SC-trait are likely to perceive themselves as being competent in a variety of sports. Confidence in one's ability in a particular sport is termed *sport confidence-state* (SC-state). Achievement goal theory is also concerned with ideas of demonstrating competence, by mastery and/or competition. Indeed, all of the theories appear to be based around the need to demonstrate competence and/or avoid failure.

Practical implications

The first problem facing the coach is to determine the intensity and persistence of the motivations of their athletes. I am assuming that they have chosen to take part in the activity because their directional motivation has led them that way. It would also be useful for the coach to know whether the person is high or low in Ms and Maf and whether they are mostly mastery or competition motivated. There are questionnaires that can be used for this purpose (see Table 1.1 for a list of questionnaires), but most athletes are uneasy with filling in questionnaires for coaches. They have less of a problem with sports psychologists, but there is often a wariness concerning the reasons why the coach wants to know this information. It is therefore probably best if the coach simply observes the athletes' behaviour. Athletes will provide information

Table 1.1 Questionnaires for determining motivational type of athletes

Task and Ego in Sport Orientation Questionnaire (TEOSQ) (Duda, 1989)
Perception of Success Questionnaire (POSQ) (Roberts, 1993)
Sport Orientation Questionnaire (SOQ) (Gill, 1993)

about their motivation by what they do and what they have to say. The coach can find out the latter by talking to the athletes. These discussions can be casual or formal and in private or in team meetings.

Setting goals for the season (see Chapter 3 for a lengthier discussion of goal setting) can provide valuable information to the coach concerning the performers' motives. If they are competition motivated they will want outcome goals concerned with winning medals and championships. If they are mastery motivated they will want goals concerned with the development of skills and fitness. Those high in Maf will shy away from heavy competition, while those high in Ms and low in Maf will want to compete against the best. Allowing the athletes to partake in the goal setting will help to fulfil their need to demonstrate self-efficacy. By taking part in the goal setting process, the athletes perceive the goals as being theirs; therefore, success is down to them more than to the coach.

The main problem for the coach is changing the motivations of those athletes whose type of motivation is inappropriate. As we have seen, those highly competition motivated but with little interest in mastery are prone to drop out, while those high in mastery and low in competition are likely to perceive losing as less of a problem than the coach would like. Choosing the right goal can help this. The coach can try to get the competition motivated individuals to set some goals that are linked to mastery. It can be pointed out to them that they can only win if they are willing to develop their skills. Also, the coach can get competition motivated athletes to work at skill acquisition by introducing extrinsic rewards such as 'most improved athlete' or 'best trainer'. This use of extrinsic motivation can, and does, sometimes result in the athlete becoming intrinsically motivated. While the person may have set out to improve in order to demonstrate ability compared to others, they get satisfaction by simply demonstrating improvement to themselves. Similarly, the mastery motivated person can be persuaded that the real test of their mastery is how they perform against others. Knowledge of other aspects of the athlete's character can help the coach in his/her approach. With some mastery motivated individuals, whom I knew had a sense of responsibility to others, I pointed out that unless they were competitive they were letting their team-mates down. This, of course, will not work with everyone.

Many of the problems with motivation can be dealt with if the coach has a good relationship with the athlete. As we have seen, the performer has a need to demonstrate competence and some form of self-importance; i.e., they have to feel that success was due, at least partially, to their own efforts. Many, however, are also afraid of failure. These two factors together affect what Vealey would term SC-state or self-confidence in that activity at that moment in time. The coach needs to be ready to *praise* the athletes. This praise must be earned, however. Praise for something that has not been worked for is meaningless. Research has shown that unexpected praise is particularly useful. The athletes expect to be praised when they have just won a competition or achieved a goal, but praise for something that the athlete thought had gone unseen, e.g. a decoy run in basketball that led to a shot at basket for someone else, can have a major effect on self-confidence. If the coach is trying to alter an athlete's motivations they can make sure that they always praise activities that might lead to the individual altering their type of motivation. For the competition motivated athlete praise for practising hard, or praise for an unsuccessful but valiant attempt by an athlete high in Maf, may lead to a change in attitude.

One of the most effective ways of developing motivation in athletes is by the coach's own example. If the coach is enthusiastic it generally 'rubs off' onto the athletes. Coaches who encourage mastery of skills will tend to produce performers high in mastery motivation. Those who do not demonstrate fear of losing are less likely to produce athletes high in Maf. The opposite, of course, occurs. Coaches low in mastery motivation and high in competition motivation tend to enhance similar motivations in their athletes. Those coaches who constantly demonstrate their fear of losing will instil that into their athletes. We must not, however, think that all that the coach needs is to set a good example. Athletes have their own personalities and the coach is only one 'significant other' in their lives. With children, parents are more important than coaches. With adults, partners and friends can also be a factor. Nevertheless, the coach is an important influence and setting a good example is vital.

While changing an athlete's type of motivation over a period of time is difficult, there are many simple ways of affecting motivation in the short term. Many coaches put signs up around the changing rooms. These might emphasize an upcoming game or championship. They might show scenes concerning previous successes. Comments by opponents about the team's prowess, or alleged lack of it, can also be useful motivators. Some coaches use quotations from famous people about achieving success and working hard. The use of humour, especially cartoons, can be helpful. It is important that these signs and posters are changed quite frequently. Leaving the same ones up leads to the athletes actually seeing them but not perceiving them. With younger performers posters of star athletes or quotes about effort and ambition can be useful. The former football manager Brian Clough once took his players down a coal mine so that they could see the type of job they would have if they did not keep performing to the best of their ability.

One of the most negative parts of being a sports performer, especially for team games players, is training. Coaches can help to improve motivation to train in a variety of ways. The use of fitness testing at different stages in the season can be useful, especially if the results are displayed. They must, at least, be fed back to the individual athletes. Competitions between groups of athletes during training in the long and short term can help training to be more pleasurable. One coach I played for held competitions between the English and Scottish born players. No need for any further motivation. The use of a variety of training activities, rather than using the same drills day in day out and week in week out, can also be motivational. Even a simple change of venue, like going to train at the seaside or a trip to a foreign country, or bringing in a visiting coach or trainer for a day or two, can have the desired effect.

Task 5 *You are the coach of a team or group of athletes who are high in mastery motivation but comparatively low in competition motivation. How would you go about increasing the latter?*

Summary

Coaches can have a major effect on the motivation of their athletes by the example that they themselves set. Mastery motivated coaches tend to produce mastery motivated athletes while competition motivated players often come from groups coached by individuals with the same type of motivation. The ideal appears to be someone highly mastery motivated but also having a fairly high competition motivation. Coaches can develop this kind of athlete by judicial use of goal setting and by subtle use of praise. The mastery motivated athlete can be led to see the advantages of competition and how it can help improve mastery, while the competition motivated athlete can be shown that mastery is necessary if one is to demonstrate competence. Similarly, coaches can show athletes that Ms can only be achieved if we can eliminate our Maf. Coaches who allow their athletes to try things and who are slow to criticize when things go wrong tend to produce athletes low in Maf.

Key points

- motivation describes the direction, intensity and persistence of behaviour
  - direction refers to choice of activity
  - intensity refers to how hard the person is willing to work
  - persistence refers to the length of time that the person is willing to work at the activity

- motivation can be intrinsic and extrinsic
  - intrinsic motivation is a desire to perform the activity for its own sake
  - extrinsic motivation refers to the need for social recognition
  - intrinsically motivated individuals tend to have greater intensity and persistence than extrinsically motivated individuals
  - extrinsically motivated people are more likely to drop out than intrinsically motivated individuals, especially if they are not successful

- achievement motivation theory refers to the need to achieve (nAch)
  - the intensity of one's nAch is dependent on the interaction between motive to succeed (Ms), motive to avoid failure (Maf) and the probability of success (Ps)
  - people high in Ms and low in Maf like tasks with low Ps
  - a person high in Ms and high in Maf will choose tasks with moderate Ps
  - people low in Ms but high in Maf will choose tasks where Ps is high
  - some individuals have a motive to fail (Mf)

- according to achievement goal theory individuals are task or ego oriented
  - task oriented individuals possess mastery motivation
  - ego oriented people are competition motivated
  - mastery motivated people tend to show greater persistence than competition motivated individuals
  - competition motivated people tend to drop out more than mastery motivated individuals

- according to self-efficacy theory, we are motivated to demonstrate competence

- according to sport confidence theory, some individuals are high in sport confidence trait (SC-trait)
  - those high in SC-trait are likely to demonstrate sport confidence state (SC-state) in several sports
  - some people are high in SC-state in only one or two activities

- coaches can manipulate motivation by
  - setting mastery or competition goals
  - ensuring that their athletes achieve some success in practice and competition
  - providing praise to their athletes
  - setting an example in which the right attitudes are shown

- mastery motivated coaches tend to produce mastery motivated athletes and competition motivated coaches tend to produce competition motivated athletes.

2

Leadership and Cohesion

Learning objectives

At the end of this chapter, you should

- understand what we mean by cohesion
- understand the difference between task and social cohesion
- understand the factors that affect cohesion
- understand the nature of leadership
- understand how coaches can develop cohesion
- be aware of the major ethical issues facing coaches.

When examining cohesion, we normally think of the inter-relationship between team members, and that of coaches and teams. In this chapter, we will also examine the relationship between the coach and athlete in individual sports. Furthermore, we discuss how leadership styles affect these relationships. The first part of the chapter is concerned with team or group cohesion. Before we examine what we mean by team cohesion, it is necessary to identify exactly what we mean by teams. To most of us when we talk of teams we mean those groups taking part in what have been described as '*interactive sports*'. Interactive sports are those in which the players cooperate in a coordinated way to produce performance. They

Coaching Science   Terry McMorris and Tudor Hale
© 2006 John Wiley & Sons, Ltd

are mostly *invasion* sports, such as football, rugby, American football and basketball. The *team* attacks and defends. *Everyone is working together against everyone in the opposition.* The team wins or loses. Individuals can play well or badly but the result is a purely team affair. This is different to *co-active sports*, such as golf, lawn bowls and tenpin bowling. In these sports *individuals play against one another*. The team result is a combination of all of the individual scores. An individual can win or lose as well as the team winning or losing. The player does not have to cooperate with a team-mate during the competition. In fact, these sports can be, and are, played purely as individual sports.

A third type of sport is one in which interaction and co-action both occur. The best examples of this are cricket and baseball. When fielding the cricketers and baseball players must work interactively. When batting, they act like a co-acting team. However, the result is a team affair not an individual one. The effect of cohesion is far greater in the interactive and interactive/co-active combined sports than in the purely co-active. From a performance perspective, the aim of coaches in these activities is to ensure that *the sum of the whole is greater than the sum of the parts*. In teams that are well organized strengths are accentuated and weaknesses are hidden. Moreover, the composition of the team is balanced. Cricket teams have fast bowlers and spin bowlers; baseball sides have right handed batters, left handed batters and switch-hitters. Football teams have defensively minded midfield players and attacking midfield players. Our interest in this chapter, however, is more with the interpersonal relationship between team members than their technical abilities.

> **Task 1** *Answer this question before reading the rest of the chapter. How important do you think cohesion is in interactive, co-active and mixed interactive/co-active sports? Check your answers again after reading the chapter. Have you changed your mind?*

As well as understanding what we mean by the term 'team', we need also to know what we mean by team cohesion. Albert Carron (1984) described team cohesion as being 'a dynamic process that is reflected in the group's tendency to stick together while pursuing its goals and objectives'. He divided team cohesion into *group integration* and *individual attraction*. Group integration refers to the way in which the group operates as a whole. Individual attraction explains how being a member of the group satisfies the needs of the individual and team. Carron further sub-divided each component into *task* and *social* aspects. Task aspects are concerned with the way the team performs, while social aspects refer to the rapport between team members.

Individuals differ in what they perceive as being the most important factors, depending on their motivation and personality. People with personality types that are independent will perceive social aspects as not being very important. Those high in dependence will view them as being vital. Similarly, those high in Ms will wish to join teams that are high in task cohesion and may care little about social cohesion. Most performers will perceive all of the factors as having some relevance.

> **Task 2** *How important is cohesion to you? Is task cohesion more important than social, as far as you are concerned? How are your answers to these questions affected by your motivation type and personality?*

Carron and his colleagues have identified a number of factors that are thought to determine the nature of cohesiveness. Task cohesion requires that the team members know their roles (*role clarity*), accept their roles and those of others in the team (*role acceptance*) and are able to perform their roles well (*role performance*). This, of course, would ensure that the sum of the parts was greater than the sum of the whole. The word teamwork may well describe these qualities. Probably the factor most likely to cause a lack of cohesion would be role acceptance. If an athlete feels that he/she is worthy of a more important role this could cause disharmony.

On the social side, cohesiveness appears to depend on a sense of belonging to the group and valuing that belongingness. In other words, the athlete must believe that it is worth being a part of the team. It appears that this sense of belonging is helped if the group is relatively stable, in other words turnover of players is low. How well team members are willing to conform also affects the level of cohesiveness.

The level of cohesiveness will be affected by the pressure placed on each of the factors outlined above. We have already mentioned how a failure to accept one's role might affect cohesion. The inability of one or more team members to perform their roles adequately can disrupt task cohesion. Similarly, if players are unsure as to what is required of them, with regard to performance, cohesion will be affected. I am writing this shortly after the death of the great Dutch football coach Rinus Michels. Among the many comments made about Michels' coaching, I noticed that several of his former players pointed to the fact that they always fully understood what he wanted from them. This was said as a compliment and as an explanation for his success.

Role acceptance can come not only through one's perception of one's own worth but can also be related to tactics. If players perceive tactics as being inadequate or unsuitable, role acceptance will be compromised. Team selection issues can also affect role acceptance. By this I am not only talking about how non-starters perceive selection but how starters perceive it. If the majority of starters see one or two other starters as not being able to fulfil their role performance (in other words, they are not good enough) this will cause problems.

On the social side, research shows that players who are homogenous tend to behave cohesively. This will be affected by the group size. In large groups, it is difficult to have homogeneity. In large groups, one tends to get sub-groups. This is fine as long as they do not become cliques. I played for one football team where there were large differences in age between two sub-groups. There was no problem, however, as each group respected the other. Socially we did not particularly wish to mix because we had different interests. On the other hand, I played for another team that was split into a sub-group of ex-professionals and a group of amateurs. These two groups, in effect, became cliques. There was a great deal of disharmony and each blamed the other for defeats. Interestingly, the former team was successful while the latter was not.

As we have seen above, age and playing background can affect inter-relationships. The list of what can disrupt or aid cohesion is almost endless. Table 2.1 shows some possible factors. They are by no means exhaustive. We should not see these problems as being insurmountable. During the worst years of the recent 'Troubles' in Northern Ireland the national football team managed to perform cohesively despite being made up of Catholics and Protestants. In the former Yugoslavia the national sports teams performed admirably and Serbs, Croats and Muslims worked cohesively.

The most important factor affecting team cohesion, however, is *success*. Most coaches aim to get cohesion in order to achieve success. There is some evidence to say that cohesion can lead to success. It is most likely to be task

Table 2.1 Factors affecting group cohesion

Factor	Effect
Success level	Success leads to cohesion
Size of group	Smaller groups are more cohesive
Leadership style of coach	Coaches can enhance role clarity: self-efficacy: a sense of belonging
Motivation types	Homogeneity leads to better cohesion
Social class	Homogeneity leads to better cohesion
Personality type	Athletes with a desire for power can disrupt coach–athlete cohesion
Gender of athletes	Males and females differ in their preference of leadership styles and need for democracy within the group
Age	Children have different needs to adults

cohesion. However, the majority of the evidence suggests that success leads to cohesion. While this may appear to be obvious, if we compare it with other parts of life it is not so straightforward. As we see in wartime, cohesion often comes from people seeing themselves as victims or as being in some form of danger. So one might think that sports teams would 'rally round' when they were having a hard time and work together to improve their situation. This does not appear to be the case.

Task 3 *Look at Table 2.1. Can you think of any other factors that might affect cohesion?*

Leadership

One of the main factors involved in team cohesion is the interaction between the coach and the team. This is generally studied under the title *leadership*. Barrow (1977) described leadership as being 'the behavioral (sic) process of influencing individuals and groups toward set goals'. House's (1971) *path–goal theory of leadership* puts forward a very similar viewpoint. House sees the role of the leader as being to provide the athletes with the necessary support to achieve their goals. According to House, there are four different styles – *directive, supportive, achievement oriented* and *participative*. Directive refers to the giving of instructions and orders, while supportive leadership is concerned with helping the team members towards their goals. Achievement-oriented leaders place the emphasis on outcomes. Participative leaders are more interested in the taking part. House believes that the key is to use the most appropriate leadership style for any given situation. This is not unlike Fielder's (1967) *contingency model of situational control*. The difference is that Fiedler believes that individuals cannot alter their leadership styles, while House thinks that they can adopt different styles.

The best known theory of leadership in sport is Packianathan Chelladurai's (see Chelladurai and Saleh, 1978) *multidimensional model of leadership*. Chelladurai identifies five leadership styles or types of behaviour – *training and instruction behaviour, democratic behaviour, autocratic behaviour, social support behaviour* and *rewarding behaviour*. Leaders demonstrating training and instruction behaviour are similar to those using House's achievement-orientated behaviour. They are interested in developing skills, tactics and teamwork. With regard to developing team cohesion their major strength is that they clarify role orientation. Athletes with such leaders tend to be strong on role acceptance because roles are normally explained clearly. Those demonstrating democratic behaviour normally strengthen cohesion though a sense of belonging and having responsibility. Autocratic behaviour refers to independent decision making by the coach. This should also aid task cohesion as role clarity is normally straightforward. However, role acceptance may be compromised because it is dictated from above. Social support behaviour and rewarding behaviour should both improve social cohesion, although the latter can also aid task cohesion if the reward is related to task factors.

Chelladurai argued that comparison between three factors – *prescribed behaviour*, *actual behaviour* and *preferred behaviour* – would affect athlete performance and athlete satisfaction. Prescribed behaviour refers to what the sporting sub-group, in that particular activity, would expect of a coach. A basketball coach is expected to behave differently to a cricket coach. The latter has much less to do with tactics and decisions during the game because the sub-culture of cricket expects this to be the role of the captain. Preferred leader behaviours are what the athletes would like to see. Research has shown that the closer the relationship between preferred behaviours and actual behaviours, what Chelladurai termed *congruence*, the better the chance of good performance and high athlete satisfaction.

> **Task 4** Which type of leadership style do you prefer when you are the athlete? Is this different to when you are the coach? How does your personality affect the answers to these two questions?

Theories of developing cohesion

Perhaps the best known theory of developing cohesion is that of Tuckman (1965). Like all cohesion theorists, he sees cohesion as being dynamic in nature. To Tuckman, cohesion develops linearly through a process of *forming, storming, norming* and *performing*. The forming stage is, as it says, the beginnings of the process. Team members get to know one another and the group's goals. The storming stage is one of some disruption, with conflict and even rebellion. The norming stage is characterized by the members becoming aware of one another's strengths and weaknesses. In this stage, the disruption slowly dissipates and some form of cohesion is developed. There is co-operation between members. In the performing stage, the team works as a unit to achieve its goals.

Opposed to the linear type model of Tuckman are the *pendular* models, which state that the level of cohesion fluctuates, or swings backwards and forwards, between cohesion and disharmony. Whether the group is feeling united or disunited will depend on the level of conflict between the individuals' goals and the team's goals. Individuals trying out for a team and competing against one another for a place will not show team cohesion. Once the team has been selected, they will begin to work together to achieve their joint goals.

Coach–individual athlete interaction

So far, we have dealt with cohesion between athletes in teams, and coaches and athletes in a team situation. However, the coach–athlete relationship in individual sports is equally important. All of the factors outlined in the above sections apply to the coach–athlete relationship in individual sports. However, there are some specific problems in individual activities. This coach–athlete interaction is often referred to as the coach–athlete dyad. Horne and Carron (1985) examined what they termed *coach–athlete compatibility*. Horne and Carron followed the ideas proposed by Schutz (1966) with regard to relation orientation-behaviour. Schutz identified three positive factors – *affection*, *control* and *inclusion*. Affection refers to how close the two people feel with regard to their relationship. Control is concerned with power, dominance and authority, while inclusion concerns communication between the two and the level of interaction in such factors as decision making. Horne and Carron found that, where there was a sense of inclusion, both the athlete and coach felt as though they were compatible. That does not mean that affection and control were not important, just that inclusion was the major factor.

More recently, Sophia Jowett and colleagues have put forward a model of coach–athlete relationships. Using a method of research called factor analysis, they highlighted three main areas – *closeness*, *commitment* and *complementarity*. Closeness is similar to Schutz's affection and refers to 'feeling emotionally close with one another' (Jowett and Ntoumanis, 2004). This means such things as feeling liked and valued. Complementarity is similar to Schutz's inclusion. It refers to whether or not coach and athlete interact in the making of decisions, particularly regarding training. The third dimension, commitment, refers to the coach's and athlete's intention to continue their relationship. Jowett has also argued that a fourth dimension, *co-orientation*, exists, although her factor analysis failed to identify this mathematically. Jowett has defined co-orientation as representing the shared beliefs and goals of the athlete and coach. This is not vastly dissimilar to her notion of commitment. This theory is only in its infancy and more research is necessary to support Jowett's claims.

Ethics

One of the most important responsibilities of any coach is the adoption of a code of ethics, which will underlie their relationships with their athletes. It is not the role of a coaching science book to examine the philosophical development of such a code but it is important that we are aware of the practical implications of the ethical approach that we adopt. One's coaching philosophy, and hence one's code of ethics, will be determined by many factors. The law of the land and the rules of the particular sport will have a major effect but perhaps of greater importance is one's own set of moral principles. As we all know, laws and rules can be broken or not adhered to. This is especially so if our own moral values differ from those of the government or sport ruling body. Many coaches who advise their athletes to use drugs do not see anything wrong with this. To them the rules are due to petty bureaucracy, or the coach takes an 'everyone is doing it' approach. This latter mentality comes about from a 'winning is everything' philosophy. This philosophy is often referred to as the Lombardi approach or ethic, after the American football coach Vince Lombardi. This is unfair on Lombardi, as his statement was taken out of context and his own behaviour as a coach does not support such an ethos.

Although I have stated that the coach's own philosophy of life will have a major effect on his or her coaching code of ethics, the American social psychologist Brenda Jo Bredermeier (see, e.g., Bredermeier and Shields, 1986) has highlighted a phenomenon that she calls 'games reasoning'. Bredermeier noted that many individuals perceive sport as being separate from 'normal' life. The normal rules of behaviour do not necessarily apply but rather the unwritten conventions of the sport. We see this, in particular, with the so-called 'professional foul' in football. Many coaches see fouling someone in order to stop him or her from scoring as part of the game. Indeed, a player who does not foul the opponent and lets him or her score is likely to be dropped from the team. The same coaches, however, would not defend deliberately hurting a player through a vicious tackle. Similar practices can be seen in most sports. Many Rugby Union coaches teach their front row forwards to deliberately collapse the scrum, something not only illegal but also dangerous. A friend, teaching physiology on a Canadian National Coaching Certification Program course, told me that one of the ice hockey coaches in the class spent most of his time trying to get a boxing coach to give him some tips that he could pass on to his players when they got into a fight during an ice hockey game. If you have a 'win at all costs' mentality, your code of ethics will be insensitive to cheating. At best this will mean that you will accept minor rule infringements, while at worst you are likely to promote the use of drugs and violence that can maim.

A 'grey area' for coaches is the use of 'gamesmanship'. Gamesmanship refers to following the letter of the law but not necessarily the spirit of the law. Many coaches see nothing wrong with this, although they are often quick to criticize when it is done to them. Personally, I do not like gamesmanship. Moreover, I am far from convinced that it works very often. It is very likely to backfire. Some tactical decisions are sometimes called gamesmanship. For example, a tennis player who knows that his/her opponent likes to 'get on with the game' might deliberately take time between serves. I think the morality of this depends on how far one goes. If you simply make sure that you do things in your own time and are not rushed that appears to me to be good play. Stopping to wipe your racket every two minutes is ridiculous. It is also likely to disrupt you as much as your opponent.

Ethical issues in sport

In this section, I will highlight some of the major ethical issues that coaches face today. Tragically I have to state that sexual abuse is an ethical issue in many sports. That sexual abuse, particularly of minors, is unacceptable in all societies goes without saying. However, there are some areas that some coaches may feel are not 'black and white'. Most sport governing bodies frown on sexual relationships between coaches and athletes, even if they are adults and consenting. The rationale behind this is that the coach is in a privileged position, which brings the consent into some doubt. This is not an issue limited to sport alone. Any employer–employee or boss–worker relationships have the same problem. Most businesses and organizations, like the sports governing bodies, frown on such relationships. Of course, there are some husband–wife coach–athlete relationships. In most cases they were married before joining up as coach and athlete, although not always.

Two other areas that are also obviously wrong are racial and religious discrimination. These can be problems in team sports with regard to team selection. Some of this comes about simply through bigotry but often it can be due to racial stereotyping. It is not many years since almost all black football players in England played in wide positions because they were considered not have the tactical acumen to play in so-called 'key positions'. This practice, known as '*stacking*' in the United States, is less prevalent today, but does exist in some teams.

We have already mentioned the 'win at all costs' mentality and how it promotes cheating, including drug taking. The latter is a major issue in many sports. A defence put forward by many coaches for advocating the use of drugs is that they do not really do any harm if used properly. This is a common argument for the use of many steroids. Some coaches perceive the use of drugs that allow shortened recovery periods in training as acceptable because the athlete still has to do the work. Coaches who go along with this line of reasoning should be very careful because we are limited in our knowledge of the side-effects of many drugs, particularly if they are taken for long periods of time.

The issues we have dealt with so far are fairly straightforward; however, there are some ethical problems that are less obvious. It is obvious to most people that coaches who hit their athletes are in breach of human rights. However, there are many other forms of physical abuse that are less obvious. Coaches who get athletes to perform when they have injuries often cause many problems. The overuse of pain killing drugs can result in major injuries. I know a number of physiotherapists in football who tell me that they have been put under considerable pressure to declare a player fit enough to play when in fact he was not. We must also be careful in having performers continue when injured. The temptation to leave a performer playing following a head injury, which may have resulted in concussion, is too great for some coaches. Such action can never be condoned. You are literally risking that player's life. Even lesser injuries may have long term consequences. In the 1966 World Cup the Brazilian superstar Pelé suffered a knee injury while playing against Portugal. Pelé begged for a pain killing injection so that he could continue playing. The Brazilian doctor and coach refused despite the fact that this meant that the unanimously recognized greatest player in the world would be lost to them. The doctor knew that this was a serious injury and wanted to ensure damage limitation. How many other coaches and doctors would have taken that attitude?

Abuse can also be mental and/or verbal. Many coaches like to belittle their athletes. Some coaches argue that this is necessary to force them to obey orders but one is left wondering the extent to which it is more a way of showing their own power. Coaches should be particularly careful how they talk to the press about their players. I have seen many coaches, particularly those whose jobs may be in question because of poor results, put the blame on the players to take the pressure off themselves. I have even seen coaches of individual athletes blame their performer. I accept that with some very egotistical athletes public criticism may be necessary but very rarely so. What the coach says to the press and what they say in private may be very different. Another form of mental abuse is not speaking to the athlete. Athletes performing badly are sometimes totally ignored by the coach. This can have a major effect on the athlete's self-confidence and self-esteem. I feel that this way of behaving is very childish.

When you ask athletes what they admire most in a coach the word 'honesty' is probably the most commonly heard. Coaches who 'play games' by telling lies to players are soon found out. They become mistrusted not just by the athlete to whom the lies were told but also to those who witnessed the fact. Honesty and fairness from those in positions of authority over us are characteristics we all admire. If athletes perceive the coach as being honest and fair they will accept decisions even if they think that the coach is wrong. If the coach is perceived as having favourites or being inconsistent, coach–athlete cohesion is jeopardized.

Coaches have a responsibility to their opponents. They should learn to win graciously. Being magnanimous in victory is not difficult. Similarly, when they lose they should be slow to complain about the officials, the weather, state of the pitch or track and saying that the opposition were lucky. You may well think those things but in public that is not the attitude to take. I am writing this in the middle of the football season in England. I have just seen a number of coaches of losing teams blame refereeing decisions. I agree that the decisions were poor but so was the defending. The coaches would be better employed looking at the weaknesses in their defences rather than blaming the referee.

In this section, I have refrained from preaching to you. Personally, I hope that you will opt for very high ethical standards. Without such standards your sport is likely to suffer. I also believe that some unethical actions are tactically counterproductive. Take the professional foul in football. It is not unusual to see an attacker fouled in the penalty area when he/she has only the goalkeeper to beat. This results in a penalty. So the opposition can call on their best penalty taker and the goalkeeper has to stay on the goal line. Had the attacker not been fouled, the keeper would have left the line to narrow the angle. Furthermore, more often than not the attacker in possession was less likely to score than a specialist penalty taker.

Summary

It is natural to assume that cohesion is important and even necessary in teams. Moreover, one would expect social cohesion to be the more important. Research, however, shows that social cohesion plays little, if any, part in success as measured by performance. It does not appear to be necessary for players to like one another. What is important, however, is task cohesion. Athletes need to know their roles; understand the roles of others; accept their roles and those of others; accept the type of leadership used by the coach and agree with the goals set and probably have had some part to play in the setting of those goals. However, there appears to be something of a circular effect between success and task cohesion. Success leads to greater task cohesion, while task cohesion can lead to success. It would appear that the move from success to task cohesion is stronger than the other way round.

This is not to say that social cohesion has no value. There is some evidence to show that teams high in social cohesion get a great deal of satisfaction in attempting to perform well. It would appear that, to some extent, good social cohesion can make up for a lack of success in terms of outcome. One must be cautious with this statement because the evidence is limited. It may well be greatly affected by the players' motivational types and personalities. It may also be affected by the level of competition. For amateurs, social cohesion may be more important than task cohesion but for professionals this cannot be the case because of the nature of their job. The aggressive, success chasing, type A personality individual will also be much less likely to perceive social cohesion as meaning very much. One of the main problems with regard to cohesion is where the athletes in a team differ from one another in their perception of the importance of task and social cohesion. This can be particularly important in teams where the players spend a great deal of the time 'on the road'. If some players perceive a need for the team to socialize while others want to be 'left alone', there is the potential for conflict.

Leadership also appears to affect team cohesion. The major factor appears to be whether there is a discrepancy between the style of leadership preferred by the athletes and the actual style of the coach. The problem is exacerbated by the fact that the coach's actual style is often different to what they imagine. While different personalities and motivational types will prefer different types of coach, we can generalize to some extent. Those athletes performing in inter-active sports are more likely than those in coactive teams to prefer coaches who use training and instruction behaviour. This is probably because such teams need to be well organized. There are, however, gender differences as well. Males prefer an autocratic style of leadership. Females prefer a democratic coach enjoying the input of all members in the group. Males also prefer more social support from the coach. This may be to make up for their lack of say in decision making due to the preference for an autocratic leadership style.

Practical implications

For a coach taking over a new team, the first stage is to determine the actual level of team cohesion at that moment in time. This can be done by the use of questionnaires (see Table 2.2 for a list of possible questionnaires). Athletes are

Table 2.2 Questionnaires that can be used to determine level of cohesion

Sports Cohesiveness Questionnaire (SCQ) (Martens and Peterson, 1971)
Team Cohesion Questionnaire (TCQ) (Gruber and Gray, 1981)
Sport Cohesion Instrument (DCI) (Yukelson *et al.*, 1984)
Group Environment Questionnaire (GEQ) (Widmeyer *et al.*, 1990)

likely to complete such questionnaires honestly if they are anonymous. This, however, is not the only way to monitor team cohesion. Coaches can hold team meetings and discuss cohesion matters, particularly those of task cohesion. It is important to remember that cohesion does not mean 100 per cent agreement. Burke and Collins (1996) point out that conflict can be good and can, if handled properly, lead to an improvement in task cohesion. If the coach is not happy dealing with such conflict him/herself, a sports psychologist can be called in. Coaches can also use assistant coaches and captains to help them be aware of any cohesion issues.

Most teams have rules concerning team conduct pre-, during and post-competition. These matters range from minor points, such as dress code for travel to and from venues, to major factors such as discipline during competition. Coaches are advised to devise these rules in conjunction with the athletes. Performers who perceive the rules as belonging to themselves, rather than being imposed on them by the coach and team management, adhere to the rules more readily. Some teams also have fun type regulations such as a small fine for making minor errors. This money can be collected by one of the players and used for an end of season social event. Coaches should make sure that these are for minor actions, e.g. being voted the worst performer during a training session.

Along with the setting of rules we can include goal setting in teams as a way of developing team cohesion. Individual goals are useful in helping to develop the desired type of motivation and controlling anxiety. The same applies to team goals. Team goals must be set by the whole team for the athletes to consider them as being theirs. Coaches, of course, can include the right to veto any aspect that they feel is unacceptable. Good coaches will structure the discussion to make sure that nothing is decided that they cannot accept.

While the above measures are more concerned with task than social cohesion, a popular method of trying to develop the latter is the use of 'bonding' exercises. These can be such as going away to a training camp, taking part in an outdoor adventure week or simply going out together for a meal. The literature in adventure education tends to be strongly supportive of adventure activities;

however, it is far from being unequivocal. I have seen such bonding exercises backfire. Similarly, while social evenings can be fun and useful they can also lead to a drink culture within a team, which is not conducive to fitness.

Bonding exercises away from the home environment, however, can allow the coach and coaching staff to observe relationships more closely than they can at home, when players 'disappear' after training and games. Coaches can determine whether there are any cliques or not. They can also see who the leaders are among the players. Formal leaders, e.g. captains, may not be the informal leaders to whom the athletes look for advice and whose example they follow. These informal leaders may or may not have a good effect on team cohesion and coach–team relationships. The presence of leaders who are disruptive can cause a lack of cohesion. One head coach, for whom I worked, decided to release his best player at the end of the season. When I asked him why, he said that the player was a disruptive influence in the dressing room. He continuously questioned the coach's decisions and, on some occasions, had deliberately ignored the coach's instructions and led others to do the same.

While informal leaders have an effect on cohesion so too do formal leaders. Formal leaders can include assistant coaches. Some head coaches deliberately use their assistants as 'sounding boards' for the players; in other words, they encourage athletes to go to the assistants with their complaints. These are then passed on to the head coach, without any names being used. Team captains can also be used in this way. This will only work if the athletes trust the assistants and the captain. The choice of captains is a very important factor. One of the best coach–captain relationships was that of the England Rugby Union World Cup winning coach Sir Clive Woodward and his captain Martin Johnson. Their task cohesion was almost 100 per cent and the team's record speaks for itself. The relationship between Woodward and Johnson worked because not only was there mutual respect between the coach and captain, there was also respect for the captain from the other athletes. The team readily accepted Johnson as captain. The whole idea of role acceptance is crucial to cohesion. Role acceptance, however, only occurs when there is clear role identification and the players feel that the individuals are capable of carrying out their roles. Role identification can be as simple as giving someone a position in a team, e.g. someone is a starting pitcher in baseball or an opening bowler in cricket. However, sometimes, particularly with younger performers in interactive team games, role identification is not so readily clear. The players need to know the value of one another to the team. Coaches must not only praise individuals but also do so in the presence of the other players. It may be necessary to point out exactly what an individual has done to deserve the praise. The hockey defender who works hard in an unglamorous role may need the coach to explain to team members what he/she had actually done for the team. This is generally not necessary with experienced players but can be crucial with youngsters, whose knowledge of the activity is not all that great.

Most of what we have been discussing, so far, is intrinsically related to performance and task cohesion. However, more extrinsic factors have a role to play. Most athletes like the idea of a team uniform for pre- and post-game occasions, e.g. team tracksuits and blazers. Squad photographs clearly shown in prominent places within the training and competition environments also aid the feeling of belonging.

So far, we have been talking about how the coach can develop cohesion between team members. We must not, however, forget how coaches can influence cohesion between themselves and their athletes. This may be in a dyad or a coach–team relationship. Figure 2.1 shows the kinds of factor that the coach must consider. It is obvious that the personalities of the coach and his/her athletes will interact but the problem facing coaches is whether they can

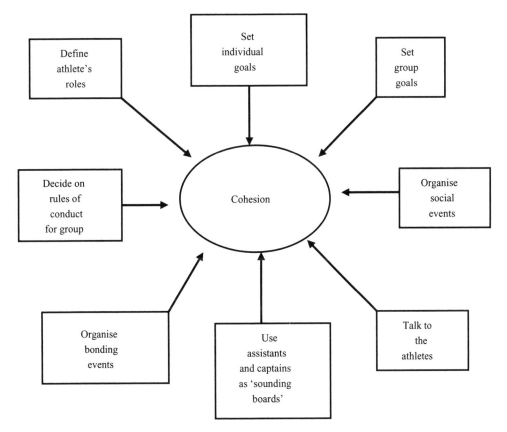

Figure 2.1 How the coach can affect cohesion

adapt to the personalities of the performers. In order to do this, the coach must be realistic and decide to what extent they actually would wish to change. Communication between coaches and athletes can lessen the effects of personality clashes. Acceptance of one another's failings and idiosyncrasies can improve cohesion. With one swimming team with which I worked as a sports psychologist, the coach had a high need for control. Unfortunately, so did one of the swimmers. By discussing this fact, both were able to see the other's point of view. They then came to a compromise over how training schedules were decided. Neither was fully satisfied, as both wanted full control, but they were able to achieve a working harmony. More importantly, the swimmer improved his times and went on to win several medals.

Different tasks will affect the way in which the coach must act. For example, a field hockey coach interested in technique, tactics and teamwork will probably take a more task oriented approach than a coach of a 800 m runner. The latter is more likely to be concerned with increasing self-confidence in the athlete, although tactics will be a factor. Similarly, the situation will have an effect on the choice of leadership style. A successful team or individual is unlikely to need too much in the way of social support, while a less successful team may need a great deal of confidence building and, hence, a coach demonstrating rewarding behaviour and social support behaviour.

It is, of course, very easy to say these things and to point out which problems require the coach and/or athlete to change their normal pattern of behaviour. Actually doing that is much more difficult. Some people find it very difficult to suppress behaviour that is natural to them. Some do not wish to do so under any circumstances. Coaches must be honest with their athletes about what they see as open to compromise and what they will not alter. It may be that some coaches and athletes have to agree to go their separate ways.

Task 6 *You have just taken over as coach to a team that is noted for its poor cohesion. How would you set about improving task and social cohesion?*

Key points

- sport can be interactive, co-active or a mixture of both
  - in interactive sports, players cooperate in a coordinated way in order to defeat their opponents
  - in co-active sports, individual team members play against individuals from the other team but the result is decided by a combination of the scores of the team members

♦ sports such as cricket and baseball include interactive and co-active elements

- cohesion is 'a dynamic process that is reflected in the group's tendency to stick together while pursuing its goals and objectives' (Carron, 1984)

- cohesion can be divided into group integration and individual attraction
  ♦ group integration refers to the way in which the group operates as a whole
  ♦ individual attraction refers to the way in which being a member of the group satisfies the needs of the individual and the team

- cohesion can be divided into task and social
  ♦ task cohesion refers to the group working together in order to perform well
  ♦ social cohesion refers to the rapport between group members

- team cohesion is dependent on
  ♦ role clarity – team members knowing their roles
  ♦ role acceptance – team members accepting their roles and those of others
  ♦ role performance – the ability of team members to perform their roles

- success affects team cohesion and cohesion affects success
  ♦ success tends to affect cohesion more than the other way round
  ♦ task cohesion appears to be more important than social

- leadership refers to 'the behavioral (*sic*) process of influencing individuals and groups towards set goals' (Barrow, 1977)

- according to path–goal theory, there are four types of leadership, namely directive, supportive, achievement-oriented and participative
  ♦ directive refers to leaders giving instructions and orders
  ♦ supportive leaders help team members to achieve their goals
  ♦ achievement-oriented leaders are interested in outcomes
  ♦ participative leaders are interested in the 'taking part'

- according to path–goal theory, leaders can change their styles to suit the situation, but according to the contingency model of situational control theory, they cannot

- according to Chelladurai's multidimensional model of leadership, there are five leadership styles

- ♦ leaders using a training and instruction style are interested in developing skills, tactics and teamwork
- ♦ leaders using a democratic style induce a sense of belonging and responsibility
- ♦ those using an autocratic style make all of the decisions independently
- ♦ those demonstrating social support behaviour develop social cohesion through friendships within the team
- ♦ those showing rewarding behaviour develop cohesion by ensuring that the athletes receive tangible recognition for their efforts

- athlete satisfaction is determined by a comparison between prescribed behaviours, actual behaviour and preferred behaviour
  - ♦ prescribed behaviour refers to what the sporting sub-culture would expect
  - ♦ actual behaviour is what really happens
  - ♦ preferred behaviour is the type of behaviour the athletes would like to see
  - ♦ when actual and preferred behaviours coincide the group is said to experience congruence
  - ♦ congruence improves athlete satisfaction

- according to Tuckman (1965), cohesion is developed by 'forming, storming, norming and performing'
  - ♦ the forming stage is an introductory one and the athletes get to know the team goals
  - ♦ in the storming stage, there is disruption, conflict and rebellion
  - ♦ in the norming stage, team members become aware of one another's strengths and weaknesses: disruption and rebellion dissipate
  - ♦ in the performing stage, team members work together as a unit

- according to Horne and Carron (1985), individual coach–athlete inter-relationships depend on affection, control and inclusion
  - ♦ affection refers to the closeness of the relationship
  - ♦ control refers to the dynamics of power, dominance and authority between the athlete and coach
  - ♦ inclusion refers to the way in which the athlete and coach interact to make decisions

- according to Jowett and Ntoumanis (2004), the individual coach–athlete inter-relationship depends on closeness, commitment and complementarity
  - ♦ closeness refers to the level of the emotional interaction between the athlete and coach

- ◆ commitment refers to the intensity of motivation of the athlete and coach
- ◆ complementarity refers to the interaction between the athlete and coach in making decisions

- coaches' ethical values are normally related to their moral values in everyday life
  - ◆ some coaches see sport as being separate to everyday life; this is called game reasoning
  - ◆ gamesmanship is a form of game reasoning

- coaches can affect cohesion by
  - ◆ developing rules for behaviour with their athletes
  - ◆ setting team goals
  - ◆ using 'bonding' exercises
  - ◆ making use of influential individuals in the team, e.g. captains
  - ◆ ensuring that communication between them and the athletes is good.

3

Anxiety, Arousal and Performance

Learning objectives

At the end of this chapter, you should

- understand the nature of arousal
- know the meaning of and types of anxiety
- understand the major theories concerning the arousal–performance interaction
- understand the major theories concerning the anxiety–arousal–performance interaction
- know some of the methods coaches can use to control anxiety and arousal
- understand the factors affecting goal setting.

Anyone who has ever played sport knows that anxiety and arousal affect performance, but rarely are they sure exactly what we mean by these terms or what is the difference between anxiety and arousal. Elsewhere, I have defined arousal as being 'the physiological and/or cognitive readiness to act' (McMorris, 2004). This definition is somewhat different to some of the early theories, which concentrated on physiological factors. Humphreys and Revelle

Coaching Science   Terry McMorris and Tudor Hale
© 2006 John Wiley & Sons, Ltd

(1984) used a similar definition, stating that arousal is a 'peripheral somatic or physiological response to a situation and/or biochemical central response to a situation'. The 'biochemical central response' is what I have termed 'cognitive readiness'. The physiological changes that we observe when arousal level rises are increased heart and respiratory rates, sweating, increased blood pressure and increases in plasma concentrations of adrenaline and noradrenaline. In extreme cases there will be firing of antagonist muscles, which can lead to a lack of coordination.

Changes in arousal are caused by any type of emotion – positive or negative. Anxiety is one of the negative emotions that causes increases in arousal. The physiological changes are identical to those outlined above. Anxiety is generally divided into two types – cognitive and somatic. *Cognitive anxiety* occurs when we assess situations negatively. Feelings such as 'I am going to lose', 'My opponent is too good for me', 'I will get hurt' and so on are examples of negative thoughts that result in anxiety. More scientifically, we might say that anxiety is provoked by thoughts that suggest that *our motivational needs are not going to be met*. *Somatic anxiety* could be described as negatively induced arousal. It is the physiological response to cognitive anxiety.

Task 1 Make a list of things that make you anxious when performing.

So far we have been really talking about what Spielberger (1971) would call *state anxiety*, i.e. anxiety resulting from the situation in which we find ourselves at that moment in time. It is a passing experience. Anxiety is something that we all feel from time to time, especially in sport. The other kind of anxiety described by Spielberger is *trait anxiety*. Trait anxiety is an *enduring negative feeling often related to a lack of self-confidence*. Indeed, the American sports psychologist Rainer Martens (1977, 1982) included self-confidence as a measure of anxiety in his Competitive State Anxiety Inventory (CSAI). There is strong evidence to say that those high in trait anxiety are likely to suffer from state anxiety regularly, while those low in trait anxiety are less likely to find situations anxiety provoking.

Although we have talked of arousal as being the result of positive or negative emotions and anxiety as being a negative emotion, recent research has suggested that anxiety can have a positive effect on performance. Although anxiety is a negative emotion and comes from negative appraisal of the situation, it is sometimes necessary if the athlete is to perform well. We have all seen poor performance when an athlete thinks there is no problem, no chance of defeat. In such situations some fear of defeat would have a positive effect on the athlete's performance. In such cases, the positive effect is due to anxiety increasing arousal. In most cases, however, anxiety has a negative effect.

Arousal–performance theories

Yerkes–Dodson theory

Although it was first postulated in 1908, the theory of arousal by Yerkes and Dodson, more commonly known as *inverted-U theory*, is still the most widely known and accepted arousal–performance theory. According to this theory, when arousal is low, performance is poor. When arousal rises to a moderate level, performance becomes optimal. If arousal continues to rise, however, performance deteriorates until it eventually returns to a level equal to that shown during low levels of arousal. When plotted graphically, performance demonstrates an inverted-U curve (see Figure 3.1). The theory by Yerkes and Dodson has intuitive appeal. We all know that it can be difficult to try one's hardest in games that one expects to win easily. As a result one plays poorly. In important games, however, one can become too excited and, as a result, play equally poorly.

Yerkes and Dodson also believed that the nature of the task would interact with arousal levels to affect performance. They claimed that if a task were easy the performance curve would be skewed towards the higher end of the arousal continuum rather than being a perfect U-shape, while if the task were complex it would be skewed the other way (see Figure 3.2). In other words, *easy tasks require high levels of arousal* for optimal performance, while *complex tasks require lower levels of arousal*. This has major implications for performers. Forwards in rugby and linemen in American football need to be more aroused than scrum halves and quarterbacks. This makes the team talk for the coaches difficult. It is often best to segregate the players during preparation.

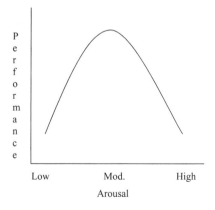

Figure 3.1 The inverted-U model by Yerkes and Dodson of the arousal–performance interaction (based on Yerkes, R. M. and Dodson, J. D. (1908). The relation of strength of stimulus to rapidity of habit formation. *Journal of Comparative Neurology and Psychology, 18*, 459–482)

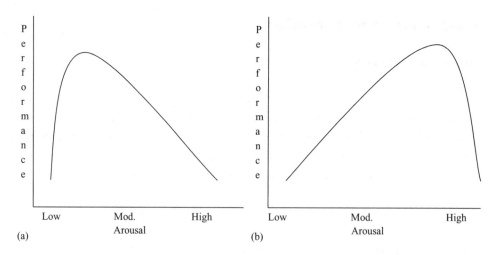

Figure 3.2 The inverted-U model by Yerkes and Dodson of the arousal–performance interaction when tasks are (a) simple or (b) complex (based on Yerkes, R. M. and Dodson, J. D. (1908). The relation of strength of stimulus to rapidity of habit formation. *Journal of Comparative Neurology and Psychology, 18*, 459–482)

> **Task 2** *Make a short list of activities that might require low levels of arousal for optimal performance and some that will require the opposite.*

Easterbrook's cue utilization theory

Although the theory by Yerkes and Dodson was and still is widely acclaimed, it was criticized for failing to explain why and how arousal affects performance. As a result, Easterbrook (1959) developed *cue utilization theory*. According to Easterbrook, when arousal level is low people attend to *too much information or cues and attend to irrelevant as well as relevant cues*. As arousal rises, attention reaches an optimal level, when only relevant cues are processed. This corresponds to the top of the curve in the theory by Yerkes and Dodson. If arousal continues to rise, however, attention will narrow further and even relevant cues will be missed, hence deterioration in performance with high levels of arousal.

Drive theory

An alternative to inverted-U theories was put forward by Hull (1943), and later developed by Spence (1958). It is called *drive theory*. Drive theory developed from Hull's observation that high levels of arousal do not always result in a deterioration in performance. Similarly, moderate levels of arousal do not always result in optimal performance. Indeed in some cases arousal has no effect on performance whatsoever. According to drive theory, *increases in arousal will result in an increase in performance if habit strength is high. If habit strength is low then increases in arousal will either have no effect or will result in a breakdown in performance*. Hull and Spence claimed that the equation is further complicated by the *incentive value* of completing the task. They stated that there would be an *interaction between arousal, habit strength and incentive value*. This interaction could be explained by the formula

$$P = D \times H \times I$$

where P is performance, D is drive or arousal, H is habit strength and I is incentive value. By 'habit strength' Hull and Spence mean *how well learned a skill is*. If their theory is correct, this has a major impact on the arousal–learning inter-relationship. If high levels of arousal were likely to lead to a breakdown in performance, it would be foolish to have beginners practise while in a highly aroused state. On the other hand, experienced performers need to produce optimal performance when highly aroused. So coaches must gradually increase the arousal levels as their performers improve their skill level. This can be done by introducing competition or spectators or both.

Drive theory is often depicted graphically by a straight line; see Figure 3.3(a). This is incorrect. A straight line will only be demonstrated if the task is well learned. If not, it may act as in Figure 3.3(b). Drive theory is in many ways the 'forgotten theory' of arousal and performance.

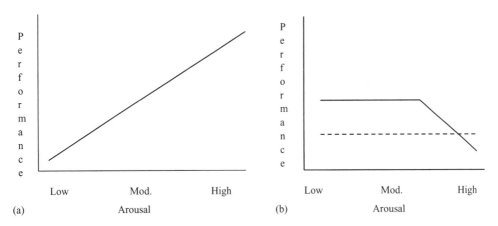

Figure 3.3 According to drive theory, (a) shows the arousal–performance interaction for a task high in habit strength, while (b) shows the possible results for a task low in habit strength

Allocable resource theories

Like drive theory, *allocable resource* theories accept that the interaction between arousal and performance is affected by factors other than simply the arousal itself. The first of these theories was put forward by Kahneman (1973). Kahneman believes that individuals have a limited number of resources. The amount is not fixed but flexible. Kahneman claims that, as arousal rises, the number of resources available within the brain increases. Like Yerkes and Dodson, he argues that this increase is beneficial for performance up to a certain point, after which there will be a return to baseline levels of performance. To Kahneman, increase in arousal is not the only factor affecting performance. The increase in the number of resources, as arousal rises to a moderate level, will only result in improvements in performance if the person *allocates* the resources to the task in hand.

The allocation of resources to task relevant information is said to be undertaken by *cognitive effort* (often just referred to as *effort*). Kahneman believes that performance, even at low levels of arousal, can be optimal if cognitive effort allocates resources to task relevant information. This can be seen when we perform well because we are composed and not emotionally aroused, e.g. the experienced tennis player who swiftly defeats an inexperienced opponent in the first round of a tournament. Similarly, Kahneman does not see high levels of arousal leading to narrowing of attention. Rather he sees the problem as not being able to allocate resources to the task. For example, the person starts to focus on the feelings of distress or excitement. Kahneman believes that, at high levels of arousal, cognitive effort cannot overcome the emotional factors and so is unable to allocate resources effectively.

Task 3 Which of these theories do you think best explains the arousal–performance relationship? What are the reasons for your choice?

Anxiety–arousal–performance theories

The theories examined in the last section are concerned with the arousal–performance interaction when arousal is induced by any kind of emotion. In this section, we deal with the interaction when the cause of the increase in arousal is due to anxiety. For many years inverted-U theory or drive theory was used to explain this three-way interaction. In other words, theorists thought that anxiety was unidimensional in nature and had a unidimensional effect on performance. More recently, theories have used a multidimensional explanation for the effect of anxiety on performance.

Catastrophe theory

John Fazey and Lew Hardy at the University of Wales, Bangor, began applying catastrophe theory to sport in the late 1980s and Hardy and a variety of colleagues (e.g. Hardy and Parfitt, 1991) have continued this work since then. Hardy and company were particularly concerned with the interaction between cognitive and somatic arousal. They tend to use the word physiological rather than somatic. When the performer is low in cognitive anxiety, somatic anxiety is seen as affecting performance in the classical inverted-U fashion. However, if cognitive anxiety is high, performance will improve from that at low levels of arousal as somatic arousal increases to just beyond the optimal level (the top of the inverted-U curve). Once somatic arousal has risen above this level, the athlete will suffer a catastrophe effect. Performance will not slowly deteriorate, as the inverted-U theorists claim, but will disintegrate. The only way to recover is to stop performing, have a break from the activity (could be a small period of time) and start again. We should remember that if cognitive anxiety is high but somatic anxiety low performance can still be optimal.

Processing efficiency theory

Eysenck and Calvo (1992) developed processing efficiency theory from the allocable resources theory of Kahneman. In particular, they were interested in how allocation of resources could affect the way in which the brain deals with problem solving. If you remember from the last section, according to Kahneman increases in arousal above the optimal will result in effort being unable to allocate the resources to the task. Eysenck and Calvo argued that, even under high levels of anxiety and arousal, effort can allocate resources to the task, which can then be performed optimally. They termed this *performance effectiveness*. However, in such cases optimal performance would be at the cost of *performance efficiency*. Performance efficiency refers to how hard the individual has to work to achieve the result. The more difficult it is for effort to allocate resources, the lower the efficiency.

Eysenck and Calvo also argue that anxiety and arousal will not affect tasks that are not complex. The types of complex task Eysenck and Calvo refer to are undertaken by higher centres of the brain and these appear to be most vulnerable to a lack of resources. Simple tasks need fewer resources, therefore are not disrupted even by high levels of arousal.

Task 4 Which of these theories do you think best explains the anxiety–performance relationship? What are the reasons for your choice?

Practical implications

In this section, we examine (a) how to assess anxiety levels; (b) how to control the likelihood of anxiety arising; (c) how to ensure that the athletes are optimally aroused before the start of competition and (d) how to maintain control during performance. Unlike sports psychology texts that cover these points from a sports psychologist's perspective, we will examine what the coach can and should do.

Assessing anxiety

Sports psychology texts always recommend the use of the major sports anxiety questionnaires when attempting to assess anxiety. The reality for the coach is somewhat different. Few athletes, especially team sports players, like to complete questionnaires, which their coach can peruse at his/her leisure. They feel intimidated by this. However, it is useful for the coach to know whether the athlete is high or low in trait anxiety, suffers more or less from cognitive or somatic anxiety and is high or low in self-confidence. The first and most important thing for the coach to do is observe the athletes. There are many signs that let us know whether the athlete is anxious or not. Over time the coach can work out whether showing signs of nerves is an indicator of good or bad performances. One player I had always played well if pre-game he was constantly talking and moving around the changing room. He was a nuisance to the rest of us but we knew that it was a good sign. Even the other players recognized this without being told. If he was quiet and sat in one place I knew that I had to psyche him up. For other performers, of course, the opposite is true.

Task 5 Do you have any idiosyncrasies that manifest themselves when you are anxious? Are you aware of similar behaviours in others?

Table 3.1 Questionnaires that can be used to determine level and/or type of anxiety

Trait questionnaires
Cognitive Somatic Anxiety Questionnaire (CSAQ) (Schwartz *et al.*, 1978)
Sport Anxiety Scale (SAS) (Smith *et al.*, 1990)
Sport Competition Anxiety Test (SCAT) (Martens, 1975)
Competitive Trait Anxiety Inventory (CTAI-2) (Albrecht and Feltz, 1987)

State questionnaires
Competitive State Anxiety Inventory (CSAI-2) (Martens *et al.*, 1990)
Competitive State Anxiety Inventory for Children (CSAI-2C) (Stadulis *et al.*, 1994)
Competitive State Anxiety Inventory including directional scale (CSAI-2D) (Jones & Swain, 1995)

With some athletes, particularly in individual sports, the coach may find using questionnaires useful (see Table 3.1 for a list of questionnaires that can be used). While most of the questionnaires simply provide information about state or trait anxiety, the Test of Attentional and Interpersonal Style (TAIS) provides information concerning how the performers will react. This, of course, is valuable information for the coach. The TAIS was developed by the American Robert Nideffer (1976), who was a student of Oriental philosophies and combined what he learned from the East with his training as a psychologist in America.

Nideffer identified four attentional styles, broad external (BET), broad internal (BIT), narrow external and narrow internal. A BET attentional style is indicative of someone who can handle a great deal of information in the environment without becoming overloaded. BIT describes a style that allows the person to integrate many mental thoughts. Narrow external describes the ability to focus on a single external cue, while ignoring other information. Narrow internal is similar except that the information is cognitive rather than physical. Nideffer found that individuals who were good at narrow internal were also good at narrow external, therefore he decided to simply classify them as having a narrow (NAR) attentional style. On the negative side, however, Nideffer recognized than we can also become overloaded by information. Those easily overloaded by external cues were described as having an overload external attentional style (OET). Those overloaded by many internal cues were described as having an overloaded internal attentional style (OIT). These people become confused if they have too much to think about. Nideffer described people who, under stress, focus on negative thoughts as having a reduced attentional style (RED).

Nideffer claimed that, under optimal conditions, we are able to switch to the most appropriate style. However, under moderate stress we would favour our strongest style. Under high anxiety, we would demonstrate a RED style. This information, in itself, is useful to a coach and can be obtained from Nideffer's TAIS. However, understanding the TAIS is not as simple as some people think. Nideffer never intended the TAIS to be used as an end in itself. It needs to be interpreted by someone who has been trained to do so. The TAIS, as its name implies, does not merely test attentional style; it also examines interpersonal factors. According to Nideffer it is these factors that will greatly affect the stress the person perceives. Nideffer identified nine interpersonal factors. These can be seen in Table 3.2 and are commented on in the next section.

Task 6 What is your dominant attentional style? Which of the interpersonal factors outlined by Nideffer cause you the most problems?

While the TAIS can provide valuable information concerning how the athlete will respond to anxiety, the use of the positive versus negative addition to the CSAI by Jones *et al.* (1993) is useful. This measures the extent to which the person feels that the anxiety is positive or negative with regard to its effect on

Table 3.2   Nideffer's interpersonal styles

Style	Description
Information processing (INFP)	Ability to use a great deal of information or cues
Behaviour control (BCON)	Tendency to be impulsive and engage in anti-social behaviour
Control (CON)	Need to be in charge (control) of situations
Self-esteem (SES)	Having a positive self-image
Physical orientation (P/O)	Capacity to enjoy physical activity
Obsessive (OBS)	Tendency to worry over an issue without solving the problem
Extroversion (EXT)	Need to be with others
Introversion (INT)	Need to be alone with own thoughts and ideas
Intellectual expression (IEX)	Willingness to express thoughts and ideas
Negative affect expression (NAE)	Tendency to express negative feelings towards others
Positive affect expression (PAE)	Tendency to express feelings of affection to others

performance. Knowledge of this would allow us to know whether to psyche up or psyche down an athlete. Indeed the German sports psychologist Yuri Hanin (1989) has proposed that there is an optimal zone of arousal for every participant; this he calls the *zone of optimal functioning (ZOF)*. Several researchers have tried to provide empirical evidence for this theory but with only limited success. The theory has intuitive appeal but, from my own personal experiences, I could not honestly say that I had a ZOF. Maybe I did but just could not recognize it. What about your own experiences?

Preventing anxiety

The easiest way in which to prevent anxiety is to remove the likely causes. This, of course, is not always possible. However, planning ahead and trying to foresee problems and how to deal with them is vital. Good coaches often make a list of 'What ifs'. These are all the possible causes of anxiety that might arise. A knowledge of what is likely to cause anxiety in your athletes helps with this task. The interpersonal factors highlighted in the TAIS provide some good examples of personality factors that can cause anxiety.

> **Task 7** *Your team is playing away in a major competition. There has to be an overnight stay in a hotel. Make a list of 'What ifs' that might help you to stop problems before they begin.*

Nideffer saw self-esteem as being a major issue. Individuals low in self-esteem can easily become anxious and the coach needs to be constantly reassuring them. Those high in self-esteem may need very different treatment. It is sometimes necessary to be somewhat verbally aggressive when dealing with such people. This can be particularly the case in team activities, where they may perceive themselves as being better and more important than their team-mates. This is particularly a problem if they are outspoken. They can become critical of team-mates and cause anxiety in others.

Nideffer also identifies depression as an interpersonal factor. Mild depression will occur in most athletes at some stage in their careers. Thankfully, most of the time it is a temporary state. However, if you think that an athlete is having problems that are causing more than mild depression, particularly if they are not being caused by the sport, you should recommend that they seek assistance. I have unfortunately experienced this a few times in my coaching career. It is difficult to deal with and you must remember that you are not qualified to start giving advice other than telling the person to see a doctor or clinical psychologist.

Perhaps the two best known interpersonal styles are extroversion and introversion. Extroverts enjoy the company of others and like to be active before a game or a competition. Introverts prefer a quieter existence and often like to be alone or, at least, enjoy quiet before a competition. Having extreme extroverts and introverts in a team can be problematic. In one team, with which I worked as a consultant sports psychologist, we found that by separating the extroverts from the introverts in the changing rooms we lessened individual anxiety and improved team cohesion. Luckily most people are not at the extremes on either scale, therefore this type of action is rarely necessary.

The factors outlined above definitely cause anxiety but can mostly be dealt with by good organization. The main cause of anxiety in athletes, however, is fear of failure, i.e. fear of playing poorly and/or losing. This cannot be removed by organization. The first and best way to prevent this kind of anxiety is through education. We can attempt to get the athletes to place success and failure in their correct perspective. However, we do not want them to begin to believe that winning or playing well does not matter at all. We can, nevertheless, keep it in perspective. One of the best ways to do this is to use goal stetting.

Goal setting

Goals represent what we aim to achieve and so are related very much to motivation. Research has shown that by using goal setting we can educate the individuals as to what they can realistically achieve. This in turn relieves much of the anxiety because the person is attempting to achieve something that is within their grasp.

Research has highlighted several major rules concerning goal setting. Goals should be *challenging*. They should, in other words, inspire the athletes to develop their skills. Although they should be challenging, they must also be *attainable*. If the athletes think 'I will never be able to do that', they are very unlikely to even try. Goals need to be both *long term* and *short term*. Long-term goals are what they say they are, what you are aiming for in the long term. This time span may be anything from a few weeks to a year or more. With most of my teams, we set goals for the end of the season or even for the beginning of the following season. Short-term goals should be stepping-stones to the long-term goals. It is important with short-term goals that the athletes can obtain success. Also, they need to have some way of *measuring* whether or not they are achieving their goals. This does not have to be objective or quantitative measuring. It can be a subjective assessment of performance. However, it does help if some quantitative value is given. With my football teams when we set goals about improving positional play, for example, I give each player a mark out of ten at the end of each game. Thus, they can see how well they are doing. One of the problems with short-term goals is that one does not always achieve them and sometimes extraneous circumstances intervene. As a result, we need to be able to change our goals, particularly our short-term goals. They need to be *flexible*.

Most of the literature about goals suggests that we should set *performance* goals. These are goals concerning the quality of the performance. However, recent research suggests that we should also set *outcome* goals. These are goals regarding our performance with respect to others, e.g. we will win the league or a particular championship. If we wish to use goals to reduce anxiety it is best to employ performance goals, as the athlete has more control over these. Performance goals are not affected by the opposition as easily. Outcome goals are greatly affected by your opponents' performance. They are even affected by luck. Outcome goals are best used with successful athletes and teams.

One of the most important factors in goal setting is to include the athlete or athletes in the process. This way the coach will get some idea of the athlete's motivation and, more importantly, *the goals will belong to the athletes as much as they do to the coach*. If coaches set the goals themselves, they are the coaches' goals not the athletes'. Goals can be *group goals* or *individual goals*. In teams individual goals should be compatible with the group goals. Moreover, the athlete should be able to focus on his/her individual goals during training and competition without this hindering group performance.

Task 8 *Draw up a set of goals for yourself with regard to learning to be a coach.*

Performance profiling

The idea of performance profiling was developed by Richard Butler (see Butler and Hardy, 1992), working with the British Olympic Boxing team. It is in many ways similar to goal setting and can be used without any specialist training, hence its usefulness to coaches. The first stage is to decide what factors are necessary to be a good performer in a particular sport. These can be drawn up by individual athletes, or teams, or athletes and coaches. Younger performers will need a lot of help. The second stage is for the athlete to rate him/herself on each of the factors. This can be done for all factors involved in a performance or you may choose a specific area, e.g. fitness components or technical factors. Butler suggests dividing areas into physical, technical, psychological, coordination, strategy and character.

The coach should also evaluate the athlete on each factor. The coach and player can then discuss areas of difference. The main point in profiling is for the athlete and coach to decide which areas need improving and by how much. In order to do this, Butler recommends drawing up a profile like that in Figure 3.4. As you can see, each factor has an optimal score for that particular athlete and a score for where they are now. The aim is to reach the optimal. Butler particularly stresses the use of this visual profile, as he believes that this helps the athletes to picture where they are and how well they are progressing.

Task 9 *Set out a performance profile for yourself as either a performer or coach.*

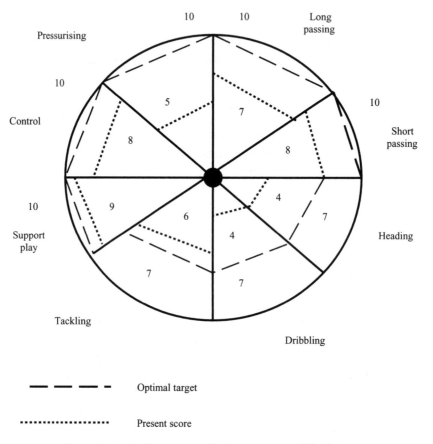

Figure 3.4   Performance profile for a soccer midfield player

The pre-competition speech

Pre-competition speeches by coaches can be inspiring, deflating or down right hilarious. They are, of course, meant to be the former. One football coach for whom I worked used to say 'We may not be as good as them but we can work harder than them'. This may well have been true but he could not see that he was being negative in the first part of his sentence. It is, however, important to be realistic. Coaches who tell performers that they are better than they really are, or that the opposition is poor when in fact they are good, are not doing anyone any favours. Pre-competition speeches need to have the emphasis on what the athletes *can* do. The second part of the quote above, concerning work rate, is positive and achievable. What the coach has to say must follow the rules of goal setting. What the coach is asking the athlete to do is, in fact, a form of setting short-term goals.

Another problem with pre-competition instructions is the amount of information given to the athlete. Most people can only deal with a limited amount of information. Information processing theorists claim that we can only handle 7 ± 2 bits of information at any one time. Given all that the athlete has to think about and all of the other thoughts vying for attention, it is best if instructions are very limited. Coaches will soon see which performers can deal with a lot of information. In team games, these people become captains. Those whose short-term memory is very limited may need help from team-mates. One of my football players could not remember his role at free-kicks and corners, so the captain had to remember this player's job as well as his own.

Mental rehearsal

I spent some time thinking about whether or not to include this in a coaching book. The measures we have covered above can all comfortably be carried out by coaches without special training. Mental rehearsal is also not difficult to use; however, it does require some training. Some argue that you can learn it from books or tapes but I am not convinced of that. I have decided to include a brief description of what can be done but I strongly suggest that you undertake some form of training before setting out to use it systematically with your athletes. Advising athletes to use mental rehearsal and imagery tapes, by themselves, is a little different as they are responsible for what they do. Once you begin instructing people in the use of mental rehearsal it is your responsibility and, as we will see, there can be some problems. I presume that those who are working for degrees will probably learn how to use mental rehearsal as part of their course.

At its most basic level, mental rehearsal is simply thinking about what you are going to do. There is, of course, no problem in asking your athletes to do that. Day dreaming is a form of mental rehearsal. Most forms of mental rehearsal are preceded by relaxation. There are many different ways of inducing relaxation and performers can follow instructions on tapes quite easily. Some use muscle tensioning followed by release of the tension, others are closer to the ways that hypnotists induce relaxation. Relaxation is normally followed by the use of imagery. Imagery can be in two forms, *external* or *internal*. External requires the person to image themselves performing a skill as though they were looking at a film of themselves. Internal imagery means that the person sees and feels the movement 'from within' their body. It is generally thought that the latter is the more powerful.

Although most of the time the use of imagery is harmless, it is best to let athletes use tapes and do the imaging by themselves until you have some training in how to take charge of a session yourself. Some forms of imaging, especially visuomotor behaviour rehearsal, are very close to hypnosis and occasionally can result in bad reactions by the athlete. I would, however, encourage all coaches to develop the skill of taking control of imaging sessions as it can be very useful.

Working with a sports psychologist

Above we have dealt mostly with methods of preventing anxiety that the coach can use or can soon learn to use themselves. Of course, there are often problems that require the use of a sports psychologist. Table 3.3 gives a list of possible treatments that sports psychologists can use. These require specialist training. Some of you will be training to be sports psychologists, as well as coaches, and this raises an interesting point in itself. Even if you are a trained sports psychologist there can be conflict of interest in your role as coach and that of sports psychologist. In my own teams, I never acted as both coach and psychologist because of this. If a performer requires a sport psychologist it is because there are problems. The athlete–coach relationship may be one of these problems. The athletes need to have someone to whom they can speak in confidence, i.e. the sports psychologist. Even if relationships with the coach are not a problem, performers may feel that they cannot discuss all of their problems with their coach. This can particularly be the case in team games where the coach chooses the team. The athletes may feel

Table 3.3 Typical treatments used by sports psychologists

Treatment	Effect
Relaxation	Controls somatic anxiety: mostly used in conjunction with imagery
Imagery	Increases self-confidence: sets positive mood
Visuomotor behavioural rehearsal (VMBR)	A combination of the effects of relaxation and imagery but thought by some to be more intense in nature
Hypnosis	Similar to VMBR but thought to have a greater effect on the sub-conscious
Rationalization	Puts cognitive anxiety into perspective: can aid self-confidence
Implosion	Person has to confront fears
Biofeedback	Helps athlete to 'read' the symptoms of somatic anxiety: can lead to athlete controlling some symptoms

that to tell the coach some of their anxieties might lead to the coach not choosing them.

If you bring in a sports psychologist then the roles of coach and sports psychologist must be laid out in no uncertain terms. The athletes must know that they can speak to the sports psychologist without fear of what they say being reported to the coach. Similarly, the coach must be able to talk to the sports psychologist in confidence. It is normal for the sport psychologists to agree with the athletes what they can tell the coach. In some situations, especially in team sports, the sports psychologist, coach and players actually meet to discuss their problems. This can be very useful but as coach you must let the sports psychologist take control of such meetings. You cannot suddenly decide that now you are in charge because something is said that you do not like. While all of this may seem like commonsense, I can assure you that some coaches find it difficult to relinquish complete control.

Setting arousal levels

Even when anxiety is controlled, we need to ensure that arousal is optimal at the beginning of performance. Knowledge of the athletes and observations of their arousal levels allow the coach to decide whether they need to be psyched up or psyched down. It seems to me that the need to *psyche up* is the less common of the two. Occasionally, however, athletes for some reason or another are below optimal level of arousal. This can happen in unimportant events, e.g. an end of season game with no real relevance for league or championship position. It can also occur if a team or individual feels superior to their opponent. An 'easy' first round tie in a Grand Slam tennis tournament can be a case where a player is under-aroused. In such circumstances, the coach needs to psyche up the athlete. This is the time for the rousing speech or the curt reminder of what the press will say if the 'star' loses.

In most cases, athletes are too highly aroused and need to be calmed down. *Psyching down* is best done by playing down the chances of defeat and concentrating on performance factors. The athletes may need to be reminded of past good performances, especially those against the present opponents. The use of humour by the coach can also help to calm players down.

When psyching up and psyching down, coaches can use the warm-up to help. A great deal of research has shown that physical activity affects performance. It is thought that physical activity of about 70 per cent of the individual's maximum volume of oxygen uptake can be used to help the performer achieve optimal arousal. Exercise induces the secretion of the neurotransmitters noradrenaline and dopamine in the brain. These neuro-transmitters are involved in cognition and emotion and, at optimal concen-trations, they aid arousal. There is some evidence also to say that warm-up should include tasks that are very similar to the ones to be used in the actual performance. It is thought that such activity improves the individual's *psychological* or *activity set*. Activity set means the person's readiness to perform a particular skill. Another way of putting it is that, following allocable resources theory, when the activity set is optimal the person's cognitive effort is able to allocate resources to the task. It should be noted, however, that there is also research that has shown that warm-up has no effect on performance of skills.

Maintaining optimal arousal

Once a performance begins there is no guarantee that the athlete can maintain optimal arousal. This can be a particular problem if things go wrong. Robert Nideffer suggests the use of a process called *centring*. If the athletes find themselves becoming under or over aroused or anxious they will centre. In order to centre, they breathe in and slowly let the breath out. Immediately they focus on their pre-chosen thoughts or words. These can be task oriented or mood oriented. This is similar to the use *self-talk*, i.e. to repeat words that will regain your focus. These need not even be proper words. All you need to do is get your focus back to the task and away from your negative thoughts. Such words are often mood words, i.e. they are aimed at getting the person into the optimal arousal state.

Another method is to use routines at key points in performance. One of the most famous of such routines is Jonny Wilkinson's pre-penalty kick routine. Most cricket and baseball batters have routines, as have most tennis players pre-service. These routines get the person into the correct activity set. The routine acts as a trigger to the activity set.

Warm-up decrement

Another problem facing performers in many games, such as basketball and ice hockey, is having to come off for a break and then return to the game. Research has shown that, following a period of rest, performance will show a temporary decrease. This happens due to the phenomenon known as *warm-up decrement* (*WUD*). Nacson and Schmidt (1971) claimed that WUD was the result of the person losing concentration or changing their activity set. When the player resumes the activity, it takes time for cognitive effort to re-focus the mind to the task. Some players try to maintain the correct activity set by following the game closely or by using imagery to ensure that arousal is optimal. The Manchester United manager, Sir Alex Ferguson, claims that Ole Gunnar Solksjaër is a good player to send on as a substitute because, when he is on the bench, he follows the game very closely.

Summary

We have seen that anxiety affects arousal, which in turn has an affect on performance. Education and goal setting can help lessen the chances of anxiety occurring but they are unlikely to eliminate it. Methods such as mental rehearsal and imagery are excellent aids to controlling anxiety. They also help with the control of arousal. Good use of warm-up can produce the correct activity set, while centring, self-talk and set routines can all help maintain arousal once performance has begun.

Key points

- arousal is the physiological and/or cognitive readiness to act

- arousal can be positive or negative

- anxiety is a negative emotion, which induces changes in arousal

- anxiety can be divided into cognitive and somatic
  - cognitive anxiety refers to negative thoughts
  - somatic anxiety represents the physiological responses to a situation

- anxiety can also be divided into trait and state
  - trait anxiety is an enduring negative feeling
  - trait anxiety is often linked to weak self-confidence
  - state anxiety is a negative response to a particular situation
  - state anxiety is not permanent

- although anxiety is a negative emotion, it can have a positive effect on performance

- according to Yerkes and Dodson, arousal affects performance in an inverted-U fashion
  - at low levels of arousal, performance is poor
  - at moderate levels, it is optimal
  - at high levels, it is poor

- task complexity affects the arousal–performance interaction
  - complex tasks are performed best when arousal is low
  - easy tasks are performed best when arousal is high

- according to Easterbrook's cue utilization theory, attention narrows as arousal increases
  - at low levels of arousal, we attend to too much information: both relevant and irrelevant
  - at moderate levels of arousal, attention is on relevant information only
  - at high levels, attention is on relevant information but some relevant information is missed

- according to drive theory, performance depends on the interaction between drive (arousal), habit strength (how well learned the task is) and the incentive value of performing the task
  - ♦ at low levels of arousal, performance will be poor
  - ♦ if the task is well learned, performance will improve as arousal rises
  - ♦ if habit strength is weak, arousal will have a negative effect or no effect on performance

- according to Kahneman's allocable resources theory, the number of resources available to the person increases as arousal rises
  - ♦ this is good up to a point but too many resources can have negative effect on performance

- according to Kahneman, how arousal affects performance will depend on cognitive effort
  - ♦ cognitive effort is responsible for allocating resources to the task
  - ♦ at low levels of arousal, performance can be as good as at moderate levels if effort allocates resources to the task
  - ♦ at high levels of arousal, effort cannot overcome the negative effects of too many resources and performance is poor

- according to catastrophe theory, if cognitive anxiety is low, changes in somatic arousal will affect performance as shown in inverted-U theory
  - ♦ if both cognitive and somatic anxiety change, performance will improve as arousal rises to just beyond the optimal level then there will be a catastrophe effect
  - ♦ if cognitive anxiety is high but somatic low, performance can be optimal regardless of arousal level

- according to processing efficiency theory, effort can allocate resources to the task even under high levels of arousal, but only if the task is well learned: this is called performance effectiveness
  - ♦ however, this will only occur with a great deal of effort and the process will not be as efficient as at optimal levels; this is called performance efficiency

- according to attentional and interpersonal style theory, we have a dominant attentional style or focus
  - ♦ a broad external style refers to focusing on a great deal of information in the environment

- ♦ a broad internal style refers to focusing on a great number of thoughts and emotions
- ♦ a narrow style refers to focusing on one or two pieces of information, internal and/or external
- ♦ under little stress, we can switch styles to suit the situation
- ♦ under high levels of stress, we revert to our dominant style
- ♦ under very high levels of stress we adopt a reduced (RED) attentional style

- coaches can help avoid anxiety by increasing athletes' self-esteem

- goal setting can eliminate many of the causes of anxiety

- goals should be long-term and short-term
  - ♦ short-term goals are stepping stones towards the long-term goals

- goals should be
  - ♦ challenging but attainable
  - ♦ able to be measured
  - ♦ flexible

- goals can be outcome (results) or performance (how well we play compared to our previous performances and ability)

- performance profiling can aid goal setting

- mental rehearsal can help overcome anxiety

- warm-up can help set arousal levels

- substitutes should be aware of warm-up decrement, i.e. a short, temporary decrease in performance following a period of inactivity.

4

Coaching and Learning Styles

Learning objectives

At the end of this chapter, you should

- understand what is meant by coaching styles
- understand what is meant by learning styles
- know the basic coaching and learning styles
- understand some of the factors affecting the coaching–learning style interaction.

This chapter could easily have been included in Part III, examining skill acquisition; however, I decided to place it here as it refers not only to skill acquisition but also to coach–athlete relationships. Coaching styles are linked to leadership behaviours. Unlike leadership, very little has been examined with regard to coaching styles. This is, in fact, so much the case that in this chapter I have borrowed from work on teaching styles in physical education. At one time teaching styles would have been seen as having no bearing on coaching. Teaching was seen as being concerned with the development of the individual as a whole, while coaching was thought to be concerned only with outcome, i.e. winning and losing. This attitude has changed greatly over the years and coaches perceive their roles as being concerned with the individual's welfare as

Coaching Science   Terry McMorris and Tudor Hale
© 2006 John Wiley & Sons, Ltd

well as their performance. In reality, the gap between what was considered to be purely the domain of physical education and that which was looked on as being concerned with coaching has merged.

Coaching styles

One of the early attempts to highlight coaching styles was undertaken by Rainer Martens (1987). Martens divided coaching into two styles, *command* and *cooperative*, although he accepted that, to some extent, it is a command–cooperative continuum. The command style is characterized by the coach taking responsibility for all aspects of learning and performance. The athletes simply have to do what the coach tells them. The coach organizes practices, team tactics and motivation. Such coaches are thought to favour extrinsic motivation and use many reward and punishment systems. Also, they tend to place outcome as being the most important of their goals. Cooperative coaches are almost the opposite. They see their role as that of a facilitator, making it possible for the athletes to achieve their goals. They prefer to develop intrinsic motivation and put the athletes' welfare ahead of outcome. This does not mean that they are not interested in winning but that they see social factors as being the more important.

Martens believes that there are personality reasons for coaches adopting each of the styles. He believes that cooperative coaches are high in self-esteem and are able to empathize with their athletes. One would have to have high self-esteem to let the athletes have the major say in training and practice sessions, and team tactics. The coach, when using such a style, has to be willing to 'take a backseat' and not be in the limelight. To Martens, the command style coach is low in self-esteem, hence the need to be seen to be in control. Often such coaches will try to take the praise for performances. Also, they are low in the ability to empathize with their athletes.

More recently, John Lyle (1999) has taken a similar stance to that of Martens. Lyle divided coaching styles into *autocratic* and *democratic*. He points out that we should not get mixed up between these styles and those of leadership. He claims that it is possible to be democratic with regard to communicating with athletes (the leadership role) while being autocratic during practice and training sessions (the coaching role). The autocratic style is like Martens' command style. The coach is 'in charge' of everything. Practice and training are organized by the coach and the coach tells the athletes what to do. They have no say in the matter. The democratic style is similar to Martens' cooperative style, with the coach involving the athletes in organization and decision making concerning what is to be done and even how it is to be done.

Task 1 Do you prefer an autocratic or democratic style of coaching? What are the reasons for your answer?

Coaching styles based on Mosston's teaching styles

The physical educationist Muska Mosston identified nine teaching styles used in physical education. Observation of these styles shows that they are also employed by coaches. In this section, I have adapted Mosston's teaching styles to a coaching role. I have also taken the liberty of simplifying some of the concepts, particularly those that are more involved in educating the person as a whole. Table 4.1 outlines each of the styles and gives their major characteristics. Here I will expand a little on the content of the table.

The *command* style is almost identical to Martens' command and Lyle's autocratic styles. The coach is very much in charge. Content is chosen by the coach and the methods of practice and training are decided solely by him/her. There is no ambiguity in the role of the coach, assistants and individual athletes. This style can be particularly useful when the activity involves an element of danger, e.g. coaching the javelin or discus. It also has some advantages with large groups. One of its major advantages is that it is the easiest of all of the styles in which to maintain discipline. Coaches who feel threatened by a lack of athlete discipline often resort to this method of coaching. Obviously its lack of input

Table 4.1 Mosston's teaching styles

Style	Description
Command	Coach makes all decisions and instructs learners during practice: everyone practices the same tasks, at the same level of difficulty
Practice	Coach makes all decisions but learners progress at own rate depending on their ability level
Reciprocal	Athletes coach one another
Self-check	Athletes assess their own success and failure
Inclusion	Athlete and coach decide on what is to be learned and the coaching methods to be used
Guided discovery	Athlete makes all decisions guided by the coach
Divergent	Coach sets problems for athletes to solve
Individual programme-learner's design	Learner decides on what is to be coached
Learner's initiated style	Coach only helps when asked
Self-teaching	Athlete takes sole responsibility for all aspects of learning

from the athletes can alienate some of them. For coaches to use this style successfully they need to be particularly well respected for their knowledge. The style has major limits if the athletes are at different levels of ability and development. It tends to be a style more suitable for homogenous groups.

Mosston claims that, for this style to be successful, the coach must be aware of the emotional state of the athletes. If the athletes are getting bored or not achieving success they are powerless if the coach is using such a style. Coaches who successfully use command style, and there are many, constantly monitor their athletes and alter practices, or even abort them, when they feel that it is necessary. Perhaps the most successful users of this style are individuals who have strong and charismatic personalities, what some people call the 'X' *factor*. In reality though, I think that few coaches actually use a pure form of command style. Most seem to include other styles as well.

Most coaches who believe that they use the command style in fact use the *practice* style. As with the command style, the coach is very much in charge. The athletes do what the coach tells them. However, the speed and type of progression during the session will vary from athlete to athlete depending on their ability levels. Unlike in the command style, not everyone is practising and progressing at the same rate. This is called *differentiation*. The coach lets the athletes practise as individuals, or in groups, and goes round providing individual and small group coaching. This style does allow for small inter-individual differences in ability and developmental stage.

The *reciprocal* style is sometimes called *peer coaching*. The coach sets the agenda, i.e. chooses the topic or topics to be coached, but splits the team up into groups of twos or threes and so on. Then each group goes off and practises. They provide one another with feedback. It can be particularly useful when the athletes know the tasks well and can help one another. Some athletes like this because they feel that making mistakes will not lead to the coach seeing them as being poor performers. Good coaches will move around the groups, as with the practice style. Athletes can progress at their own rate and each can work on aspects of their own performance rather than simply everybody doing the same thing. Obviously this can only be used if there is good discipline and the athletes have a sound knowledge of the activity. Care must be taken with choice of groups. Individuals who do not get on together can end up arguing in such situations, while some athletes will not be critical of people whom they see as being better than themselves.

The *self-check* style is similar to the reciprocal style in that the coach sets the agenda but, instead of being 'coached' by a peer, the athletes actually 'coach' themselves. The athletes practise by themselves, or in small groups, and assess their own success and failure. They attempt to put problems right and try out changes in technique or tactics. The coach can go around checking on them. As well as allowing the athletes to work on their own problems and progress at their own rate, it increases athletes' self-esteem and independence. This can be very important. Many individual athletes, in particular, need to learn to compete without their coaches being there to give them feedback. With beginners, who have little knowledge of the activity, this can end up as being trial and error learning. With more advanced performers, however, the athlete has some knowledge to draw upon and the trials will be more than hopeful guesses.

The *inclusion* style is the first of Mosston's styles that involves the learner in the decision of what to learn. The learner and coach together agree on what the athlete should work on, the level at which they should begin and the rate of progress they should make. Thus this level takes care of individual differences with regard to ability level and experience. However, lazy athletes can opt for an easy time. The coach needs to be a good communicator to get success. They must be good motivators. Some athletes want to do too much. The coach needs all of his/her diplomacy skills with such an athlete to get them to work at a more suitable level. This must be done without damaging the athlete's self-esteem. Not an easy task.

We cover the *guided discovery* style in Chapter 8, when examining practice. Suffice it to say here that guided discovery requires the coach to help the athlete to make the correct decision concerning what they are to practise, how they are to practise, what the results of the practice tell them and how they are going to change in order to perform better. This sounds like a difficult task for the coach and it is. It is far easier to take a command approach and tell them that they have done this incorrectly and this is how to improve. It is more difficult to get the athletes to work it out for themselves. However, the ability to come to the conclusions yourself, albeit under a lot of guidance, aids the memory process. The memory trace is stronger because of the cognitive processes that one must use to decide what the problem is and how to correct it. In other words, the learner is not only finding out how to do something but also why it should be done this way. More parts of the brain are involved and reasoning is deeper. All of this aids learning.

The *divergent* style could be termed a *problem solving approach*. The coach sets a problem, or task, and lets the athletes work out a solution or solutions for themselves with or without help from the coach. The use of this style demands a great deal of self-esteem from the coach, as the coach is letting the performers 'take charge' of their own learning. It does, however, lead to some great moments of innovation. It also allows for an increase in independence and self-esteem in the athlete. Where the athletes have developed a tactical ploy of their own they are more likely to want to implement it than one that has been forced upon them by the coach. In team sports different parts of the team can be working on different problems. I have seen this style used extremely successfully in professional football. The main issue for the coach is to set realistic problems and to explain the scenario succinctly to the athletes. Players do need a lot of experience to use this method successfully.

The *individual programme-learner's design* refers to where the learner decides on the main area to be practised, e.g. receiving serve in tennis. In many individual sports this is very common. Many tennis players and golfers highlight their strengths and weaknesses then decide what they wish to work and on and go to a coach for help. The coach takes care of the actual practice. The *learner's initiated* style takes the individual programme-learner's design a stage further, with the coach merely giving advice when asked. The athlete decides not just on the area to be worked on but also the type of practice to be utilized. Mosston's final style is the *self-teaching* style, which does not require a coach.

Task 2 *Which of Mosston's styles is closest to that which you use? Are you capable of switching style? If not, why do you think that is? If yes, are there any styles that you cannot use?*

Learning styles

While coaching styles are very important, so are the styles used by the learner. Furthermore, as we will see in the final section of this chapter, the interaction between coaching and learning styles is an important one. There are four types of learner, *activists*, *reflectors*, *theorists* and *pragmatists*. Activists, sometimes called *accommodators*, are characterized by open-mindedness and a willingness to became involved immediately in trying out the new skill. They like to be given a challenge and love to 'have a go'. Activists are not afraid to make mistakes. Males tend to be more activist than females.

Reflectors, or *divergers*, prefer to think through a problem before trying to perform a skill. They are willing to listen to what the coach has to say about how to perform a skill. They tend to be cautious in approach but will work out alternative methods of performing a skill. They like to work in small groups or pairs. Females tend to be more reflectors than males. Theorists, or *assimilators*, are similar to reflectors and like to take their time in working out how to do something. They are more analytical than reflectors but less cautious, although they will only try out movements that theory suggests will work. They like to work alone. People using a pragmatic, or *convergent*, style are more like the activists, in that they enjoy trying things out without too much reflection or theorizing. However, they use some theorization in that they like to see if ideas will work. However, unlike the theorists and reflectors they are willing to do this with a minimal amount of cognitive questioning. These people like to find out the answers using action rather than reflection.

Task 3 *Which learning style do you think that you use? Do you find that some coaches make it difficult for you to use your preferred style?*

Practical implications

I will be surprised if any coaches completing Task 1 are out and out autocrats or democrats. I will be even more surprised if they are very accurate in knowing which style they actually use. Thinking about how you deal with coaching sessions and how you behave during competition will help you make an educated decision on your style. However, research has shown that coaches are notoriously poor at actually knowing how they behave. Finding out is simple. You can make up a checklist. You can divide activities into those that would be displayed by an autocrat, e.g. giving instructions and commands; and those that a democrat would use, e.g. asking questions, listening to suggestions. Get someone to observe you coaching and put a tick or cross next to each of the types of behaviour as you use them. Table 4.2 gives an outline of autocratic and democratic behaviours that you could use to help you make up your checklist. There are now sophisticated computer packages such as *Sports Coach*, which use video evidence and computer print-outs to determine your coaching style. In essence, they are only checklists using technology. However, they are useful in that you can see yourself doing the coaching. Not always a pretty sight.

Task 4 *Draw up a checklist to examine your coaching style. Get someone to watch you coach and score you on each item. Did you expect these results?*

Table 4.2 Behaviours used by autocratic and democratic coaches

Autocrats	Democrats
Decide what is to be coached in each session	Discuss with athletes their needs and agree on content of session
Tell athletes what to do and how to do it	Provide options on the best ways to perform a skill
Have all athletes working on the same task and progressing at the same time	Use differentiation based on individual abilities
Dictate tactics	Discuss with athletes the tactics to be used

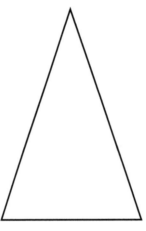

Athlete
Ability
Experience
Age
Motivation
Personality
Emotional
Strength
Intelligence
Gender
Learning style

Coach
Knowledge Experience
Motivation Personality Gender

Task
Cognitive demands Physical
demands Technical demands

Figure 4.1 Factors to be taken into consideration when deciding which coaching style to use

Mosston does not recommend one style over another; he says that the style used should depend on the interaction between the coach, the athlete and the task. Figure 4.1 shows this diagrammatically. As you can see from Figure 4.1, the coach brings much to this interaction. While personality factors are obvious, what is less straightforward is whether we can alter our natural behavioural patterns. For many people, reacting to different tasks and athletes is not too difficult; they will naturally empathize with nervous athletes or be more patient with beginners than experts. Some coaches can easily flip from being high on technical information to being motivational with little technical input. However, most individuals cannot change so readily. In one of our coaching courses at Chichester, the staff deliberately try to adopt a specific coaching style in order to give the students an example of what it looks like in practice. We all find this very difficult to actually do. I normally choose to use a command style. This you would think is easy but I always find myself drifting into guided discovery and problem solving (divergent style) approaches. Some coaches have to simply accept that they have only one style. It is normally not fully one of Mosston's styles but is more likely to be something of a mixture. This mixture can include a wide range of Mosston's styles.

If possible, coaches should alter their styles when appropriate. Although most of us do not like to use the command style, it can be necessary if discipline is an issue. The command style allows the coach to remain in charge. This may be necessary if the task is a dangerous one, e.g. javelin throwing in groups. While guided discovery is my favourite style because it gets the learners to think their way through a problem, it may not be the best with tasks that have a element of risk. 'There are four ways of getting from the bottom of the swimming pool to the top, see if you can find them' is obviously inappropriate and equally obviously a joke. However, letting people try to work out how best to pack down in a rugby scrum is also inappropriate. At the other extreme, I have often seen people use command or practice styles when teaching dribbling in hockey, football and basketball or running past defenders in rugby. Dribbling is a skill that depends on the person using their own strengths to outwit an opponent. Moreover, great dribblers are innovative. How can you be innovative if someone is telling you what to do? Two of the best runners with a Rugby ball are Josh Lewsey and Jason Robinson, but they go past defenders using different strategies and styles. Lewsey attacks at speed and begins his move a comparatively long way in front of the defender. He swerves around the defender while already running at speed. Robinson gets closer to the defender before beginning his move and relies on his ability to change direction and accelerate in limited space. To teach Lewsey and Robinson to use the same strategies would be stupid.

Task 5 *Make a list of four or five skills and decide which coaching style would be best suited to the acquisition of these skills.*

One of the major factors in Figure 4.1 is motivation. We have said much about this in Chapter 3 but its importance cannot be underestimated. Highly motivated individuals will spend long periods of time doing what, to others, is repetitive and boring practice. They can, and will, work alone. They are able, and willing, to use the individual styles set out by Mosston (individual-learner's design and learner's initiated styles). The coach must be careful, however, and take into account the skill level of these athletes and the task they are learning. The great ice hockey player Wayne Gretsky spent hours, as a child, practising by himself. Learning the basic skills using this individual approach was fine, even for a child. However, more advanced skills may need greater input from a coach, especially with younger performers. Experts may be best left to themselves and may well come up with something new when left alone in these situations. Innovative plays in many sports have come about from this kind of practice. Similarly, some of the best vaults in gymnastics and jumps in trampolining are the result of such practice.

So far, we have not talked about the role of the athlete's learning style in the decision of how to coach. While there are questionnaires that can be used to determine individuals' learning styles, these are designed for classroom studies and may be inappropriate. More importantly, in team games, players are reluctant to give such information to coaches who select the team. With individual athletes the coach can find out how the athlete learns by simply talking to them about the process. In team situations, it may be safer to assume that all of the learning styles are represented; therefore, variety in your use of style will help. When introducing a new skill activists like to 'have a go' before any instruction is given. This can unnerve reflectors and theorists, however. When dealing with males I tend to let them have a go first because males are more likely to be activists than females. With females, I point out what we are going to do and why. Pragmatists also like the idea of having a go but they want some time to work out an answer for themselves. Activists do not mind having a go then being stopped, told how to do it and then returning to the practice. Activists, and to a lesser extent pragmatists, are happy with command and practice styles of coaching. Pragmatists prefer self-check and inclusion. They also do not mind reciprocal coaching but that will also depend on their relationships with the others in the group.

I must say that I am not keen on reciprocal coaching. I have seen it work very well with experts but have major problems using it with beginners. Mosston included it in his teaching styles because, as an educational tool, it is useful in helping the peer 'coach' to understand the skill better. However, if the peer does not get it right the coaching is incorrect. Reflectors and theorists are happier with guided discovery and problem solving. Coaches can set problems and help the athletes to solve them. Many reflectors and theorists like to spend time inactive physically but very active mentally. Activists hate this and even pragmatists are not too happy. These differences can cause problems in teams.

Summary

Martens and Lyle identified coaching styles along a continuum from autocratic to democratic. The physical educationist Mosston saw teaching styles as falling into very similar types. Unlike Martens and Lyle, he divided teaching styles into 10 sub-groups, ranging from command (autocratic) to self-coaching, which goes even further than a democratic style. More importantly, Mosston claimed that the style of choice should be made depending on the coach–athlete–task interaction (see Figure 4.1). One of the factors that coaches should take into consideration concerning the athlete is his or her learning style. Although four styles have been identified, in essence one could argue that there is a continuum from the activist to the theorist. Males tend to be more activist and females more theoretical in approach. The difficulty in adopting different coaching styles to suit different situations is the coach's personality. Can he/she really change? This appears to be possible for some but not for all.

Key points

- according to Martens, coaches work on a command/cooperative style continuum
  - command style coaches make all the decisions
  - cooperative style coaches act as facilitators to help the athletes make their own decisions

- according to Lyle, coaches follow an autocratic/democratic continuum
  - autocrats take all decisions
  - democrats involve the athletes in decision making

- according to Mosston, there are 10 styles
  - command style coaches make all decisions
  - practice style coaches are similar to command style but the athlete has some input into what should be practised
  - reciprocal style coaches set the agenda but the athletes coach one another: sometimes called peer coaching
  - self-check style is the same as reciprocal except that each individual coaches him/herself
  - inclusion style refers to coaches who give the athletes some say in deciding what they are to learn
  - coaches using a guided discovery style help the athlete to make decisions about how and what they are to learn
  - coaches using a divergent style set the athletes a problem and let them try to solve it

- ♦ in the individual programme-learner's style, the learner decides what they are to be coached and asks the coach for help with specifics
- ♦ in the learner's initiated style, the athlete decides what he/she wants to learn and only asks the coach's opinion when needed
- ♦ self-teaching style refers to the individuals taking responsibility for all aspects of their own coaching

- there are four learning styles, activists, reflectors, theorists and pragmatists
  - ♦ activists (or accommodators) get involved actively immediately
  - ♦ males tend to be more activist than females
  - ♦ reflectors (or divergers) are cautious and like to 'think through' a problem before acting
  - ♦ females tend to be more reflective than males
  - ♦ theorists (or assimilators) are analytical and like to use hypotheses to solve problems
  - ♦ pragmatists (or those using a convergent style) act quickly but do use some theorizing
  - ♦ coaches should try to change their style to suit the situation but this is not always possible
  - ♦ incompatibility between coaching style and preferred learning style can cause problems with task cohesion.

II

Skill Acquisition

Introduction

In the following chapters, we examine the theory and practice of how athletes acquire skills. Helping their athletes to acquire skills is a major part of the task of the coach. Seeing your athletes perform a skill that you have taught them is arguably the most rewarding aspect of coaching. Just think of the immense pleasure that Sir Clive Woodward must have had when he saw his team win the Rugby World Cup in 2003. It does not, however, need to be a World Cup that brings pleasure to the coach and performer. Seeing someone you have coached perform well on the local recreation ground can be very rewarding.

Before moving on to examine the factors affecting skill acquisition, it is necessary to define exactly what we mean by skill. Skill is 'the consistent production of goal-oriented movements, which are learned and specific to the task' (McMorris, 2004). So we are not born with skill, but rather we develop it through practice. Only when it is consistently produced can we be said to be skilful. Although it is debatable as to what limits the skill level that we reach, one thing for certain is that we must *practise* if we are to reach any standard at all. If you are to be a successful coach, it is vital that you ensure that your athletes are going to practise properly and often. Too many athletes think they practise a great deal but, when we compare the time they spend practising with that of Tiger Woods or Michael Jordan or Maria Sharapova, we realize that they are simply deluding themselves. To repeat an old cliché, 'there is no substitute for practice'.

As we will see later in this part of the book, skill acquisition cannot be studied in isolation from the socio-psychological factors that we have covered in Part I. The developmental issues examined in Part IV also affect skill acquisition. Skill acquisition is not the end goal of coaches, that is performance, but without it performance cannot be successful. Performers who lack skill do not win much. Perhaps more importantly, it can be argued that the greater our skill level the more we enjoy performing even when we do not win.

In this part of the book, we begin by examining the nature of learning. Then we briefly look at some of the basic theories of learning. The bulk of this part, however, is based on factors affecting practice and feedback, which are the essence of skill acquisition. Without practice, we cannot and will not learn. The better the feedback, the faster and more accurately we will learn. Organizing practice and providing feedback is the day to day concern of the coach. It is of little use being a great motivator or tactician if your athletes are not skilful.

Additional reading

Carr, G. (2004). *Sport mechanics for coaches*, 2nd ed. Human Kinetics: Champaign, IL.

Hay, J. G. (1993). *The biomechanics of sports techniques*, 4th ed. Prentice-Hall: Englewood Cliffs, NJ.

Knudson, D. V. and Morrison, C. S. (2002). *Qualitative analysis of human movement*, 2nd ed. Human Kinetics: Champaign, IL.

McMorris, T. (2004). *Acquisition and performance of sports skills*. Wiley: Chichester.

5

Learning

Learning objectives

At the end of this chapter, you should

- understand the nature of learning
- understand the difference between learning and performance
- know how to measure learning
- have an understanding of motor programs
- understand some of the major theories of learning
- understand the nature of instruction and demonstration.

Before examining the nature of learning, it is necessary to define what we mean by the term. Kerr (1982) defined learning as being 'a relatively permanent change in performance resulting from practice or past experience'. The key words here are 'relatively permanent'. One cannot claim to have really learned a skill until one can perform it *consistently*. We have all seen cases of 'beginners luck', e.g. when a novice golfer hits the ball long and straight from the tee. The next shot, however, is likely to go anywhere. The first shot was not the result of learning. It is, in fact, an example of what we call performance. Performance is 'a temporary occurrence fluctuating from time to time: something which is

Coaching Science   Terry McMorris and Tudor Hale
© 2006 John Wiley & Sons, Ltd

transitory' (Kerr, 1982). The fact that it is temporary and fluctuating means that we cannot judge learning based on one performance. We need to be sure that our athletes can repeat the skill with some consistency. This consistency can only come about by practice or experience. It is the role of the coach to ensure that his or her athletes practise sufficiently to obtain that consistency.

Types of learning

It was, until quite recently, thought that learning could not take place unless the learner consciously set out to acquire the skill. This is called explicit learning. *Explicit learning* refers to what we might call the 'normal' way of learning. We are given overt, or explicit, instructions and told to concentrate on the task at hand. Recent research has shown that, in fact, we can learn subconsciously or implicitly. Researchers such as Richard Magill (see, e.g., Magill, 1993) and Richard Masters (see, e.g., Masters, 2000) found that we can, and do, improve our level of expertise simply by repeating a task even when we are not consciously attending to what we are doing. This is what we mean by *implicit learning*.

Possibly more surprising than the fact that learning can take place implicitly is that research has shown that we do not have to practise physically in order for learning to be demonstrated. In Chapter 3, we examined the use of the various forms of mental rehearsal in order to help performers control their anxiety. It has been shown that mental rehearsal can also result in learning. However, most researchers believe that, as a learning tool, mental rehearsal only works in *conjunction with physical rehearsal*. Research has shown that individuals who use mental rehearsal, as well as physical rehearsal, do learn more quickly than those using physical practice only. One theory put forward to explain the advantages of mental rehearsal is that, by thinking about the skill, we build up a picture or model in our central nervous system (CNS) of how the skill should be performed. The CNS, which includes the brain, reacts to this mental process in a very similar way to when we actually practise physically. Thus, if we *think about doing something, the CNS learns the same, or almost the same, as when we actually carry out the task.* Bruce Hale (1982) provided some experimental support for this. He had people mentally rehearse doing a task. While they were mentally rehearsing, he had electromyographs (EMGs) fitted to the muscles that would be used if they were physically performing the skill. He showed that there was some neural activity even though the person never overtly moved.

Before moving on, we should note that, so far, we have assumed that learning is always *positive*, i.e. through practice and/or experience we improve.

This is not necessarily the case. Learning can be *negative*. We can develop inappropriate responses.

Measuring learning

The fact that performance fluctuates can make it difficult for coaches and athletes to measure the amount of learning that has taken place. Strictly speaking we cannot actually measure learning; we can only infer it based on performance. The three most commonly used methods for inferring learning are the use of retention tests, transfer tests and the plotting of performance curves. *Retention* is *the persistence of performance over a period of no practice*. As such, it measures consistency.

The use of retention tests provides the coach and performer with quantifiable information about how well they are developing their skills. When using retention tests, coaches and sports psychologists normally have their athletes perform a pre-practice test first. Following this, they have the athletes practise the skill and then perform a post-practice test. *This is not the retention test*. It is a performance test. Learning takes time to occur. The retention test takes place some time later. This can be a matter of hours or preferably days. Figure 5.1 demonstrates the learning of two netballers taking shots at the net. Player A shows that she has retained what she learned over the period of no practice, while player B demonstrates some loss. She is still better than she was pre-practice, however. Figure 5.2 shows the performance of a third netballer on the skill test. Notice that she actually improves over the period of no practice. This phenomenon is called *reminiscence*. As we stated above, it takes time for learning to be manifested. Why and how this occurs is examined later.

Another method of testing for learning is to use *transfer tasks*. The use of transfer tasks to infer learning is based on the assumption that if a skill is truly learned it can be performed in a number of different environments or situations. A method of transfer might be changing the task demands, e.g. learning the set shot in basketball and then moving on to the jump shot. Another method is by changing the environment, e.g. moving from playing short tennis (tennis on a modified small court) to playing on a full-size court. Coaches do this automatically when they progress from one practice to another.

Task 1 Choose two skills, one that you do well and one at which you are weak. Work out a transfer task in which you can perform the skills. See if the stronger skill is transferred more readily than the weaker.

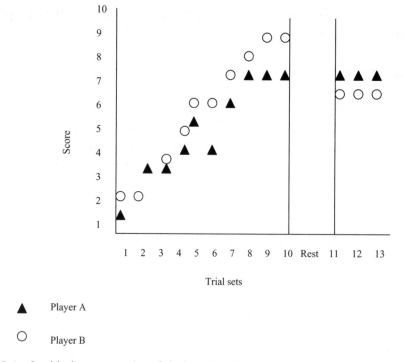

Figure 5.1 Graphical representation of the learning of two netball players over a series of trials. Each set of trials represents 10 shots at the net

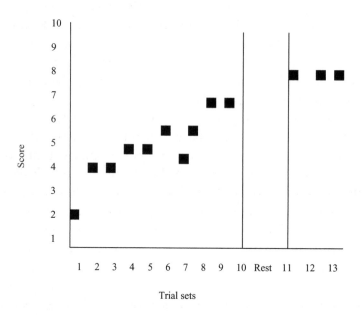

Figure 5.2 Graphical representation of a netball player over a set of trials. Each set of trials consists of 10 shots at net. The post-rest results show an effect of reminiscence

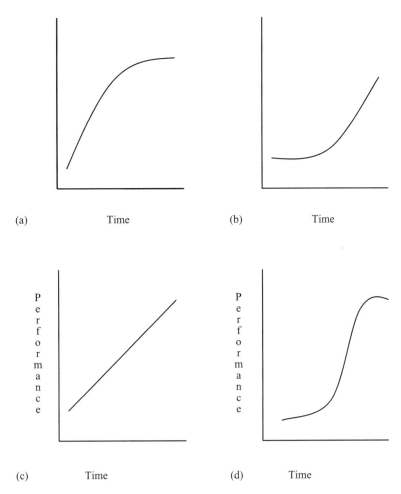

Figure 5.3 Typical learning curves: (a) shows a negatively accelerated curve, (b) a positively accelerated curve, (c) a linear 'curve' and (d) an ogive or S-shaped curve

Performance curves are, also, used to measure learning. The calculation of performance curves can be useful. In order to do this, the performance of the learner is plotted over a period of time and/or a number of trials and is shown graphically. There are four common types of curve that have been found by researchers. Figure 5.3(a) depicts a *negatively accelerated curve*. There is an early improvement but then performance tapers off somewhat. Figure 5.3(b) shows a *positively accelerated curve*. There is an overall general improvement but, as we can see, it is slow at first and then accelerates. Figure 5.3(c) shows a *linear* improve- ment with practice, while Figure 5.3(d) demonstrates an *ogive* or *S-shaped curve.*

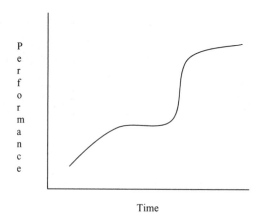

Figure 5.4   A graph showing a plateau in learning

Task 2 *Choose a skill that is new to you, preferably one which is easy to score. Plot your own performance curve. Which type of curve is it?*

The curve in Figure 5.4 demonstrates the effect of what we call a *plateau* in learning. This is quite a common occurrence and is probably something you have experienced yourself. There comes a point when practising does not appear to be having any effect. This is the plateau. If we keep on practising, there is a break-through and more learning is demonstrated. Of course, sometimes what appears to be a plateau is in fact the limit of our capability and no more improvement is demonstrated, regardless of the amount of practice we undertake. There are a number of reasons why plateaus might occur. It is possible that boredom, or reactive inhibition, is causing a temporary hold on performance. There is, also, the possibility that the problem is in the limitations of measuring performance. Evidence from studies using biomechanical methods of assessment shows that there are changes in the way in which the skill is being performed, which do not produce an immediate quantitative change in outcome and are not easily seen by the naked eye.

A more likely explanation, however, lies in the nature of memory. There is no specific part of the brain that is memory. Rather memory is demonstrated when we form neural interconnections in our CNS. These interconnections take time to form. The formation of these connections can be likened to the development of a path across a field of high grass. At first, it is difficult to get from one side to the other. After time, however, we wear down the grass in certain areas to produce a clear pathway across the field. It is this phenomenon that also explains reminiscence and why retention tests are better than post-practice tests as measures of learning.

Cognitive approaches to learning

The examination of learning outlined above is based on a cognitive approach, i.e. it is assumed that the CNS plays the key role in learning. This has been hotly disputed by the dynamical systems theorists, and we will examine their arguments later in this chapter. Here we will outline the theory that has dominated our beliefs about learning over, at least, the last 40 years. This is information processing theory.

Information processing theory

Information processing theory was developed at the same time as computers and owes much to computing technology. Although there are many information processing models, they are basically the same. The model that can be seen in Figure 5.5 is a simplification of Welford's (1968) model.

The *input* to which the information processing theorists refer is all of the information present in the environment. It is sometimes referred to as the *display*. The display contains a vast amount of information, some relevant to the task and some irrelevant. This information, from the display, is relayed to the CNS by afferent or sensory nerves. According to the information processing theorists, the role of the CNS is explained by the boxes or divisions shown in the model.

The first task for the CNS is to interpret the incoming information. If we have normal senses we will all actually see, feel or hear the same things. However, the way in which we interpret them will differ. You only have to hear two people's accounts of the same incident to verify this. How we interpret the incoming information is the role of *perception*. Perhaps the major role of perception is to focus attention to task relevant cues at the expense of irrelevant ones. This is known as *selective attention*. Good selective attention is demonstrated by playmakers such as quarterbacks in American football or stand-offs in rugby. Some individuals such as the former ice hockey player Wayne Gretsky possess selective attention skills of the highest order.

The information processing theorists place great importance on the role of *memory* to aid perception and selective attention. Perception, according to them, is what we call *indirect*, i.e. it is dependent on our interpretation of the incoming information. This interpretation is based on a comparison between what we hold in *short-term memory* (STM) and what we hold in *long-term memory* (LTM). As you can see from Figure 5.5, there are arrows going from

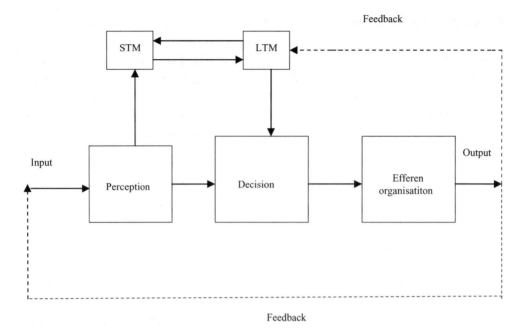

Figure 5.5   Model of information processing (adapted from Welford, A. T. (1968). *Fundamentals of skill*. Methuen: London)

STM to LTM and, also, arrows going the other way. The arrows going from STM to LTM represent the passing of information that we see, hear or feel to LTM, where it can be stored for future use. In other words, *this is how we learn*. The arrows from LTM to STM are concerned with performance rather than learning. By comparing what we hold in STM with past experiences held in LTM we are able to decide what action to take. This is represented by the decision-making box in Welford's model. This interaction between perceptual information held in STM, information retrieved from LTM and decision making is referred to as *working memory*.

Once a decision of what action to take has been made, the CNS has to organize the movement (*efferent organization*). The information, concerning movement organization, is sent from the CNS to the peripheral nervous system (PNS), by the efferent or motor nerves, so that the movement can take place. Once we start to move, we begin to process *feedback*. Feedback can be information about the nature of our movements. In Figure 5.5, this is depicted by the bottom feedback arrow. In slow movements, we can use this information to alter or refine our actions as they are being carried out. The top feedback arrow represents information about the success or failure of our actions, and is fed back to LTM. This information is stored and is responsible for learning. The more we practise a skill, the stronger the neural connections in the CNS become. When these connections are fully formed we are said to have established a motor program (the American English 'program' is normally used rather than the UK English 'programme'). The existence and nature of these programs are a contentious issue in sports psychology at the moment; therefore, we will take some time to examine them.

Motor programs

Keele (1968) defined a motor program as being *a set of muscle commands that allow movements to be performed without any peripheral feedback*. In other words *the movement becomes automatic*. This is, of course, what coaches want their athletes to achieve. According to Keele, the person sees a movement and stores a *template* or *model of the task* in their LTM. When the athlete practises the skill, he or she constantly compares the outcome and the nature of the movement with the template. During practice, *corrections are made until the action matches the template*, then the motor program is established. Examples of motor programs are basically any skill that you can think of. Playing a forehand drive in tennis or doing a somersault are both examples of motor programs. So, too, are more simple tasks like walking or running. Furthermore, when motor programs are established, they are performed smoothly and consistently. Watch Tiger Woods playing a drive from the tee or Maria Sharapova making a forehand drive.

There is a marked difference between our efforts to perform the skill before and after a motor program has been developed. Performance while we are developing the program is comparatively uncoordinated, looks crude and lacks consistency. Compare the beginner golfer to the effortless ease of Tiger Woods and Anneka Sorenstam.

Although motor program theory has intuitive appeal, it is not without its weaknesses. Early motor program theorists believed that we store the specific *sequencing, timing and range of movement*. Observation of people performing skills, however, shows that motor programs are not always repeated at the same speed or indeed in exactly the same body position. Look at Figure 5.6. Here we see a football goalkeeper catching the ball in four different positions. According to early motor program theorists, he would need four separate motor programs. Few of today's information processing

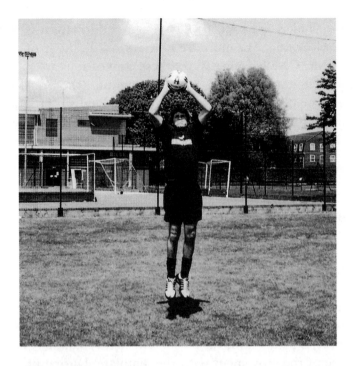

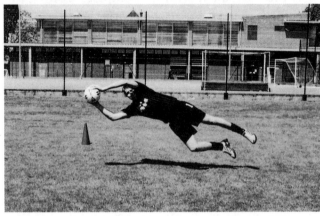

Figure 5.6   The goalkeeper is using the same generalized motor program to catch the ball in four different positions

theorists accept the notion of specific motor programs. This theory has been superseded by the idea that we form a series of *generalized motor programs*. In other words, our goalkeeper has stored a set of basic rules about how to catch a ball. He is able to alter the specifics of his movements to meet the particular situation in which he finds himself.

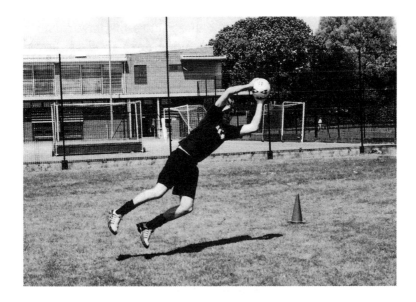

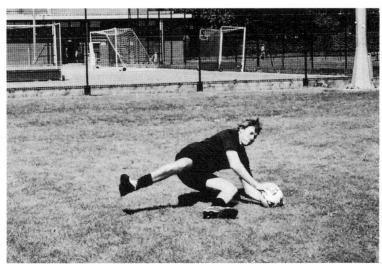

Figure 5.6 (*Continued*)

Cognitive theories of learning

At this stage, it would be beneficial to examine some cognitive theories of learning. There are numerous such theories but I have decided to examine only four, the three stage theory of Fitts and Posner (1967), Schmidt's (1975) schema theory, Anderson's (1982) adaptive control of thought (ACT) theory and Bandura's (1977) observational learning theory. I chose these because they are the most commonly cited in the literature and have major practical implications. It is up to the readers to decide, for themselves, how well each of the theories explains learning.

The three stage theory of Fitts and Posner

Probably the most cited cognitive theory is that of Fitts and Posner (1967). They claimed that learning takes place in three stages, the cognitive, associative and autonomous. In the *cognitive* stage the person tries to make sense of instructions. He or she make a great deal of use of verbal labels. This does not mean that instruction needs to be verbal, but simply that the individual uses verbalization to aid memory. In skills requiring perception and decision-making, there are often mistakes made and the person attends to irrelevant as well as relevant stimuli. The motor component is characterized by crude uncoordinated movement.

With practice the individual develops the knowledge of what to do. When someone is at this stage they are said to be in the *associative* stage (sometimes called the intermediate stage). At this stage, practice is required to perfect the skill and develop the consistent coordinated movement that demonstrates learning. When the person can perform consistently and with little overt cognitive activity, they are said to have reached the *autonomous* stage. Although performance at this stage is rarely affected by distraction and stress, it is difficult to alter. This can be negative if the person has developed responses, or aspects of the response, that are inappropriate.

Schmidt's schema theory

Richard Schmidt developed his theory due to his dissatisfaction with motor program theory. If motor programs were specific then we would need very large brains to hold all the programs we use. Moreover, motor program theory was unable to explain how we are able to perform a large number of variations of the same skill. Even more alarming was its inability to account for that fact that we are able to perform novel skills, i.e. we are able to improvise when we need to produce a movement for which we have no specific motor program. Schmidt (1975) set out to rectify these difficulties by developing Schema Theory.

A schema is a *set of generalized rules or rules that are generic to a group of movements*. Schmidt believes that we develop two kinds of schema, these he called the recall and recognition schemas (or schemata). The *recall schema* is responsible for the choice and initiation of action, while the *recognition schema* evaluates the ongoing movement and makes appropriate changes in the action. Schmidt stated that the learning of the recall and recognition schemas is brought about by the development of the general rules, which evolve during performance. In developing the recall schema, we remember the *desired outcome, the initial conditions, the response parameters and the sensory consequences*. An example of initial conditions would be the position of the individual's body parts when preparing to play a forehand drive in tennis. The speed, line and length of ball flight would also be initial conditions. Response parameters, sometimes called *response specifications*, are changes in the specifics of the action that are necessary if we are to be successful. These parameters will depend on the situation in which we find ourselves. The parameters will be different if the initial conditions change. For example, if we wish to play a forehand drive in tennis and we are stationary, the response parameters will be different to those when we are running across court. Or if we want to kick a football hard at the goal, the parameters will be different to those when we want to pass it softly to a team-mate. We do not need to have previously experienced the exact initial conditions or response parameters. If a recall schema has been developed, the CNS can automatically adjust the interaction between the two.

Similarly, with the recognition schema, we remember the desired outcome, initial conditions and the sensory consequences. It is the latter that are the most important for the recognition schema. The sensory consequences are what the movement feels like. As with the recall schema, we do not need to have experienced the exact same sensory consequences to know if we are performing the movement as desired. The development of the schema allows us to know if we are within the correct boundaries. Those of you who play striking games, like tennis, cricket, golf or baseball, will all have known that a strike was good, without having to see where the ball went, just from the feel of the movement. You also know when you have underhit or overhit a shot.

Task 3 Choose a skill and write down the desired outcome, the initial conditions, the response parameters and the sensory consequences.

The development of the schemas is controlled by *error labelling*. For fast movements sensory information is fed back to the CNS after the completion of the action. Any mismatches between the desired and actual outcomes are labelled as being errors and are used to alter the schemas, ready for the next time the individual needs to achieve the desired goal. This, also, occurs for slow movements until the recognition schema has been developed, then the sensory information is fed back to the CNS and the movement is continually altered during performance in order to achieve the desired outcome.

Adaptive control of thought (ACT) theory

According to Anderson's (1982) *adaptive control of thought (ACT)* theory the period of time when we learn what to do in any given situation is said to be the time taken to develop *declarative knowledge*. Declarative knowledge is knowing *what* to do. Anderson believes that we acquire declarative knowledge prior to what he terms *procedural knowledge*. Procedural knowledge is not merely making the correct decision but knowing how to ensure that the goal of our action is met. It is difficult to argue against a claim that there is a difference between knowing what to do and being able to do it. Many coaches are very good at the former but were not as good as their athletes at the latter. There is, however, no proof that declarative knowledge precedes procedural knowledge in sport. It may well be that greater exposure to the sport means that the expert has picked up more declarative knowledge. They may not, however, use this when acquiring procedural knowledge. Indeed, recent research examining implicit learning suggests strongly that we can obtain procedural knowledge without ever having declarative knowledge of the skill (Masters, 2000). The former Manchester United and Northern Ireland football star George Best openly admitted to not having been aware of why and how he beat opponents. He just did. Moreover, he did so very often.

ACT theory is particularly good at explaining how we learn to make decisions during games. Anderson believes that when we are learning to make decisions we predetermine what we will do in any given situation. He claims that we solve problems by saying 'if this happens, then I will do that'. This is declarative knowledge. As we practise more and more we need to do this less and less until we respond automatically when we perceive the situation. This is procedural knowledge.

Task 4 *Choose someone whose style of play you know well. Then pick out some common decisions that need to be made in his/her sport. See if you can decide what action they will take in each of these situations. Try to watch them in action and see if you were correct. How often do they deviate from your expected response?*

Observational learning theory

Bandura's (1977) observational learning theory is not an attempt to replace other learning theories but is more an explanation of how we learn from observing demonstrations. According to Bandura, we learn by *observation of the behaviour of others and the consequences of that behaviour*. Bandura believes that this observation can be *deliberate or incidental*. Deliberate observation is when we explicitly, or overtly, attend to the action being demonstrated. The demonstration can be given by a coach for us to copy or by observing someone else performing a skill. Incidental observation is probably how we learn implicitly. We are not overtly aware of observing the skill but nevertheless we do become able to perform it.

To Bandura, the key to successful observational learning is *reinforcement*. If the model is reinforced, the observer is most likely to imitate the movement. Therefore, if the person sees that the action brings success, they will try to do it themselves. However, if the model is unsuccessful, they are unlikely to copy it. This is self-evident, but Bandura found with social behaviour that unsuccessful behaviour is sometimes learned even though the learner has consciously rejected it. This has major implications for learners because it means that exposure to incorrect movements, in the early stages of learning, may result in the acquisition of bad habits.

Bandura stresses the advantages of the use of *mental imagery and verbal coding* when acquiring skills. He, also, points out the need to observe complex skills several times before imitation is possible. From what we have so far said, it may look as though Bandura is saying that all we need to do is observe a skill a number of times and then we will be able to repeat it. In fact, he is not. For a skill to be learned, Bandura asserted that physical practise is essential. Mental imagery can aid learning but cannot replace what Bandura calls *motoric reproduction*.

Summary

To summarize, I will outline the areas of agreement between the cognitive theories. According to these theories the aim of learning is to develop one's LTM store. In learning we set out to memorize *what* we should do in any given situation and *how* we should do it. The theories also generally agree that, in the early stages of learning, we try to verbalize or intellectualize what it is we are trying to do. However, recent research into implicit learning has brought this into question. Whether implicit or explicit, however, it is unanimously believed that practice is necessary for skills to develop. When a skill is fully developed it can be performed *automatically*, with little recourse to consciousness. At this stage it is said that a motor program has been developed. Although originally it was believed that these programs were many and specific, it is now believed that they are generalized and can be adapted to different situations.

Dynamical systems theory and learning

If I were writing a situation comedy, at this stage I would probably say 'And now to something completely different'. Dynamical systems theory is an ecological psychology theory. To the ecological psychologists, memory is of little use in the learning and performance of motor skills. Ecological psychology places great emphasis on the interaction between humankind and the environment. The environment dictates what opportunities for action are available, at any given time, in any specific situation. J. J. Gibson (1979), one of the founding fathers of ecological psychology, called these opportunities for action 'affordances'. Moreover, no two situations are exactly the same, therefore affordances may be similar but never identical. While affordances are present at all times, they will not be acted upon if the individual is unaware of their existence. The person must *actively search* the environment or display for the presence of affordances. Thus, perception of the affordance is dependent on movement, as much as receiving sensory information. This is very obvious when a golfer is about to play a shot. He or she will examine the possibilities from many angles, not merely stand there and expect the information to come to him or her. The existence or non-existence of an affordance will be obvious to the performers; they *do not require the use of memory*. This is called *direct perception*.

Sport provides many examples of direct perception. As long as you know the aims or goals of the game, the environment provides the necessary opportunities for actions. If you had never played tennis before but saw that your opponent was at one side of the court, you would not need past experience to see the affordance of playing a shot to the other side of the court. I am sure that you can provide similar examples from your own sports.

Until recently, the ecological psychologists rarely talked about learning. To them every time we perform a skill is the same as the first time. The organization of movement is not dependent on memory but is the result of the interaction between limbs that are obeying scientific laws. Thus, it is said that the organism is capable of 'self-organization'. Therefore, there is no need for motor programs. However, ecological psychologists accepted that the evidence that experience affects performance is overwhelming. Therefore, the dynamical systems theorists began to examine the nature of learning. To them, the key to learning is to *become attuned to affordances*. This means that, as we gain experience, we automatically know where in an environment to search for affordances that will allow us to achieve our goal. The hockey centre-forward, when in the D, will look for opportunities to get a shot at goal. The learning of this will occur naturally by *trial and error*. Taken to its logical conclusion, all the coach would need to do would be to tell the learner what they should be aiming to do in any given situation. The cricket coach could say 'hit the ball' or 'score runs'. By experimentation, the learner would eventually become attuned to the affordance and play the correct shot. This may, of course, be very time consuming. The coach can shorten it by helping the learner to perceive the affordances. To the dynamical systems theorists, the best way to achieve this is not to say 'do this' but to guide the learners toward perceiving the affordances for themselves.

Before leaving dynamical systems theory of learning we should briefly mention some other important factors. One of these was called 'bootstrapping' by Lev Vygotsky (1978). Bootstrapping means stretching the learner beyond what they can already do. A good example of bootstrapping is when a coach progresses from a relatively simple practice to a more complex one.

One of the effects of bootstrapping is what Michael Turvey (1992) calls *'freezing' and 'unfreezing' the degrees of freedom*. The degrees of freedom are all the muscles, joints and nerves that we must control in order to perform a skill. When we first learn a skill, it is difficult to control the many muscles and joints that are used. As a result, we naturally overcome this by freezing many of the degrees of freedom, e.g. we ensure that some joints are kept locked. Watch someone learning a backhand serve in table tennis. They will lock their wrists and limit the movement of their elbow. When they become proficient, however, they realize that simply getting the ball across the net is not good enough. They must apply spin. This is not possible if the wrists are locked and the elbow rigid. At this stage, the learner must 'unfreeze' the degrees of freedom in order to perform the task properly. For example, in order to impart backspin, the wrist must be loose so that the bat can be swept underneath the centre of the ball. Golfers provide a good example of freezing and unfreezing degrees of freedom. Beginners try hard to keep muscles and joints still so that they do not slice or hook the ball. Experts will deliberately allow free movement of specific joints so that they can deliberately make the ball alter its trajectory in mid-air.

Task 5 Can you think of any skills that require freezing of degrees of freedom early in learning and unfreezing at expert level?

Practical implications

Most of the practical implications of the theoretical aspects of learning outlined in the previous section are manifested during practice and are therefore covered in the next chapter. Indeed, to the dynamical systems theorists, practice is learning. There are, however, some implications that we can examine before we move to the chapter on practice. One of the most important factors is the decision of what to coach at any given time. This is a factor that is far too often treated lightly by coaches. In Chapter 13 we examine the development of annual programmes, and these are closely linked with the decision of what to coach. However, as Chapter 13 is more concerned with the rules of developing a programme of work over a year, in this section we will look at the more basic stage, which precedes this. Figure 5.7 shows the major factors that must be taken into account when deciding what to teach to any group of learners. As you can see, the areas stated are not only those covered earlier in this chapter but also factors examined in Parts I, III and IV of this book.

When determining what factors we need to consider, I have followed a cognitivist approach. Most of these areas, however, would also be considered to be important by dynamical systems theorists. As dynamical systems approaches are covered in some detail in Chapter 8, I thought it best to use an information processing approach in this section. Therefore, the key issue is the past experience of the learners. We need to decide what they bring to the learning situation. We may know this already if we have coached this individual or group previously. However, we may equally need to find out. This can be done by some form of test. In activities such as track and field this can be simple. Just let the athlete perform. Times or distances can be measured. With team games, it is less clear. Simply observing someone perform can be useful in such circumstances. However, some coaches prefer to have quantifiable data from skills tests. This can, also, act as a motivator for the learner.

Whatever we decide to coach, we should take into account bootstrapping. It is up to the coach to instil in the learner a desire to improve on their performance. As we have seen in Chapter 1, the extent to which the athletes wish to develop is determined by their motivational level and type. It is not always possible to actually measure this using psychometric tests. Indeed, some would question the use of such tests, as the performer will normally tell the coach what they think the coach wishes to hear. In most real life situations it is up to the coach to determine, by observation of what the athlete does, what their motivation is. The ability to do this is, in itself, a skill. The coach should not be afraid to try different approaches and see which is most appreciated by their athletes. This can be a good guide to what the athletes want.

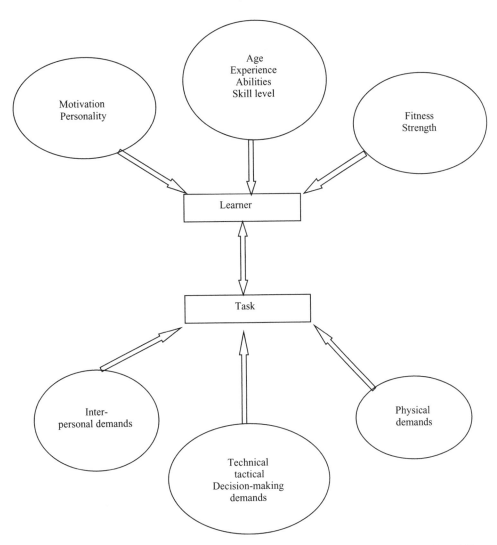

Figure 5.7 Major factors that a coach needs to take into account when deciding what skills to coach at any given time

Instruction/demonstration

Once the coach has decided what to coach, he/she needs to determine what kind of instruction to use. To the cognitivists, instruction is vital when learning is to be explicit. The instruction can take many forms and can, in fact, be in the form of demonstrations, hence the title of this section. As with deciding what to coach, the stage of cognitive development of the learners needs to be taken into account. The coach must not *overload* the working memory of the learners.

The number of schemes that can be dealt with at each age group have been outlined by Pascual-Leone (see Chapter 13) but it must be remembered that each person develops at his or her own rate. Therefore, these can only be used as guidelines.

There does appear to be a general difference between children and adults with regard to when they receive instruction and the amount of detail provided. Children like to have a go at the skill before receiving any instruction. Moreover, they like instruction to be brief and to the point. The older adults get, the more detail they want. Regardless of age, however, there are certain concrete rules about instruction. Even adults have a limited working memory capacity, therefore the coach must not provide too much information. Coaches must, also, be careful with the words they use. Jargon should be avoided where possible or only used if the coach knows for sure that the athletes understand it. When dealing with children, in particular, one should be careful even with words that appear to be in common use.

The problems of using verbal instructions have been known for some time. As a result a large amount of research has examined the comparative strengths of *verbal, visual* and *verbal plus visual* instruction. Based on the 'a picture paints a thousand words' idea, most researchers have hypothesized that visual instruction or demonstration will be better than verbal. In general, this has been found to be the case but not unequivocally. We would expect visual instruction to be superior to verbal because it is not possible to verbally articulate many skills.

Task 6 Choose a skill from your own favourite sport and try to write down an explanation of how to perform it.

While it is possible to verbally articulate some skills, the notion that a demonstration is easy to follow is something of an exaggeration. There is no guarantee that the learner is focusing on the cues that are important if they are going to acquire the skill.

Task 7 Look at Figure 5.8. Do not dwell on it too long. Try to perform the skill yourself.

I would expect most of you to get somewhere near doing the turn correctly. But what did you do with your arms? The role of the arms is important in this skill (the Cruyff turn). To carry out the skill properly defenders must think that the player is going to kick the ball rather than turn. The deception is greatly advanced by the use of the arms. I have chosen this skill because the use of the arms is often missed by observers. They become obsessed with the feet.

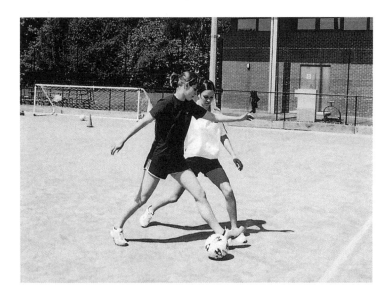

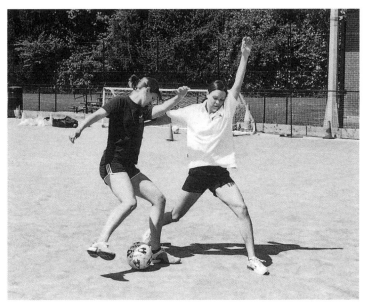

Figure 5.8   An example of the Cruyff turn

The problems with demonstrations, outlined above, support the research findings that verbal plus visual instruction has been shown to be the most productive. It is important that the coach *draws the learner's attention to the key points*. It should be of no surprise that research supports Bandura's assertion that the learner needs to observe more than one demonstration.

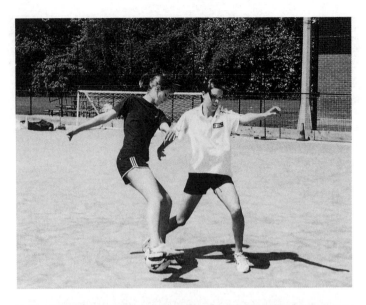

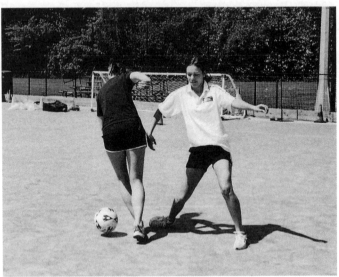

Figure 5.8 (*Continued*)

Look at Figure 5.8 again and concentrate on the arms. It is very unlikely that, at this second time of looking, you had any difficulty in seeing what the player is doing with her arms.

Task 8 *Choose a skill and write down which key points you would have the learner look at during a demonstration. Try to get the points in order of priority.*

If we want people to learn by observation the demonstration needs to be correct, especially as Bandura believes that incorrect demonstration may be subconsciously copied. There will be some skills that the coach cannot demonstrate, because their own performance level is not good enough. In such cases there has to be some kind of compromise. The coach needs to decide whether their level of performance is satisfactory to demonstrate the skill. The demonstration needs to be adequate, not necessarily perfect. Some people overcome limitations by demonstrating in slow motion. There are problems with this. If you are to use this method, you must make sure that speed is not an essential factor in the performance of the skill. For example, dribbling in football, basketball or hockey requires the player to accelerate when going past their opponent. If learners have only seen a slow motion demonstration, this key point may be missed. If the learner does not see an accurate demonstration then the template they need to use in order to develop their own motor program will be incorrect. If they continue to practise the skill incorrectly, they will develop an inaccurate motor program. Once a motor program is developed, it is very difficult to change it.

Slow motion demonstrations may, however, be necessary in some cases even when the instructor can demonstrate at normal speed. Some skills are performed too quickly for the learner to see exactly what is happening. The hand actions of pitchers in baseball and spin bowlers in cricket can be so quick that the learner cannot see what is happening. In such cases the coach will have to give a slow motion demonstration. However, this should be done only after a real time demonstration has been carried out.

As well as being instructional, demonstration can also be motivational. The learner should observe the demonstration and think, 'I want to do that'. However, they must also think, 'I can do that'. This latter point highlights a problem with coaches demonstrating skills, especially to children. The child must perceive that children can also perform this skill; it is not something that only adults can do. This has led researchers to examine the use of *peer demonstrations*. Instead of the coach giving the demonstration themselves, they get someone of the same age as the learners to perform the skill. This may be done directly or on a film, if there is no one in the group who can perform the skill.

Although we have been talking about the problems of learners being so overawed by demonstrations that they feel they cannot achieve success, it is sometimes best to show a film of a top class athlete performing a skill. This can have great motivational value. The desire to perform a skill that your 'hero' uses is appealing to most performers. Just look at how many youngsters copied Jonny Wilkinson's place kicking style following the Rugby World Cup. This desire to emulate the stars is particularly so with children.

Shaping skills

A specific form of instruction is shaping skills. This method is particularly concerned with the problems of overloading the STM. The coach instructs the performer to concentrate firstly on one small part of the skill. Once the learner is able to perform that part reasonably well, a second part is added and so on. For example, when coaching someone to kick a football with the instep, the coach might get the learner to focus on the point of foot–ball contact, then look at the approach to the ball and then the follow-through. The problem with this method of instruction is that the chances of demonstrating a plateau effect are high. Nevertheless, it can be very useful with youngsters and with complex skills.

Although this method is based on a cognitivist approach, it is also acceptable to the dynamical systems theorists, although the 'instructions' they use are more the setting of outcome goals rather than instructions *per se*. They will not tell the learner how to kick the ball but instruct them to concentrate on kicking over a distance and with some accuracy, i.e. the outcome goal. What the ecologists advocate is more akin to learning by *guided discovery*, i.e. the coach sets a problem and helps the learner to solve it. When guided discovery is used properly it has the advantage of not making all athletes perform a task in exactly the same way. The learners develop their own styles.

Key points

- learning is a relatively permanent change in performance resulting from practice or experience

- performance is temporary and fluctuates from time to time

- learning can be explicit or implicit
  - explicit learning is when we consciously set out to acquire skill and/or knowledge
  - implicit learning takes place subconsciously without intent

- mental rehearsal can aid learning when used in conjunction with physical rehearsal

- retention is the persistence of a skill over a period of no practice

- reminiscence is an improvement in performance following a period of no practice

- we cannot directly measure learning; we can only infer its presence by measuring performance

- 'learning' can be measured by
  - retention tests – a test of performance following a period of no practice
  - transfer tests – performance of the skill in a different environment or situation
  - measuring performance curves – plotting performance over a period of time

- **Information processing theory**

- the information processing theory model (see Figure 5.5) consists of
  - perception (what we make of the information around us)
  - decision making (what action we decide to take)
  - memory (short and long term)
  - efferent organization (the organization of the movements that we wish to make)
  - proprioceptive feedback (aids the control of slow movements)
  - feedback for learning

- well-learned movements become automatic and are said to have developed into motor programs
  - motor programs can be performed without recourse to feedback
  - according to schema theory, motor programs are generalized, i.e. they can be adapted to suit different conditions

- when learning a motor program we
  - form a model of the task in our long-term memory
  - compare the model to our attempts during practice
  - make corrections until the action matches the model

- **Cognitivist theories of learning**

- the three stage theory by Fitts and Posner
  - cognitive stage – use of verbal labels
  - associative stage – practice is required to refine the skill
  - autonomous stage – the skill becomes automatic

- Schmidt's schema theory
  - recall memory is responsible for the choice and initiation of action

- recognition memory evaluates the ongoing movement and makes any necessary changes
- recall schemas are based on the memory of the desired outcome: initial conditions–response parameters (changes in the specifics of the movement if action is to be successful)–sensory consequences (what the movement feels like).
- recognition schemas are based on the memory of the desired outcome: the initial conditions–sensory consequences

- error labeling (comparison of desired and actual outcomes) aids schema formation

- according to Anderson's adaptive control of thought (ACT) theory, we develop declarative and procedural knowledge
  - declarative knowledge is knowing what to do
  - procedural knowledge is knowing what to do and how to do it

- Anderson believes that declarative knowledge needs to be acquired before procedural knowledge
  - there is no definitive proof that, in sport, declarative knowledge needs to be acquired before we can acquire procedural knowledge
  - procedural knowledge may be obtained subconsciously

- Anderson believes that we decide what we will do prior to taking part in an activity
  - we follow a series of predetermined responses (if 'a' happens, I will do 'b')

- observational learning theory
  - observation of others aids learning
  - observation can be deliberate or incidental
  - successful actions are copied
  - mental imagery and verbal coding aid learning
  - physical practice is essential for the learning of motor skills

- **Dynamical systems theory and learning**

- we actively search the environment for affordances (opportunities to achieve our goal)

- perception is direct; it does not require memory, all of the information necessary is present in the environment
  - practice helps us to become attuned to affordances, i.e. to know where in the environment to search for opportunities to achieve our goals

- learning can be by trial and error

- beginners will try to limit the movement of joints and muscles, this is called freezing the degrees of freedom
  - experts will deliberately unfreeze the degrees of freedom to allow for improvisation
  - getting learners to progress to another level is called bootstrapping

- **Instruction/demonstration**

- coaches must not overload the limited capacity of the athlete's working memory

- instruction can be verbal, visual or verbal plus visual
  - verbal plus visual is the most effective
  - some skills are very difficult to put into words

- demonstrations are a particularly useful form of instruction
  - demonstrations can be given by the coach or by a peer
  - demonstrations can be motivational as well as instructive

- shaping is a way of getting the learner to focus on the key points and to prioritize them.

6

Practice

Learning objectives

At the end of this chapter, you should

- know the different types of practice
- know what to take into account when deciding on the type of practice to be used in any given situation
- understand theories concerning variability of practice, contextual interference and deliberate practice
- understand transfer of training
- understand the dynamical systems theory approach to practice.

Practice is essential if learning is to take place. To the cognitivists, practice follows instruction. It is the key factor in the intermediate and autonomous stages of Fitts and Posner, while Anderson would see it as being when we move from declarative knowledge (knowing what to do) to procedural knowledge (developing the ability to perform the task). To the dynamical systems theorists, *practice is learning*.

Coaching Science   Terry McMorris and Tudor Hale
© 2006 John Wiley & Sons, Ltd

Information processing theory and practice

To the information processing theorists, when we practise we build up our LTM store. Engrams, interconnections between brain cells, are formed in the CNS. These allow us to remember what to do and how to do it. There are significant improvements in the efficiency of working memory. Accurate selective attention is developed and making decisions becomes automatic. This is of great importance in sports that require fast decisions. Moreover, motor programs can only be developed with practice. This happens primarily in the CNS, with efferent organization becoming automatic. However, a form of memory is also developed in the PNS. This aids the smoothness of our movements. The uncoordinated and error laden actions of the beginning phases of learning are gradually replaced by smooth well coordinated movements.

Even when we have developed motor programs it appears that we need to continue to practise motor skills. With verbal skills once we have learned them there is no need to continually repeat them. This is not the case with physical skills. We need to continue to practise even after we have acquired the skill. This phenomenon is known as *overlearning*. The importance of overlearning can be seen by the fact that top class performers such as André Agassi and Justine Henin-Hardenne still spend hours and hours practising their skills.

Types of practice

In this section, we will examine the main types of practice that have been highlighted by researchers and theorists. One of the first areas of practice to be examined was massed versus spaced practice. Massed practice is where there is little or no gap between trials. Spaced practice is when work is interspersed with rest periods or breaks. Research has generally shown that there is no difference in learning resulting from the two types of practice. Spaced practice can sometimes lead to better performance because either boredom (reactive inhibition) or fatigue can set in during massed practice. Following a rest, however, there is no difference when retention tests are conducted.

Task 1 Make a list, from your own sport, in which massed practice might cause problems with fatigue.

While the evidence is that neither massed nor spaced practice is the better with regard to learning, the coach should be aware of motivational effects. To many learners, massed practice is less enjoyable, as they become bored with repeating the same task over and over again without a break. On the other hand, some performers feel that breaks are a waste of time and that they could be doing something useful in the time between trials. It is up to the coach and players to agree to what is best for them.

Whole and part practice

Whole practice, as the word implies, is practising a task in its entirety. This is straightforward enough when we examine individual skills or games, e.g. javelin throwing or tennis singles. It becomes somewhat confusing with regard to team games. While playing the full game is certainly whole practice, what about playing in a *small-sided game*, e.g. six-a-side hockey? I have seen this classed as both whole and part practice by different psychologists. The best explanation of whether it is whole or part is probably how it relates to the learner. For an adult, playing six-a-side hockey is not whole practice. For an 11-year-old, however, it can be classed as whole practice because the level of development of the 11-year-old means that playing 11-a-side is not an appropriate task.

The main advantage of whole practice is that everything happens in the environment in which it will have to be performed. The learner not only gets to practise the technique but also learns *how* and *when* to use that particular technique. In other words, whole practice develops not only technique but also decision making. To the cognitivists, whole practice is also good in helping the learner to develop schemas. They cannot simply repeat a specific motor program.

Whole practice, however, can have major drawbacks. This can be particularly so when learning team games. The amount of information with which the learner must deal when playing a full version of a game can be overwhelming for the beginner, This is particularly so if the learner is a child, with limited selective attention and past experience. Even where the perceptual and decision-making demands are not too great, whole practice can be difficult if the motor control demands are exacting. I first learned to play hockey when I was 18 years old. I had played a great deal of football and this was helpful with regard to positional play. However, it was not as useful as I had imagined it would be because I spent so much time trying to control the ball that I was not able to look around in order to make the correct decisions. In such situations, it may be beneficial to use part practice.

The strictest definition of part practice would be practising a part of a skill in isolation to the rest of the task. For example, a 100m sprinter might practice the start only or a tennis player may practice volleying, with the coach serving them, in a non-game situation. This type of practice has received a great deal of criticism, particularly in team games. It is claimed that, by taking the skill out of context, the learner concentrates only on technique and ignores the decision-making aspect of the task. In some situations this is poor coaching. However, it all depends on the needs of the learner. When I began playing hockey, I would have been better served by learning to control the ball before trying to control it and make decisions at the same time.

Even experienced performers often find value in part practice. The tennis player who is good overall but has some problems with his/her volleying may be well advised to practice that aspect of performance in isolation from the whole game. Nevertheless, the major criticism of the use of part practice is valid. This criticism is that players practise a skill or technique in isolation and are then expected to place the part into the whole game. This leads to a plateauing effect and in some cases the learner never develops awareness of when and where to perform the skill. A way of overcoming this problem is to use *part progressive practice.*

Part-progressive practice is when the task is broken down into parts and the individual practises part one, then adds part two, followed by part three and so on. The discus thrower can work on the release from the hand; then the arm movement can be added; followed by the use of the whole body; and lastly the turns. Similarly the push pass in hockey can be learned this way. Players can pass the ball in twos, while both are static. They can then begin passing and moving. This can be followed by introducing opposition and playing 3 v 1 (2 v 1 is probably too great a leap). Then 4 v 2 and 3 v 3 can be developed.

Task 2 *Choose two skills and develop a number of part-progressive practices starting at the very basics and building up to performing in a game.*

Even using part-progressive practice there can be a problem if the learner does not know to where the parts are leading. In order to overcome this problem, *whole–part–whole* practice is recommended in the textbooks. In this, we try the whole briefly in order to see where the task fits in with the real game. Then the practices are broken down into manageable parts. Gradually, we build up to returning to the whole. This is not always possible due to the nature of the task. Some skills, e.g. scrummaging in rugby, can be dangerous if the person is simply allowed to try it for him- or herself. In such cases, showing a video of the skill being performed in a real game can be very useful.

The above outlines the nature of whole, part, part-progressive and whole–part–whole practice and highlights some strengths and weaknesses of each. In the final section of this chapter, we will examine some of the issues that help us decide which type of practice is the most beneficial in any particular situation.

Variability of practice

Variability of practice means practising the skill using a variety of task and environmental demands. The most common form of variability of practice refers to asking the learner to produce different versions of a task, e.g. pass a football to an opponent 20 m away, then one 30 m away and 40 m away and so on. The tennis player may be asked to play shots across court and down the line, while the badminton player may be asked to serve short and long.

To the information processing theorists, variability of practice is vital because otherwise we cannot develop schemas and hence build up generalized motor programs. According to Schmidt's schema theory, when we use variable practice we alter the initial conditions, response parameters and the sensory consequences. When the rugby player Jonny Wilkinson practises his penalty kicks he does not kick from the same place each time. By starting at different angles and distances from the goal, he has built up a store of different initial conditions. In order to score, he must alter the response parameters. A long kick requires the application of more power and a longer leg movement. Similarly, the sensory feel of the movement will differ, albeit subtly. It is the ability to recognize these subtle differences that makes players like Wilkinson stars.

Theoretically, there is very strong support for variability of practice. However, research is less supportive. Research with children has generally supported variability. However, with adults this has not been the case. It is almost certain that the children are in the developmental process of building up schemas, whereas the adults have probably gone through these processes during their childhood. Therefore, varying practice has less of an effect.

Blocked, random and serial practice

The decision to use blocked, random or serial practice is often referred to as *practice scheduling*. *Blocked practice* is when the *learner practises one skill continually with no interference from the performance of other skills*. When undertaking *random practice* the *athlete will perform two or more skills, having random trials on each skill*. *Serial practice* is a version of random practice. The *learner practises more than one skill and practice is interspersed between the skills but in a serial order*, i.e. one skill is practised for a set number of trials, followed by practice on another skill, followed by practice on a third skill and back to the beginning. Then the cycle is repeated.

Performance immediately following practice is best when blocked practice is used. With random and serial practice it is likely that performing the other

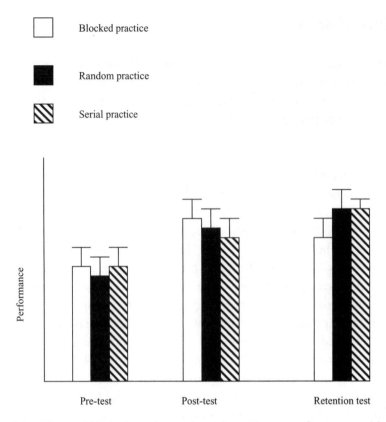

Figure 6.1   Effects of blocked, random and serial practice on performance and learning

skills has a negative effect. However, when a retention test is undertaken, random and serial practice produce better results than blocked practice (see Figure 6.1). Battig (1979) called this the *contextual interference effect*.

There are two theories that try to explain this phenomenon. Shea and Morgan (1979) claimed that, when we practise randomly and serially, we use more strategies to carry out the skill rather than sticking to one plan as in the blocked situation. They believe that all of the skills are held in working memory at the same time, thus allowing the learner to compare initial conditions, response parameters and sensory consequences of all the skills. This they called *elaboration*. Lee and Magill (1983) disagreed with this theory and put forward the theory of *action plan reconstruction*. According to them, learners experience partial or total forgetting of a skill during the periods when they are working on the other skills. On returning to the 'forgotten' skill, they have to re-plan the way in which they will perform it, i.e. re-draw their action plan. This aids the development of schemas. There is no research evidence to support one theory more than the other.

An interesting development on the effect of research into contextual interference has been to show that the effect is not always demonstrated and depends on the type of task. If two or more tasks that are very different to one another are practised then the effect is demonstrated. By 'very different' I mean where they are not using the same generalized motor program. If tasks require variations of the same generalized motor program, the contextual interference effect is not shown. Variations of the same generalized motor program are tasks such as the long pass and shooting at goal in hockey or serving and smashing in tennis.

Deliberate practice

The theory of *deliberate practice* was developed in the field of performing arts, particularly music, by the psychologist Anders Ericsson (see, e.g., Ericsson, Krampe and Teschrömer, 1993). Although I have included it in the information processing theory section, to Ericsson it is consistent with both cognitive and ecological psychology theories. Following a great amount of research, Ericsson found that elite performers had undertaken practice over a period of 10 years and/or spent about 10 000 hours undertaking deliberate practice. Deliberate practice refers to practice that includes all three of the following components. First, it requires time and energy from the learner and also access to coaches and training facilities. Second, in itself, it is not inherently motivating. In fact, it can be downright boring. The motivation must come directly from the learner. Third, deliberate practice requires effort.

Janet Starkes and colleagues (e.g. Helsen, Starkes and Hodges, 1998) have experimented on the role of deliberate practice in the acquisition of expertise in sport. They have made very similar findings to Ericsson's work in non-sports situations. However, there appear to be some factors that are specific to sport. The investment of time and the availability of facilities and coaches is the same as in other areas of life. However, much deliberate practice in sports situations appears to be enjoyable and possibly inherently motivating. This is different to Ericsson's findings. Effort remains a key issue and this has been divided into physical and mental, the latter requiring concentration.

There is nothing controversial about the idea that expertise will only be achieved with a great deal of practice. However, Ericsson argues that practice is the only consideration. Innate abilities, according to Ericsson, do not affect the acquisition of skill (he does accept that in sports such as basketball height is a factor that cannot be changed by practice). This is contrary to the ideas of most motor learning theorists, who believe that expertise is a mixture of innate abilities and the effect of practice. This is, of course, another chapter in the 'nature versus nurture' debate. This requires more research.

Task 3 *Over the last 10 years, how much practice have you undertaken? How much of it could be classed as deliberate practice?*

Transfer of training

Transfer of training refers to the effect that *practice on one task has on the learning or performance of another task*. Transfer is *positive* when the practice of one task has *a facilitating effect* on the learning or performance of another. Jason Robinson's experience of playing Rugby League has facilitated his playing of Rugby Union. Similarly, many netballers use their experience in that game when learning to play basketball. However, transfer can also be *negative*. Negative transfer is defined as being when the practice of one task has an *inhibiting effect* on the learning or performance of another. Tennis players often have difficulty when learning to play forehand and backhand strokes in squash. Individuals who are used to playing ball games are often at a disadvantage when learning to play badminton, as they expect the shuttle to behave like a ball when in flight.

Whether transfer is negative or positive, it is classed as being either *proactive* or *retroactive*. If transfer is positive, it is known as *proactive or retroactive facilitation*. If it is negative, it is called *proactive or retroactive inhibition*. Proactive transfer is when the practice on a task affects the learning or performance of a *subsequent* task. A basketball guard playing in goal in football and catching crosses is an example of proactive facilitation. The example of the tennis player having difficulty in playing forehand drives in squash is an example of proactive inhibition. Retroactive transfer is when practice of one task affects the performance of a *previously learned or practised* task. A good example of retroactive facilitation can be seen when basketball players play netball and then return to basketball. The need in netball to lose your marker often transfers very well to basketball, when the opposition is playing a full court press. Retroactive inhibition will only occur if the initial task is not well learned. One would expect professional cricketers to be negatively affected by playing golf on their days off. This rarely happens, because their cricket skill is too well developed to be affected by the new tasks. Beginners, however, would have major problems.

Task 4 *Choose six pairs of skills that you think will result in negative transfer and six pairs that will induce positive transfer. Why did you choose these pairs?*

The kind of transfer that we have been talking about, so far, is called *inter-task transfer*. This is transfer from one task to another. Of greater importance to coaches is *intra-class transfer*. Intra-class transfer is when there is transfer between *variations of the same task*. Typical examples are a football player shooting at goal and making a long pass or a tennis player playing a drive volley and a stop volley. Intra-class transfer is also used when developing skills. When learning to do a head-spring, it is normal to begin by springing from a raised surface, which makes it easier to get the necessary height. The gymnast then moves to springing from the floor. This is a case of intra-class transfer from *simple to complex*. Transfer can also occur from *complex to simple*. This can be particularly useful with experienced performers. Playing basketball on a small court can be used to help the players learn how to use space when they return to the full size court.

Transfer theories

Early transfer theories, such as Judd's (1908) *general elements theory* and Thorndike's (1927) *identical elements theory*, were developed first by Osgood (1949) and then Holding (1976). According to Holding, positive transfer will occur when *a new but similar stimulus requires the use of a well learned response*. This is called *stimulus generalization*. An example would be a football goalkeeper who is good at catching crosses playing as a receiver in the line-out in rugby. However, if a task requires a new and different response to the same or a similar stimulus then negative transfer will occur. This is called *response generalization*. We looked earlier at tennis players learning to play forehand drives in squash. The stimulus, the moving ball, behaves very similarly in the two games, but the responses, the nature of the two shots, are very different. Holding argued that there would be no transfer either way if both the stimulus and response were completely new. He also believes that the better a task is learned the less likely it is to be affected by negative transfer.

Task 5 Look at your answer to Task 4. Do you want to change any of the pairs after reading the theories? Try to account for your pairs with reference to these theories.

Bilateral transfer, sometimes called *cross-transfer* or *cross-education*, is a special form of transfer. Bilateral transfer refers to *transfer from a limb on one side of the body to another limb on the opposite side of the body, normally the contralateral limb*. Bilateral transfer does not mean that learning is easy. What it means is that the person will find acquiring a skill with the non-preferred limb *easier* than if they were learning from scratch. Most athletes, even very gifted ones, still prefer one side to the other.

> **Task 6** *Choose two skills, one you perform well and one at which you are weak. Try to perform them with your non-dominant limb. Was it easier to perform the well learned task? Did you use any strategies to aid performance?*

There are two theories concerning how bilateral transfer works. The first is that transfer is aided by *knowledge of the principles* involved in the movement. This is very much a cognitivist approach. We know how to perform the skill with our dominant limb and so can attempt to control our non-dominant limb to bring it about. This is similar to having declarative knowledge, which we need to turn into procedural knowledge. It is thought that the *better a task is learned, with the preferred limb, the better the transfer.*

The second theory came about following research using EMG. The right side of the brain controls movement of the left side of the body and vice versa. However, when a person undertakes physical activity with a limb on the right side of the body, EMG activity is shown also to occur in the equivalent limb on the left side. It is weak but, nevertheless, exists. This is because, although the neural pathways cross over in the lower centres of the CNS, there are some ipsilateral pathways. These send neural messages, albeit weak ones, to the limbs on the same side of the body. It is thought that these weak traces mean that the person is not starting from scratch when learning with the opposite limb.

Dynamical systems theory and practice

According to dynamical systems theorists, when giving instructions we merely *set the goal* for the learner. In organizing the practice we need to utilize *constraints* to help the learner achieve that goal. There are three kinds of constraints – task, environmental and organismic. *Task constraints* are limitations that the task imposes on performance, e. g the rules of a game or sport. *Organismic constraints* are what the athletes themselves bring to the performance, how strong they are or how fast or how tall, while *environmental constraints* are such factors as the weather and the size of the playing area. Newell (1986) claims that when planning a practice we should take into account all three constraints. Being aware of the three-way interaction between task, environmental and organismic constraints allows the coach to manipulate one, two or all in order to provide the kind of practice that will result in the desired effect. For example, most coaches and teachers, when introducing rugby for the first time, allow the learners to pass the ball forward. Once they are satisfied that the group is becoming comfortable handling the ball, they impose the task constraint that the ball must be passed backwards. They will probably ban tackling at the beginning. Touch or flag rugby will be played followed by the introduction of proper tackling. So the task constraints are altered. This is an example of how task constraints can be changed to help develop the practice, so that eventually the learners can play a game of rugby within the laws of the game.

Altering task constraints can, also, be used to develop team skills. If hockey coaches want to help their players to utilize the full width of the pitch they can make a rule that goals can only be scored from a pass from the wing. Basketball coaches who want to develop passing skills might not allow players to dribble with the ball. Altering the rules in this way is using what we call *conditioned games*. Conditioned games do not only mean using task constraints. Environmental constraints can also be used. Tennis coaches who wish to develop their players' backhands might play a cross-court game – from backhand court to backhand court. Badminton coaches often use long narrow courts if they want to develop overhead clears.

The manipulation of task and environmental constraints is a common practice in sport, although I doubt that coaches use the word constraint. Manipulating organismic constraints is less common. Practising while tired is a form of organismic constraint and may be very important in some activities. There is good evidence that, when we are tired, we alter the way in which we perform skills. You simply have to watch a tired person performing a skill. Often they are successful but the dynamics of the performance are different to normal. They appear laboured and lack smoothness.

Manipulating constraints can, also, help with selective attention and decision making or in ecological psychology terms attunement to affordances. A practice that I use a great deal in football is to play six-a-side on a very small pitch. This means that the players are in a shooting position most of the time but have very little time before being tackled. They soon learn that they must look to shoot as quickly as possible. This leads them to recognize the affordance of shooting. The problem with this is whether they will still look for that affordance when the constraints are taken off. The dynamical systems theorists claim that they will.

Task 7 From your own sport, see if you can devise some conditioned games with task, environmental and organismic constraints. Try to think of new ones rather than using those you have seen someone else use.

The idea that the individual can easily adapt when constraints are changed has led to dynamical systems theorists having a different attitude to transfer than information processing theorists. Dynamical systems theorists see asking someone to perform similar skills in different environments as simply altering the environmental constraints. For example, asking someone who is good at playing a drop volley in tennis to play a drive volley should result in positive transfer. All the person needs to do is alter their self-organization. In other words, the individual will automatically and naturally hit through the ball in order to achieve the goal of driving the ball. Similarly, a running back in American football learning to play rugby should be able to quickly become attuned to affordances for scoring tries, as he or she will already have a good idea of what areas of the environment to search for the affordance to run past opponents. As the ecologists believe that we have no recourse to memory when performing, negative transfer is not likely to be a problem. Changing the constraints will either have a positive effect or none at all.

Freezing and unfreezing degrees of freedom

In the last chapter, we looked briefly at the notion of freezing and unfreezing degrees of freedom. This, of course, takes place during practice. In the early stages the coach should set constraints that force the learner to freeze the degrees of freedom. As the performer becomes better, the coach can get the learner to release some degrees of freedom. When teaching the backhand in table tennis the coach will begin with a simple push, with no backspin. To do this the learner must control the degrees of freedom around the wrist, in other words keep the wrist locked. The coach will then ask the player to put backspin on the ball or hit a target that cannot be achieved unless backspin is added. Backspin requires the player to make contact with the ball using a sweeping motion, which brushes underneath the ball. This can only be achieved by unfreezing the degrees of freedom around the wrist.

Practical implications

Before deciding what we are to coach, technically, tactically and physically, we need to analyse the sport in some detail. Coaching manuals can be very useful, but one must be careful as sometimes errors in analysis are perpetuated in coaching circles. Coaches should make their own analyses. How detailed such an analysis is will depend on what is available to you. In the next chapter, we examine several methods of analysis. These are of varying sophistication but even the simplest is worth doing. It is also important to analyse your own athlete or athletes. They may have their own peculiarities. Similarly, different tactics demand different types of practice. A middle-distance runner with a sprint finish may train very differently to one who tries to break for the tape from 400+ m.

This example leads us to examine a difficult question. Do we focus on our athletes developing their strengths or weaknesses? Most coaches and players seem to favour working on weaknesses, but this can be counter-productive. Should the middle distance runner with a relatively slow sprint finish try to improve that or try to dominate races by breaking for home early in the race, thus eliminating the advantage of the fast finishers? It is pointless working on a sprint finish if the athlete does not have the inborn ability to achieve this. One football midfield player, who played for me as a youth, was an excellent passer of the ball but somewhat slow moving. However, he had exceptional antici-patory and decision-making skills, so compensated for his lack of speed to a large extent. Nevertheless, an increase in speed would have made him a better player. Therefore, I thought long and hard about trying to develop this part of his game. Watching him in training, however, it soon became obvious that his strengths physiologically were in endurance not speed. My guess was that he was high in slow twitch muscle fibres but low in fast twitch. I would have loved to have undertaken a muscle biopsy to prove my point but the club could not afford that. Given what I suspected, I decided to work more on his passing, anticipation and decision making and not worry about his lack of pace. It worked, as he went on to have a long and successful career in professional football.

Similar problems arise with teams. Do we work at strengths or weaknesses? The obvious answer is both, but which we work at most will depend on what the strengths and weaknesses are and the make-up of the team itself. First of all, however, we have to analyse the team's strengths and weaknesses. As with individual skills, there are numerous methods of analysis available. Many, however, are financially out of the reach of most coaches. In the next chapter, the relative strengths and weaknesses of these methods are discussed. One of the most reassuring facts is that even unsophisticated, cheap, often totally free, methods can provide a great deal of information.

Before leaving this topic we should state that the decision of what to coach is not simply based on perceived strengths and weaknesses. We need to set goals. As we saw in Chapter 5, these should be long term and short term. It is vital that we know to where we are going. It has never ceased to amaze me, in my time in coaching, how many coaches do not do this. They just drift along from session to session and week to week. I have come across very few coaches who use annual programmes and even fewer who have longer programmes.

Socio-psychological factors

Motivation and personality affect the coaches' choice concerning what to coach. The more intrinsically motivated the individual is the more likely he or she is to want to develop technical ability. Athletes with high mastery motivation will happily work at their skills simply in order to improve. Competition motivated individuals might need to be persuaded that working at a particular aspect will bring extrinsic rewards. The socially motivated individual will be happy to work at skills as long as the practice involves social interaction. As we saw in Chapter 3, personality interacts with motivation to affect the choice of what to practice. Some type A individuals see 'enjoyable' activities as being frivolous and not being practice at all. These characters are very willing to undertake repetitive practice. They enjoy physical training that places them under a great deal of stress. They believe totally in the 'no pain, no gain' adage. Similarly, many type A people want a large say in the choice of what to practise. A failure to include them can result in a lack of motivation. Other personality types may be happy to do as the coach says.

One of the biggest problems for coaches of team games is when there are different personality types and levels of motivation in the team. The person who wants to 'play' during practice, i.e. take part in competitive, non-repetitious activities, and the highly motivated type A personality can come into conflict. This is particularly so with regard to physical training. To the highly motivated individual training should 'hurt'. To most games players training is something that has to be done. It is to be endured, certainly not enjoyed. If the coach can make it interesting and can 'sugar the pill', by using the types of activity that we will cover in Chapters 16 and 17, they are happy. To others this kind of coaching is a sign of weakness.

Many of these problems can be overcome by communication, especially goal setting. If all of the players know to where they are going and how they are trying to get there, many of the dissatisfactions of the type A personality can be avoided. I met this problem when working as a consultant sports psychologist with a swimming team, whose coach liked to feel in command. A few of the swimmers, who were very much type A personalities, were frustrated with some of the coaching methods. They were particularly perplexed by the fact that, although they were sprinters, they spent a great deal of time working on aerobic fitness. I persuaded the coach to take some time to talk to all of the swimmers, explaining the need for a good aerobic base even in sprinters. Perhaps more importantly, I got her to include these particular swimmers in the process of deciding what training they should do. In fact, by structuring her discussions with them, she was able to make sure that they did what she wanted. However, they were convinced that they had played an integral part in the process.

Developmental factors

In deciding what to coach with youngsters the coach needs to be aware of the individuals' cognitive, motor, physical and emotional stages of development. Most physical educators and sports governing bodies now recommend the use of mini-versions of the activity. Most of these came about because people recognized the absurdity of some of the physical demands placed on children. Figure 6.2 shows a 10-year-old boy and a varsity basketball player standing on the free throw line. It is obvious that the task is very different for both of them. Not only will the problems facing the 10-year-old lead to a lack of success and probable use of incorrect techniques, but also they may ruin his confidence and motivation. Despite the obvious problems of asking children to perform on full-sized courts and pitches, we still see this practice today. Most days I pass a tennis club on my way to and from work. It is fairly common to see children as young as eight or nine years old trying to play on a full-size court with the net at full height.

The range of mini-games for any particular sport can be found in most coaching manuals or physical education texts. Suffice it to say here that the idea is that the children can physically carry out what is required them. Our 10-year-old basketballer should be using a smaller ball and the ring should be considerably lower. Child tennis players are better off playing mini-tennis – smaller court, smaller racquet, lighter ball and smaller net. These changes not only allow for better development of skill, they generally bring more enjoyment to the children because they can achieve success. In team games, the use of fewer players in each team means that the children are involved more, thus developing their skills and increasing their enjoyment. The mini-rugby player can get involved rather than be 'stuck' on the wing hoping to get a touch of the ball.

Physical factors, however, are not the only ones that cause problems for children. It can be difficult for children, even in mini-practices, to perform well due to lack of motor development. By the age of 11 or 12 years most children appear to have developed sufficient motor control to perform the majority of

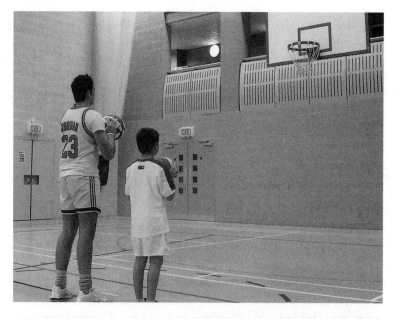

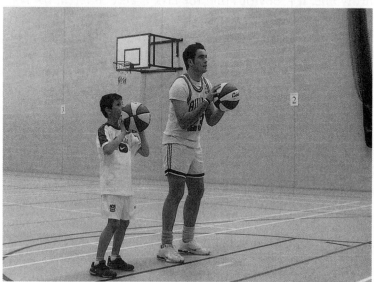

Figure 6.2 This demonstrates the differences in the 'same' task for a university basketball player and a 10-year-old

skills. Power may, however, be lacking until early adulthood. The number of skills that children can perform and the level at which they are capable of performing should not be underestimated. If children are given the encouragement and opportunity to develop skills, through good use of bootstrapping, they are capable of a great deal. I believe strongly that we do not encourage youngsters to develop sufficiently during their childhood. Children under 11 years are willing to work at basic skills and indeed get a great deal of pleasure from developing these skills. Sadly, the level of coaching and, more so, physical education teaching for children of this age is not very good, particularly in Britain.

For some time, I have held the belief that we do not 'stretch' youngsters enough with regard to their motor skills. However, until recently I was very cautious about what we asked children to do with regard to learning decision making in games. Observation of the ability of the children whom I was coaching, and recent research into age and decision making by myself and my colleagues John Sproule, Bill MacGillivary and Jane Lomax (McMorris et al., 2006), has led me to believe that children are capable of much more than I originally thought. Indeed, we have recently seen two teenage prodigies whose decision-making ability is of the highest level, the English football player Wayne Rooney and the American basketballer Lebron James. Admittedly these are exceptional players but I do believe that others can achieve very similar standards of decision making. Of course, Rooney and James also had the motor and physical development to play at top level when as young as 16 years old. Coaches, however, should be aware of the limitations that cognitive development brings. This is dealt with in some detail in Chapter 13.

Task 8 *From your own sport, devise one or two mini-games that would be useful with under-11-year-olds.*

Practice organization

Earlier in this chapter we touched on when to use massed or spaced practice, whole or part and part-progressive practices. The decision of which to use is not a simple one. The decision is based on an interaction between task, learner and coach, similar to that shown in Figure 5.1 when deciding which coaching style to use. As we will see below this interaction is far from simple.

Task considerations

We have dealt with most of these in the section on types of practice. Therefore, we will simply outline the issues here. With adults and older children we should aim, wherever possible, to use whole practice. This places the learner in the environment in which they will have to perform the skill. Specificity of practice aids intra-task transfer from practice to competitive performance. Also, in tasks that require decision making the athlete learns not only how to do something but also which technique to use in any situation. However, when an environment includes many irrelevant and distracting cues, it may be better to use part-progressive practice. In this way the perceptual demands can be delimited in the early stages of learning. This is necessary because of our limited capacity to deal with many things at once. With practice, actions become automatic and, therefore, use less and less of our limited CNS capacity. When the athletes reach this stage, more parts can be added to the practice until they are finally in a whole-practice situation.

The presence of distracting and irrelevant cues is not the only thing that can overload our limited capacity. If a skill requires much in the way of coordination it will be best to use whole–part–whole practice. The lay-up in basketball is a good example of this. It is not difficult to decide when and where to use a lay-up in a game of basketball. However, the technique requires much in the way of timing and coordination of movement. It may, therefore, be best to practise the technique in a non-game situation. Once a reasonable level of control has been established, it can be placed in a game. Thus the player sees from the whole practice where the skill should be used, practises the technique in a part practice and then returns to the whole game. In gymnastics routines, it may be best to use part-progressive practice to build up the stages before expecting the learner to carry out a difficult series of movements.

In team games, which require a great deal of decision making in complex environments, small-sided games can be useful. Dynamical systems theorists believe that in small-sided games the coach can manipulate task, environmental and organismic constraints. I gave some examples of these earlier. Allowing football players to only have only one touch of the ball before passing is an example of a task constraint. Playing Rugby Union on a small pitch to develop rucking and mauling is an example of an environmental constraint. Organismic constraints are less common in small-sided games but I have seen football coaches who say that goals can only be scored with the weaker foot. One organismic constraint that I use with hockey players is to stop them from shouting for the ball. I do this to force the player in possession to look up and not play with their head down.

The above are all examples of conditioned games. Using conditioned games is not the only way to utilize small-sided games in coaching. A common method of coaching decision making to is to use what is called the 'freeze-replay' method. Using this method, the coach shouts 'stop' when he/she wants the players to 'freeze'. They are now in a static positions and the coach can point out what action is best in that particular situation. This is a difficult form of coaching and requires a lot of knowledge on the part of the coach.

Coach considerations

Most of what needs to be taken into account with regards to the coach is dealt with in Chapter 4, which examines coaching styles. However, coaches need to take into account some more basic factors. First of all, their own knowledge level is important. As a young coach, I used to use part-progressive practices in situations in which I now use whole practice. This was because my knowledge base, in the early stages of my coaching career, was such that I could not always observe what was happening well enough. This is not a minor point. In training young coaches, over many years, I have noticed that most find coaching in whole practices very difficult. Just as there are many irrelevant cues for the performer, so there are for the coach. Selective attention is as important for the coach as the player. By using part-progressive practices the young or inexperienced coach can follow the principle of bootstrapping. As they develop their coaching skills, they can progress to more complex practices.

The coach also needs to take into account his or her own motivation. Coaches who are mastery motivated may well want to use practices that place the emphasis on learning. The coach who is more interested in the athletes having a good time and enjoying themselves may prefer whole practice.

Task 9 *What do you consider to be your own strengths and weaknesses as a coach? How easy do you think it will be to overcome your weaknesses?*

The learner

By far the most important factor when deciding what type of practice to use is what the learner or learners bring to the situation. In group practices this becomes more complex because not all learners will have the same motivations. As we saw earlier, part practice can be particularly useful with experienced mastery and/or competition motivated performers, who can see why they need to isolate a particular aspect of performance and work at it. Inexperienced learners may not be able to understand the necessity of this. To the socially motivated person this can appear pointless.

The stage of development of the individual, in particular children, will also greatly affect the choice of practice type. This is dealt with in detail in Part V. Suffice it to say, here, that the cognitive, motor, emotional and physical development of the child has to be taken into consideration. Physical factors also affect the choice of practice type for adults. Regardless of motivation, it is probably best if less fit individuals take part in spaced rather than massed practice. With fit individuals, however, massed practice can be used deliberately to induce fatigue. Performing while in a fatigued state is a form of organismic constraint and is something that most performers find themselves having to do from time to time. How many football teams practise ready for having to play extra time or American football teams prepare for overtime?

Variability and contextual interference

Variability of practice would appear to be necessary in all except the most closed of skills, e.g. shot putt, in which the conditions never change at all from performance to performance. Variability has been used by coaches for many years, long before Schmidt developed schema rheory or any research was undertaken in this area. It is, in many ways, simply commonsense. The use of contextual interference, however, is less simple. The evidence for its effectiveness, when the skills are dissimilar, is strong. However, time can be a problem. If contextual interference is used, the person actually spends less time working at each skill than if they use blocked practice. The coach has to decide whether time is best spent on one activity or on several. The use of skill circuits can aid contextual interference. Figure 6.3 gives an example of a skill circuit from basketball. This is a form of serial practice. As we will see in Chapters 14 and 15, it can be used in conjunction with physical training as well as skill practice. It should be remembered that, in many ways, contextual interference is contrary to deliberate practice, which consists of the repetition of a limited facet of performance.

Transfer

Part-progressive practice, part practice and whole–part–whole practice, by their very nature, include intra-task transfer. However, coaches rarely use inter-task transfer, although it may be used in school physical education classes. This is probably due to time factors. Most coaches have little time available, therefore must use every minute wisely. While inter-task transfer works, it is not as good as practising the actual task itself. However, skills that are similar to the one to be learned can be used in order to relieve the monotony of repeatedly practising the same thing. This can be particularly useful during

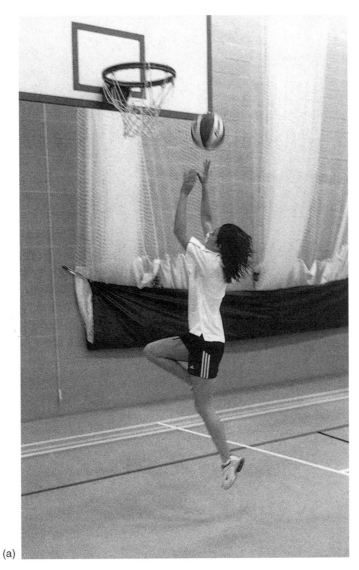

(a)

Figure 6.3 An example of a basketball skill circuit: (a) repeated lay-ups; (b) repeated jump shots; the player works his way around taking a short from each of the markers; (c) a 'dribbling' exercise; (d) working on foot-work; the player moves across and backwards and forwards to touch each of the markers (a fourth marker is out of sight on the player's right-hand side); (e) repeated rebounds; the player can act as feed for herself or someone else can feed

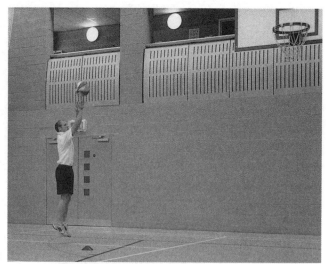

(b)

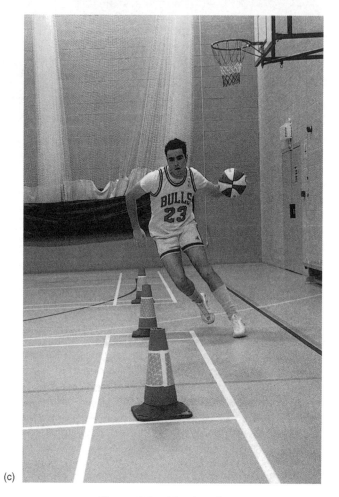

(c)

Figure 6.3 (*Continued*)

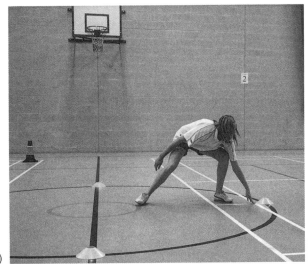

(d)

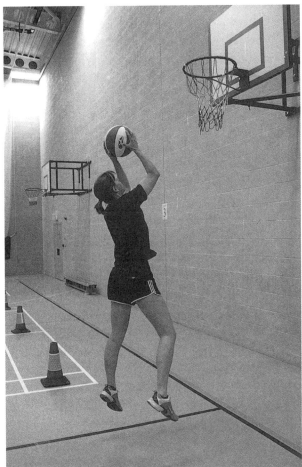

(e)

Figure 6.3 (*Continued*)

breaks between seasons or within seasons. It is helpful if the coach points out to the players where the similarities lie. It may also be worthwhile pointing out the differences.

The use of bilateral transfer in sports appears to be dependent on the sub-culture of the sport. No self-respecting basketballer would practice only with his/her preferred hand. However, it is rare to see professional cricketers throw with their non-preferred hands, even though this may be a very useful aid in getting run-outs.

Pragmatic considerations

Table 6.1 outlines a number of pragmatic considerations that must be taken into account when planning a coaching session. The facilities and equipment available can vary greatly from one situation to another. In my football coaching, I have experienced having more than one ball per player, the choice of floodlit outdoor facilities, grass or Astroturf, or large indoor facilities. In other situations, I have had to do with one ball between 20 players on a barely lit area of 40 m × 20 m. At one time, myself and a colleague found ourselves with 120 children of different ages and six footballs. Far from ideal. This was an exception and I hope that you do not have to face similar problems.

Table 6.1 Pragmatic considerations when planning a practice session

Problem	Considerations
Have you a choice of indoor and outdoor facilities? If so, which will you use?	Is the sport normally played indoors or outdoors? What is the weather like? What clothing do the athletes have? Are cold/hot drinks available?
What is the size of the practice area available?	Is it big enough to have all the athletes working at once? What is the best way to sub-divide the space? Can you see everyone easily?
How good are the acoustics?	Can everyone hear you easily?
Are there any potential dangers, e.g. slippery surface, rough edges?	If so, can you do something about them? If not, you will have to cancel the practice.
Are there any inherent dangers in the practice you are undertaking, e.g. using hockey balls, baseballs or cricket balls, throwing javelins?	How can you ensure that dangers are limited to an absolute minimum?

While the problems of having limited facilities are obvious, one should not think that having all the facilities imaginable means that there are no problems. The key issue is using the facilities properly, not merely having them available. I have seen basketball coaches working in sports halls with six rings yet practising shooting into one ring with 20 players. If the coach keeps in mind the fact that time spent practising is invaluable then such situations should not occur.

> **Task 10** *You are a basketball coach. You have a small gym with two baskets. You have four basketballs and twenty 15-year-olds, all of average ability. Choose a basketball skill and work out a practice session of 40 min for these children.*

A pragmatic consideration is the problem of safety. It is the coach's responsibility to make sure that the practice is safe. Organization must take this into account. Look at Figure 6.4(a). Can you see what the problem is? Two of the goalkeepers are in great danger of getting hit with the ball. Figure 6.4(b) shows how this can be avoided.

Finally, we should not forget the weather. Practising on hot days requires the use of spaced practice and the ready availability of water and electrolyte drinks. On cold days, it may be best to shorten practice time and, in particular, keep the athletes moving. This can especially be a problem when the players do not possess the best quality tracksuits. Of course, one must be very aware of the motivation level of the performers. I have had some excellent coaching sessions in terrible weather conditions (coming from the North-East of England this is hardly surprising), but only with highly motivated athletes.

Summary

When deciding what to practice the coach needs to analyse the sport that he/she is coaching. What are the key skills? He/she also needs to analyse the performers' strengths and weaknesses. Then the coach needs to decide whether to focus on the athletes' strengths or work at their weaknesses. In organizing the practice sessions the coach must take into account the complexity of the task. Does it need to be broken down or can whole practice be used? Similarly, the learners themselves must be taken into consideration. What is their level and type of motivation? Personality and developmental stage are also important. Finally, coaches must not forget what they themselves bring to the situation. In Part II we examined coaching styles. These cannot be ignored, nor can the coach's own level of expertise. All will affect what and how to coach your athletes.

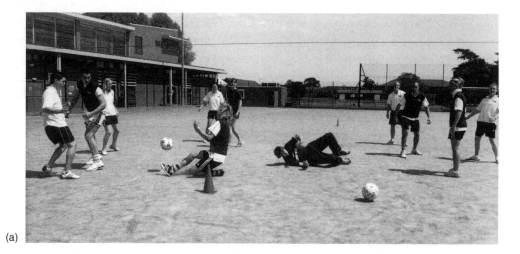

Figure 6.4   (a) A badly organized practice. Both goalkeepers are in danger of being hit by shots from the other game. (b) By one group playing North to South and the other West to East, this problem can be overcome

Key points

- practice can be
    - massed (no breaks) or spaced (regular breaks)
    - whole (practise the whole skill); part (practise part of the skill in isolation of the other parts); part progressive (practise one part of the skill, then add another part and so on)
    - whole–part–whole practice (practise the whole then break it down into parts and then return to the whole)

- according to schema theory, practice should follow the principle of variability
  - variability of practice means practising with different initial conditions; this requires different response parameters and, therefore, aids error labelling
  - research with children has shown that variability of practice results in better retention than using the same initial conditions

- random (practising two or more skills with random trials on the different skills) and serial (practising more than one skill in a serial order) practice produce better retention than blocked (practising one skill continuously without interference from the practice of other skills) practice – this is called the contextual interference effect
  - Shea and Morgan claim that this is because random and serial practice results in the learner developing more strategies to help perform the skill
  - Lee and Magill believe that it is because each time the person returns to a skill they must reconstruct their action plan
  - blocked practice produces better performance than random and serial, i.e. performance over the final set of practice trials is better than that shown by those following random or serial practice
  - the contextual interference effect is not shown if the skills are simply variations of the same generalized motor program

- deliberate practice refers to practice where
  - the learner invests a lot of time and energy
  - the practice is not inherently motivating
  - practice requires effort

- in sport, the practice can sometimes be enjoyable

- transfer of training refers to the effect of the practice of one task on the performance or learning of another task
  - transfer can be positive (aids performance) or negative (inhibits performance)
  - proactive facilitation is when the practice of a task aids the performance of a subsequent task
  - proactive inhibition is when the practice of a task negatively affects the performance of a subsequent task
  - retroactive facilitation is when the practice of a new task aids the performance of a previously learned task

- ♦ retroactive inhibition is when the practice of a new task negatively affects the performance of a previously learned task

- intra-task transfer of training is when practising one variation of a skill aids or inhibits the performance of a different variation

- Holding claims that whether transfer is positive or negative depends on stimulus generalization and response generalization
  - ♦ stimulus generalization states that positive transfer occurs when a new but similar stimulus requires the use of a well learned response
  - ♦ response generalization states that negative transfer will occur when a familiar stimulus requires a new and different response

- bilateral transfer of training is transfer from using a contralateral limb
  - ♦ this is thought to occur because we can use the same general principles to perform the skill and/or
  - ♦ because ipsilateral neural pathways mean that the contralateral limb has already experienced some learning

Dynamical systems theory and practice

- coaches can help us to perceive the affordances and make the movement efficiently by placing constraints on us

- task and environmental constraints 'force' us to learn the most efficient way of performing a skill

- constraints 'force' us to freeze the degrees of freedom when in the early stages of learning

- releasing the constraints or altering them can lead to the unfreezing and refinement of a skill in the later stages of learning

- conditioned games are a form of practice using constraints

Practical implications

- which type of practice to use in any situation depends on the interaction between the learner, the coach and the task (see Figure 5.1).

7

Observation and Feedback

Learning objectives

At the end of this chapter, you should

- understand the basic principles of observation from a motor learning perspective
- understand the basic principles of observation from a biomechanical perspective
- know which mechanical aids are available to the coach to aid observation
- understand the meaning and nature of feedback
- understand the principles affecting how and when to provide feedback
- understand some of the pragmatic factors affecting the provision of feedback.

One of the most important roles of the coach is to present feedback. Both information processing theorists and ecological psychologists believe that the presence of coaches is a major aid to learning. While the coach is not the only person able to help the learner, they are likely to be the most knowledgeable and best trained. Although the failure of many physical education teachers to

Coaching Science   Terry McMorris and Tudor Hale
© 2006 John Wiley & Sons, Ltd

provide any feedback at all has been recognized, this criticism cannot generally be levelled against coaches. To me, the main problem facing coaches comes from deciding what feedback to present. This decision can only be reached if the coach is accurate in his/her observations of the athletes' performance. Amazingly, observation is rarely commented upon in modern motor learning textbooks. Sports biomechanics texts provide much more detailed explanations of observation and much of what they have to say overlaps into the domain of the motor learning theorists.

Observation

In this section, we will examine the motor learning and biomechanical principles that affect observation. The practical and pragmatic factors will be dealt with in the section on practical implications. It is important to state, first, that observation is a skill. It can be learned. There are principles that must be taken into account if observation is to be successful.

Motor learning approach

To the information processing theorists, observation is part of the process of working memory. Observation is particularly concerned with the perception stage of the information processing model (see Figure 5.5). Of major importance is *selective attention*. Selective attention is the ability to focus on relevant information and ignore irrelevant cues. As we saw in Chapter 5, working memory has a limited capacity. If we try to attend to too many things at once we will become confused. By focusing on the relevant information we can overcome the problem of overloading working memory.

Research in the 1980s (Allard and Starkes, 1980; Allard *et al.*, 1980) showed that the selective attention of expert performers differed significantly from that of inexperienced athletes. Using eye-mark recorders, Allard and colleagues examined the search patterns of experienced and inexperienced basketball and volleyball players. They found that the experts, in both games, differed from the inexperienced players in where they looked in the environment and how long they focused on each area. According to Allard, this was due to past experience showing the experts which information was the most important.

This falls in line with working-memory theory. To the information processing theorists this occurs because the experts are able to recall from LTM which areas of the environment are likely to produce the most important information. Even ecological psychologists accept that experts are far more efficient in their search of the display, although they believe that this is due to experience leading to the experts becoming attuned to the affordances in the environment rather than memory. Whichever is correct, the main point is that we need experience, or practice, in order to develop our observational skills. This is as important for the coach as for the performer. In fact, when it comes to observation, the coach is the performer.

It is far easier for me to point out the importance of selective attention to you than it was for me to acquire that skill as a coach. Even when coaching an individual athlete, in what might appear to be a skill with not much irrelevant information, it is surprising how much the novice coach actually misses. We talked above about knowing which parts of the environment to focus on. However, observation is more difficult than that. A novice coach might be told to focus on the leg movement when someone is kicking a ball or on the hands of a basketballer throwing a free shot. What the novice coach and the experienced coach see will not differ. What they make of the information may very well do so. Seeing is not perceiving; it is sensation. Kerr (1982) described perception as being *the organization, interpretation and integration of sensory information*. In other words, it is what we make of the information that we see.

In order to make sense of information, we need to know what we are looking for. This brings us back to the point I made in Chapters 5 and 6. The coach needs to be able to analyse the skill that he/she is teaching. Once coaches know what the key points are they can refine their visual search. They will not merely focus on the foot of the kicker or the hand of the shooter but on particular parts of the foot or hand. Slowly but surely the performance of the athlete stops being a blur of rapid movement and comes to make sense.

As novice coaches develop the skill of observation, they do something similar to learning a motor program. Initially, they build up a model or picture of what the skill should look like. They can then compare what they perceive happening in any particular trial with the picture or model. It would appear that good coaches develop something akin to a schema. They are able to perceive what is and should be happening in a variety of different situations. Moreover, the good coach will take into account the fact that different performers have different abilities and will, therefore, perform the same skill differently. Bad coaches often miss this fact. Poor coaches will try to get everyone performing a skill in exactly the same way. Moreover, they will be unable to realize that different situations may need different variations of the same movement pattern. This is often called 'over-coaching'. I hate this term. One cannot be 'over-coached'. It is poor coaching, plain and simple. By using the term 'over-coaching', it appears that we are saying that the person is a good coach but is too keen. The fact is that the person is coaching badly.

Biomechanical approach

There are very few differences between the biomechanical and motor learning approaches to observation. Biomechanists like James Hay (1993) and Gerry Carr (2004) point to the importance of selective attention, although they do not use this term. They do, however, point to the building up of a mental representation of the performance of a skill. The biomechanical texts, however, go much further than coaching manuals and motor learning texts when analysing a skill. For example, Hay, when describing the front crawl, begins with simple statements about body position, and leg and arm actions similar to those you would find in a swimming coaching manual. However, he goes on to discuss such factors as propulsive forces (propulsive lift and drag forces) and resistive forces (from surface and wave drag). Also, basic algebraic formulae are used to explain the optimal way of performing the stroke.

The coaching manuals follow a cognitivist motor learning approach. This came about for two main reasons. First of all, coaching and motor learning were developed as sub-disciplines of coaching science long before biomechanics, despite the fact that the basis of sport biomechanics is the study of physics initiated by Isaac Newton as far back as the 18th century. Second, the emphasis of the information processing theorists on the role of efferent organization in the CNS led to the notion that all that needed to be observed was an overall picture of the movement. The coach could then tell the performer to make alterations and efferent organization would take care of this. To the biomechanists, this is a little too simplistic. They want to break the skill and performance of it down to a more micro-level.

The desire to dissect a skill beyond simple basics came about initially due to physicists and later biomechanists wishing to explain what was happening during the performance of skills: skills in all walks of life, not just sports skills. The initial interest was purely academic. It was a 'This is what is happening: this is how the laws of physics are being adhered to during skilled performance' approach. As sport biomechanics evolved, coaches became interested in how the sports biomechanists could help them to instruct their athletes. Sports biomechanists accept that the more basic breakdown of a skill provided in coaching texts is useful. Some even argue that the detailed biomechanical breakdown can produce information that the athlete cannot use (see Hay, 1993; Lees, 2002). However, if used properly, biomechanical analysis can be very useful to the coach and athlete.

Table 7.1 Newton's laws of motion and their implications for sport

Law	Implications
1. A body will continue in its state of rest or motion in a straight line unless forced to change that state by external forces: law of inertia	Explains how striking an object or throwing an object causes it to move. This includes not only the forces imparted by us, e.g. hitting the ball, but also the forces of nature such as gravity.
2. The rate of change in momentum of an object is proportional to the amount of force and the direction of movement depends on where the force acts: law of acceleration	How fast an object goes depends mainly on the amount of force used. The harder we strike something the faster it will move. We can alter the direction of an object by making contact at different angles.
3. For every action there is an equal and opposite reaction: law of counterforce	This explains why a runner needs to drive off the ground in order to move forward quickly. It also explains why starting blocks aid a fast start: the runner can act on the blocks thus producing a reaction, namely the start (a backward action causes a forward reaction)

Biomechanical analysis is particularly useful in sports such as gymnastics, field athletics, baseball, cricket and golf, where the athlete performs a skill that can be isolated. More importantly, these types of skill are very much dependent on technique. A knowledge of the basics of gravity, particularly how to move one's centre of gravity, is extremely useful to the coach and athlete. The roles of speed, velocity, acceleration, deceleration and force are all very important in most of the skills in these, and indeed other, sports. Biomechanists place a great deal of importance on Newton's laws of inertia, acceleration and counterforce (see Table 7.1). It is true to say that many coaches subconsciously use these laws when analysing a skill. Figure 7.1 shows a coach showing an athlete the point of release for the shot. The optimal point of release depends on the laws of physics.

My experience of observing shot putt coaches tells me that rarely do coaches fail to spot whether the angle of release is correct or not. However, many miss points such as the force that is applied in the upward thrust of the legs and body. This is probably due to a lack of knowledge of the importance of the biomechanical principles concerning changes in centre of gravity and acceleration. If the coach were explicitly aware of these principles, he/she would be unlikely to make this error. Therefore, the use of biomechanical principles in breaking down a skill is extremely helpful and is a major aid to observation.

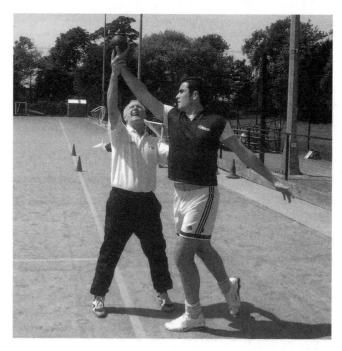

Figure 7.1   A coach using basic biomechanical principles in a simple way

The major problem with using the more sophisticated biomechanical break-down of skill, compared with the motor learning dissection, is that many of the factors highlighted are not easily seen by the naked eye. This is not only true of biomechanical analyses; it also applies to many of the areas of cognitive aspects of performance. How do we know what a player is looking at? Why are some team game players better than others when anticipating their opponent's actions? In order to answer these questions and examine biomechanical aspects of performance, we often need mechanical aids. This does not mean, however, that biomechanical analysis cannot be carried out without such aids. Duane Knudson and Craig Morrison (1997) provide some good rules for how qualitative analysis of biomechanical factors can be used. Similarly, Hay and Carr also place a great emphasis on simple visual observation. We discuss when and why to use mechanical aids in the final section of this chapter.

Mechanical aids to observation

We begin this section by briefly examining the most commonly used mechan-ical aid to observation, namely the *video* recording. Most coaches use video simply to aid their subjective analysis of the athlete's performance. They can look at an action over and over again or slow down the speed so as to lessen the chances of movement negatively affecting their observation. The use of slow motion can have drawbacks, however. If high speed film is not used, there will be periods of time between frames where a substantial amount of information can be missed. The coach needs to determine whether or not high speed film is necessary.

We have already seen that *eye-mark recorders* can be used in research to examine the athlete's visual search strategies. The areas of the environment searched, the order of observations and the time spent focusing on each cue can also provide a great deal of information to the coach. This can be particularly important with regard to decision making and anticipation. The most sophisticated form of eye-mark recorder is the *eye-tracker*. These can be used with videos or in live situations. Movement by the athlete, however, is restricted. Great improvements in eye-mark recorders have been made in the last few years and it is likely that this will continue. I would not be surprised if systems are not soon developed that allow a great deal of movement by the athlete.

Although a fairly large amount of research has been carried out in this area recently we are still a long way from being sure what the differences are between experts and novices in most sports. The differences between experts and intermediate level performers is even less well known. Nevertheless, the coach who suspects that his/her athletes are focusing on incorrect information can check this out using eye tracking systems.

Notational analysis

Notational analysis was devised in an attempt to quantify information concerning performance in team games. As far as I am aware, the first attempt at notational analysis was undertaken by Smodlaka in 1978. Smodlaka was an exercise physiologist interested in training football players. He was unhappy with the fact that there was no actual data with regard to how far players ran, what percentage of their movements were fast, medium or slow paced and so on. He, therefore, carried out a simple analysis where he subjectively assessed the distance of runs, speed of runs, distance covered sprinting, jogging etc. This was the first *time and motion* study in sport. Several years later, Tom Reilly and Vaughn Thomas carried out a number of time and motion studies (e.g. Reilly and Thomas, 1976), where they attempted to improve the objectivity by marking the surrounds of a football pitch in 10 yard (9 m) sections. This allowed for distance to be better judged.

For several years, the method of Reilly and Thomas remained the most objective and accurate. However, a number of researchers (e.g. Hughes and

Franks, 1994) decided that using video would allow for more accurate predictions of distance and speed of movement. It took some time to overcome the problems of parallax error caused by the use of video cameras. Moreover, Hughes and Franks developed customized keyboards, which allowed them to translate the information accurately and quickly into computer printouts, which could be used by the coach. Further developments allowed for trained observers to use the keyboards during an actual game, in real time, and thus provide the coach with almost instant information. These were developed for a vast range of sports from team games, such as rugby, to individual activities, such as squash. They were further developed to be used to examine tactical and skill factors involved in performance, e.g. how successful the tennis player was on his/her backhand side or how well a hockey team kept possession in midfield.

The most recent development in this field has been the digital video analysis system, which provides computerized representation of the movement of individuals in a game. Time and motion studies can be used in this way, as can analysis of positional play and tactics. These systems allow the coach to focus on specific aspects of play, e.g. in hockey, questions such as what happens when ball possession is lost or how well the team performs in midfield. It should be remembered that there still needs to be some subjective assessment with regard to use of tactics or skilled performance. The knowledge that a hockey team is losing possession in midfield does not tell us why. Was it poor passing technique, or poor choice of where to pass, or poor supporting play by the other midfielders and forwards?

Task 1 Draw up a list of performance factors that you would like to have examined by notational analysis to aid your coaching of an individual athlete or a team. These should be technical, tactical and physiological.

Summary

The first priority is to analyse the skill. The use of coaching manuals and biomechanical texts is recommended. These texts can help the coach break the skill down and observe the key points in a systematic manner. If available, mechanical aids can make it easier to observe accurately. Work on notational analysis has shown that even the use of pencil and paper can be helpful. This type of information is, however, only an aid to analysing performance. It provides quantitative data but the coach must interpret the meaning of this information. John Adams (1975) summed up this problem nicely when he said that poor coaches use such information 'like a drunken man uses a lamppost, more to lean on than to illuminate'.

Feedback

Like observation, the process of feedback is best demonstrated by the working memory. Based on perception of the current situation compared with past experience recalled from LTM, the coach makes a decision of what information to give to the athlete. Feedback, however, does not necessarily come from the coach; it can come from the performers themselves. *Feedback* is the term we use to describe *all information resulting from an action or response.*

Feedback coming from within the performers themselves is called *intrinsic* or *inherent*. It is available to the performers without outside help. This feedback can be *visual, proprioceptive, vestibular* or *auditory*. In most cases a movement will result in more than one of these senses providing feedback. We can see the results of our actions without anyone needing to tell us what happened, while the feel of a movement is intrinsic by definition. Feedback coming from the coach is called *extrinsic* or *augmented* feedback. This is normally verbal or visual but can be in other forms such as biofeedback.

There are two major forms of feedback, *knowledge of results (KR)* and *knowledge of performance (KP)*. KR is post-response information concerning the *outcome* of the action. The most obvious form of KR is visual. We see the end product of our action. In some cases, however, we need outside help to be able to make sense of our actions. A long jumper needs to have the distance they jumped measured in order to have KR. Similarly, a track athlete may need to know the time that they ran. KP, on the other hand, consists of post-response information concerning the *nature of the movement*. The most obvious type of KP is the 'feel' of the movement or, to be more technical, knowledge of the sensory consequences. KP can, and does, come in other forms, however. We can see videos of our performance. We might hear the sound of ball on bat or racket. We can also use biomechanical methods of providing KP, e.g. measuring force, using specially designed platforms (called force platforms). Table 7.2 shows a list of different types of feedback that are available to us.

Timing and precision of feedback

Feedback is a form of instruction, but it is instruction during practice and following the athlete's own attempts at performing the skill. One of the main factors is the timing of the provision of feedback following the learners' performance of a trial or trials. This is called the *feedback delay*; sometimes *KR delay* or *KP delay* are used. Research has shown that the length of the feedback delay is of little importance in learning, *but* any interpolated activity,

Table 7.2 Types of feedback (from McMorris, T., 2004, *Acquisition and performance of sports skills*, Wiley, Chichester. Printed with permission)

Verbal descriptive	qualitative, e.g. 'too far', 'spot on', 'nearly'
	quantitative, e.g. 'a foot too long', '11.2 s'
Verbal prescriptive	instructions
Motivational	e.g. 'good', 'well done', 'keep trying'
Visual descriptive	demonstration
	video or film
	computer print-out, e.g. results of biomechanical analyses
Proprioceptive	feel of the movement
Auditory	e.g. sound of bat–ball contact

activity between performance and the presentation of the feedback, can inhibit learning. In some situations, it is not possible to eliminate interpolated activity; e.g., during a game, a rugby coach must wait until half-time before he or she can give feedback.

Of more importance than the feedback delay is the *post-feedback delay*. This is, also, sometimes called the *post-KR delay* or the *post-KP delay*. This is the time *interval between the presentation of the feedback and the learner producing the next response*. As with the feedback delay, interpolated activity will affect learning. The most important factor, however, is the length of the delay. If the time period is *too short*, the learner does not have time to create a new response. The whole period between trials is called the *inter-trial interval* (see Figure 7.2).

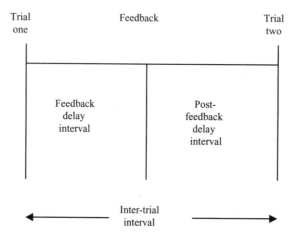

Figure 7.2 Inter-trial intervals in the presentation of feedback

Another aspect of the timing of feedback is the *frequency* of giving feedback. Commonsense would say that the higher the frequency the better. Surely 100 per cent frequency, i.e. feedback following every trial, is best? Research has failed to support this. One of the problems with giving feedback after every trial is that the athlete becomes dependent on the coach. It should be the aim of the coach to get the athlete to be able to use intrinsic feedback and not have to depend on extrinsic feedback. This, however, is not the only factor affecting the efficiency of feedback, nor is it the most important. There are other factors that determine which type of feedback is the most beneficial.

One of the first areas to be researched was *precision* of feedback. Just how precise does feedback need to be? If the coach provides very detailed feedback, e.g. 'Your point of release of the shot was 35.8°', it can be meaningless to the performer. Similarly, saying 'You missed' is of little use. The first is too detailed while the latter is lacking in any meaningful information. There is an *optimal* level for each *task* and *performer*. Some tasks require more precision than others, if we are to get them right. A dressage rider needs to be 'spot on', whereas a hurdles jockey does not require the same precision when getting over the hurdles.

The level of expertise of the performer must also be taken into account. Research has shown that beginners and experienced performers need different amounts of feedback. Beginners generally require a comparatively large amount of extrinsic feedback, with a fairly high frequency. As they develop their expertise, however, they need less and less extrinsic feedback. Therefore, the use of what we call the *fading technique* is recommended. In other words, feedback is given less and less often as the athlete improves. Ideally there will come a time when extrinsic feedback is no longer required.

Not only should the frequency of feedback alter as the performer improves, but so should the type of feedback. In the early stages of learning, the athlete requires not only KR but also KP. They need the KP to develop new movement patterns. At this stage they are not able to do this for themselves, as their knowledge base is poor. They need what we call *prescriptive* feedback. They need to be told what to do in order to improve performance. As they improve and increase their knowledge of the activity, all they require is KR. If they are making an error, they can resolve the problem themselves. So we say that they now require *descriptive* feedback.

Task 2 Choose a skill and a common fault in performing that skill. What would you say to a beginner committing the fault? How would it differ from what you would say to an experienced performer?

Recent research into feedback has examined what is termed *bandwidth* feedback. This kind of feedback developed due to problems with the precision of feedback. As we have seen, feedback can be too precise, thus making it redundant. Furthermore, we know that it is not possible to repeat motor skills precisely every time. The number of muscles, nerves and joints (what the ecological psychologists call degrees of freedom) that must be controlled means that even the great performers cannot be 100 per cent accurate all of the time. Bandwidth feedback takes this into account. The coach sets parameters for performance. If performance falls outside the parameters, feedback is given. If the performer is within the parameters or bandwidth, nothing is said. This kind of feedback has generally, although not unequivocally, been seen to be the most beneficial. It should be remembered that, by using bandwidths, the coach is in fact giving feedback after every trial. If the coach says nothing, the learner knows that he or she was within the bandwidth, which is a form of KR.

Task 3 *Choose a skill and determine what would be reasonable bandwidths for a beginner, an intermediate and an expert performer.*

Another issue that concerns the giving of feedback is whether it should be *positive or negative*. Positive feedback can be telling someone that he or she has done well. It can, also, be what we call *constructive* feedback, i.e. the coach tells the learner how to improve performance by saying 'Do it this way'. Negative feedback concentrates on errors. Sometimes coaches point out errors and then follow up with constructive feedback. Constructive feedback has been shown to be effective following either a negative or positive approach. However, negative feedback often includes 'Don't do it like that' or 'You got it wrong. You did this and shouldn't have'. This latter type of feedback can be very demotivating and is also of little use to beginners, as they need constructive, prescriptive information.

Before leaving feedback, I should point out that most of the research into feedback has been laboratory based and has used tasks that have little ecological validity with regard to acquiring sports skills. A fair amount of recent research has attempted to use ecologically valid tasks. In real life situations, there is nearly always some form of feedback available to the performer. KR is present in most tasks. We can normally see what the outcome is, e.g. if I fire an arrow at a target, I can see where it struck; or if I shoot in netball, I can see where the ball went – did I score, hit the rim or miss altogether? However, this may not always be the case for individual performance in a team game. The result of the game is obvious but KR for each individual, with regard to their own performance, is not always straight-forward. This can be because there is too much interpolated activity. It can, also, be because the player thinks that something is good when in fact it is not.

Summary

Feedback can come in the form of KR or KP. Whichever is given the coach must allow time for the learner to re-formulate his/her response. Feedback that is too precise is as useless as that which is too vague. There is an optimal level of precision for each learner and each task. Of particular importance is the level of expertise of the athletes. Experts need less feedback than beginners. Moreover, they require descriptive feedback, while the novice needs to be told how to improve (prescriptive feedback). The use of bandwidths has been shown to be particularly useful when providing feedback. By far the most important factor, however, is that the *learner must actually use the feedback to generate a new response*.

Practical implications

Based on practical experience of coaching, and the coaching, motor learning and biomechanical literature, I present a model for guidance during observation and feedback (see Figure 7.3). This model differs very little from that proposed by Knudson and Morrison (1997). In reality both my model and that of Knudson and Morrison are no more than diagrammatical summaries of what coaches, biomechanists and motor learning psychologists have recommended as good practice for many years.

The first and most obvious step is to analyse the skill. The coach should know the *key points* for good performance of the skill. This is commonsense, but it is amazing how often it is forgotten. Some coach educators insist on their student coaches pointing out the key points to the learners prior to practice. As I stated in Chapters 4 and 5, it may be better sometimes to let the learner 'have a go', without instruction before pointing out the key factors. If the coach is trying to shape the skills they may prefer to gradually add more and more key points slowly until the skill has been learned. Guided discovery methods also favour this approach. The coach, however, *must* understand how the skill is performed, if he/she is going to coach it well.

This leads us to consider the depth of knowledge that the coach will need in order to be able to claim to have analysed the skill correctly. The coach's own practical experience of performing the skill is important but on its own it is

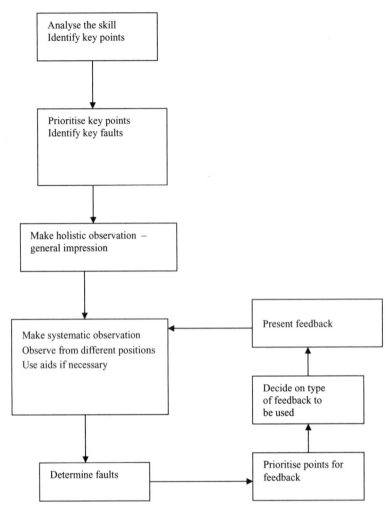

Figure 7.3   Model to guide observation and feedback

insufficient. We each have our own idiosyncrasies in the way in which we perform skills. Our way may not be the best for our athletes. We may even perform the skill incorrectly. It is necessary to examine the coaching literature. Most coaching manuals analyse the skill for you. In most circumstances, this is sufficient. However, a breakdown as recommended by the biomechanists is an added advantage. If the coach has no expertise in biomechanics, they can still use sports biomechanics texts such as those by Hay (1993) and Carr (2004). However, these texts do not cover all skills.

Analysing a skill into its key points is fine but we need also to *prioritize* the relative importance of each factor. I stated in Chapter 5 that, when instructing learners, we must be careful not to overload their working memory capacity. The same applies to our own working memories while observing. No one can take account of every aspect of a task all at once. We need to prioritize what we are going to observe first, second and so on. As we develop our observational skills, we will automatically chunk some factors together and form an overall picture or gestält of an action. If what we are seeing is not the same as what we expect, we will automatically know that something is wrong. We still may not know exactly what is wrong, however. So, even for experienced coaches, the need to break down a skill is important. This analysis does not only apply to individual performance, the same principles apply to team or group skills. For example, in invasion games we might check firstly to see if our team is penetrating the opposition's defence. If not, we will try to find out why. Are the attackers passing the ball forward when they are able? Are the players not in possession of the ball moving intelligently into attacking positions? This kind of analysis is based on what have been described as the principles of team play (most coaching manuals include a section on principles of play).

Many coaches, even experienced ones, carry a *checklist* with them when coaching. This has the key points and priorities written on them. Experienced coaches may not use a physical checklist but certainly 'have one in their head'. Table 7.3 gives an example of such a checklist. Note that not only are the key points given but also the *most common faults*. This can be a particular aid to the novice coach. The experienced coach has normally become so used to seeing these that they trigger off an automatic response.

Task 4 *Draw up a table like 7.3 for a skill that you know well. Try to check your answers by consulting a coaching manual.*

Observation

Once we have analysed the skill, we are ready to observe performance. Many coaches take a gestältist approach at first, simply getting an overall impression of performance. Then they follow a rigid ordered observation of each of the key points. If the overall picture has suggested an area that may be problematic, the coach will alter the order of observation of the key faults. When observing a football player shooting at goal, the first priority is the point of foot–ball contact. However, if the shot is accurate but lacking in power, the coach may decide to observe the movement the kicking leg, e.g. is the kicker using a long lever? Is he/she kicking 'through' the ball?

Table 7.3   Checklist used when observing performance of a soccer player kicking a ball along the ground

Check	Correct action	Common faults
1. Is the point of foot–ball contact correct?	Instep of foot contacts ball at its mid-point	Kick with toe Kick with inside of foot Contact beneath mid-point Kick with outside of foot Contact to side of mid-point Contact above mid-point
2. Is angle of approach correct?	Approach at a slight angle (about 10° from an imaginary line drawn vertically backwards from ball)	Straight approach
3. Is the follow-through correct?	Follow-through should point to where the player wants the ball to go	Follow-through to left or right of target No follow-through
4. Is the body position correct?	Shoulder on same side as non-kicking leg should be at angle of about 45° to the ball	Square on position (shoulder 90° to the ball)
5. Is the head still?	Head should be down and over the ball and remain in that position	Head jerked back on contact Head facing upwards before and on contact

This notion of following an organized pattern of search is an example of the use of selective attention. Selective attention can be a particular problem in team games. There is a great deal happening in team games and it is easy for the coach to end up observing like a spectator. The coach must be more disciplined and observe the key factors in team play. Moreover, in many team games the coach has the use of assistant coaches. In most North American sports each assistant has a particular job to do. In European sports, such as football and netball, the head coach and assistants often end up observing the same things. The use of assistant coaches needs to be organized. This also applies to observation of individual skills. Assistant coaches and head coaches can position themselves at different vantage points so that they can observe the skill from different angles. Biomechanists are particularly attentive to this when setting up camera positions, but often coaches simply stand in one place. The coach should move around to get a fuller picture of the action. The better the

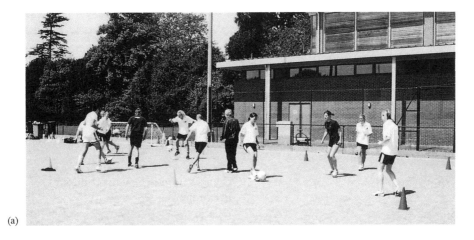

(a)

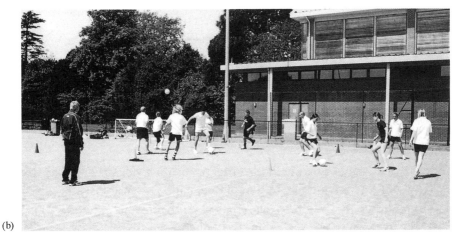

(b)

Figure 7.4 In (a) the coach (in tracksuit) is poorly positioned; he cannot see what is happening behind him. In (b) he can see all of the players

analysis of the skill, the better the choice of positions that will supply useful information.

The problem with coach positioning can be even more basic than those discussed above. Look at Figure 7.4(a). The coach is in a position that does not allow him to see all of the performers. Those behind him may be making lots of mistakes or even 'messing about'. By moving to the position he takes in Figure 7.4(b), he can see all of the performers at once.

As we saw earlier in this chapter, even if the coach does everything correctly he or she may not be able to observe sufficiently well enough to spot errors without the aid of sophisticated equipment. Table 7.4 outlines most of the equipment available. However, only a small fraction of this is available to most

Table 7.4 Mechanical aids available

Device	Uses
Video and high speed film (with or without automated systems linked to computer)	limb angles; limb speed; limb position
Force platforms	contact forces (normally foot–ground contact); changes in momentum; velocity
Electromyographs	changes in muscle activity during performance; muscle force; muscle fatigue
Isokinetic dynamometry	dynamic movement of a joint during performance; muscle function; muscle endurance
Electrogoniometry	angular position and displacement of limbs
Accelerators	acceleration of limbs; acceleration of whole body

coaches. Even where it is available the coach must decide whether its use is going to be of any advantage. Where movements are very fast, the use of high speed film allows the coach to see what is happening in slow motion. It also allows the performer to see what is happening and this may be far more important. Similarly, force platforms may provide the coach and athlete with information about the nature of changes in the exertion of power, which cannot be observed visually. The performer, however, may not be able to use such information in order to alter his/her movement. The British biomechanist Adrian Lees (2002) points out that not all biomechanical information can be used by athletes. Some of it is at such a micro-level that it cannot be acted on.

Not only must the coach decide when and what equipment to use, he/she needs to decide whether or not to bring in the help of a specialist such as a sports biomechanist or motor learning psychologist. If the coach decides to use such a person the coach must be unambiguous in what they want the scientist to tell them. Far too often coaches are very vague about what they wish to know. It may also be necessary to use a team of sports scientists specializing in different aspects of performance, especially if the coach thinks that the problem is a holistic one. The coach should also be careful to ensure that the sports scientist is accredited. In most countries this can be done easily by contacting the association of sports scientists, e.g. British Association of Sport and Exercise Sciences (BASES).

It should be remembered, however, that even if the person is accredited he or she is a *sports* scientist, not necessarily an expert in your particular sport. The coach must provide the expertise concerning what needs to be examined and how to use the resultant information. One football club with which I was associated had a player who lacked pace. They, therefore, sent him to an athletics coach. He watched the player sprint and said the problem was his style. The athletics coach then worked with the player on his sprinting style. He became much faster over 100 m but it made no difference to his short 5–10 m sprints on the football pitch. In fact, the high knee lift that the athletics coach had him develop was a hindrance at times. The player's football coach should have sought assistance from a biomechanist and shown the biomechanist the type of sprinting that is common in football. It is not the same as in 100 m sprinting.

Providing feedback

Progression

The whole aim of observation is to provide the coach with the information necessary to determine when to give feedback and what kind of feedback to give. If the athlete is undertaking part-progressive practice, the coach must also decide when to progress to the next stage. Sometimes it is necessary to regress to more basic skills before moving the learners on from what they can already do (bootstrapping). This is very easy to say. It is, also, very easy *theoretically* to know the answers to these problems. It is far more difficult in reality. I have seen many coaches constantly looking at their watches. They have decided, before starting the session, that they will spend 2 min on the first practice; move to practice two, that will take 5 min; then on to practice three and so on. This is totally unrealistic. The amount of time spent practising any task will depend on how well the learners are coping. Five minutes may be far too short. It may, also, be far too long. If the athletes are already capable of doing this aspect of the task, they may well become bored. This is particularly true with children. The only way to know when and how to move on is by observation of the performance. If the coach has analysed the skill and knows what the aims of the practice are, they are in a good position to determine when to progress.

In making this decision, the coach should be aware of motivational aspects as well as pure motor learning concerns. If the performers are becoming bored with a particular practice, they may not exhibit learning when, in fact, they have made some progress. If the coach suspects this, he/she should progress to the next stage and see what happens. If the poor performance in the previous practice was due to boredom, it will soon become obvious as the learners will show an improvement. However, if the problem was a learning one, they will not be able to cope. If this is the case, the coach can step back one or even two stages. Sometimes it is wise to have a break from that particular activity.

Such strategies as this are rarely needed and in most cases the learners progress at a steady rate. However, in team or group situations this will not necessarily be uniform in nature. Different performers will be ready for progression at different times. The coach should be aware of this and try to gear the progressions to *each* individual or sub-group of athletes. This is the process of *differentiation*.

> **Task 5** *Choose a skill and work out a number of progressions that you could use to help athletes acquire the skill. You may wish to return to Chapter 6 to look at the principles of part-progressive practice.*

When to provide feedback

As we saw earlier in this chapter, when to give feedback is not a simple factor. We noted, in particular, the frequency of providing feedback. The benefit of using the fading technique is well documented. The use of bandwidths has also generally been shown to be advantageous. By using both of these methods in tandem we can time the giving of feedback so that it can be best used by the athlete. However, we should not forget that individuals differ in their type of motivation and personality. In deciding the timing of reducing the frequency of feedback (fading technique) the coach should take into account the athlete's self-confidence and tendency towards coach dependency. Athletes low in self-confidence or being somewhat dependent in nature may need to have feedback removed more slowly than others, while the more independent personalities with higher self-confidence may find being constantly given feedback annoying.

Using feedback as a motivational tool

This brings us to the use of feedback as a motivational tool. We all like praise, in particular praise from those whom we perceive as being important. The failure of coaches to praise good performance can have disastrous effects on the athlete's self-confidence. It can also give the learners the false impression that they are not improving when in fact they are. However, overdoing the giving of praise can have negative effects. If all the athletes hear is 'well done', 'great' and 'brilliant' then these words either come to mean nothing or become so familiar to the learner that, in fact, they are not perceived by them at all. As we saw in Chapter 2, unexpected praise has the greatest effect. During practice situations unexpected praise can be particularly powerful if the learner has done something that is not outstanding and obvious to the other athletes but is seen by the coach as being significant. A quiet 'well done, I saw that' can mean a great deal to the athlete.

One of the most common errors with regard to providing motivational feedback occurs after a coach has given technical feedback. The coach tells the learner he/she has made an error. Then technical feedback is given. The learner has another trial and does well. At this stage the learner is expecting praise. Just think of the disappointment when they turn round and find that the coach has wandered off to talk to someone else.

Another important issue with regard to the motivational aspects of feedback is when to give praise and when to criticize. Most athletes can take criticism if it is sandwiched in between praise. It may not need to be actually sandwiched but should be preceded by some praise. This 'praise' might be as simple as, 'you're getting better' or 'you're getting there'. Then the criticism is made and how to put it right is added. If improvement is shown, praise must be given immediately. If there is not an immediate improvement, the learner can be encouraged to keep trying and reminded that with practice the goal can be met. It is important, however, *not to lie* to the athlete. Telling someone they are doing well when they are not can give a false sense of achievement. It will also lead to the athlete losing trust in the coach when the performance fails during a competition.

In criticizing athletes one must be very careful. As stated above, most learners need praise *before* criticism. The exception to this is the very strong type A personality with a large ego. It may be necessary, with such people, to be very critical and in fact be verbally aggressive. In deciding to take this approach one must be certain that the individual is of this personality type. Often less confident individuals try to hide their lack of self-confidence by behaving in a way which gives a false impression. I have only ever used this approach with a handful of individuals and then only after knowing them for some time (well over a year).

Precision of feedback

Earlier in this chapter, we discussed the fact that feedback can be too vague or too precise. We stated that the decision concerning how precise to be is dependent on the interaction between the task and the learner. It is pointless telling a golfer that he/she is 3 cm short. Not even Tiger Woods can reproduce shots to that accuracy. If someone is 3 cm short the coach should say nothing. This, of course, is the use of bandwidths. In using bandwidths, we can start by having quite large parameters. For example, the beginner golfer, when putting, will not receive feedback if they are within 1 m of the hole. As they improve this can be shortened.

Bandwidths are not the only factors to be taken into account. The level of cognitive development and the educational background of the learner must also be considered. Individuals with a good knowledge of skill acquisition and/or biomechanics can understand more detail than those with little background. The Olympic pursuit cycling gold medallist Chris Boardman has a good knowledge of exercise physiology. Therefore, in his preparation for the 1992 Olympics, his coach Pete Keen used sophisticated feedback. To other cyclists in the British team, Pete's feedback was at a more basic level. Everyone understood what was being said to them. This is good coaching. Children, in particular, have problems with language. Their vocabulary is limited so coaches must be sure that they are using words that the child can understand. The use of jargon can be a problem with children and indeed other beginners. With experienced performers it may be useful.

Using visual aids

The most commonly used visual aid is the video. Videos are particularly useful for skills that are qualitatively judged, e.g. gymnastics and trampolining. The performer can see what they are doing for themselves. It can also be used by the coach to reinforce his or her own observations. Often athletes are convinced that they are doing something correctly and do not believe coaches when they say that they are making mistakes in performance. In other words, KP can be greatly aided by use of video. Just as the use of slow motion can aid the coach's observation it can also help the athletes to perceive movement better. Even freezing a frame can be very helpful. I have found this particularly useful when pointing out to shot putters that their point of release is incorrect.

There are problems with using video, however. Many coaches assume that when they show someone a video the learner will automatically observe the correct areas of the display. This may be far from correct. The coach needs to point out to the athletes what to look at. It is a good practice to get the athlete

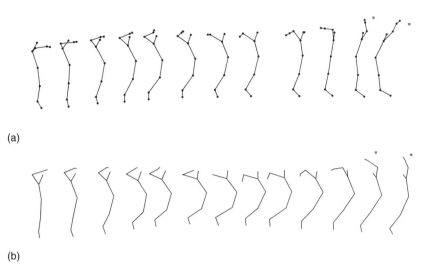

(a)

(b)

Figure 7.5 (a) shows an elite level volleyball player spiking while (b) shows a club player. The print-out can supply useful information and is easy to understand

to describe what they perceive in order to make sure that they are looking at the right areas. Also human nature being what it is, when most people are shown videos of themselves for the first time they focus on how they look rather than the technicalities of the movement. It is a good idea to let the athletes have look at themselves, give them time to get over this and then watch their performance.

A step on from the use of the video is the use of three-dimensional kinematic analysis. Figure 7.5 shows the kind of print-out produced. The feedback from this is little different from looking at a video or a series of still photographs. Figure 7.6 demonstrates the type of feedback that we get from an EMG printout. The precision of this kind of feedback is very detailed and needs to be interpreted for the athlete and coach by a biomechanist. The coach must use the information to alter the athlete's technique. Sometimes such feedback can be too detailed to be of any use to the performer.

Digital video analysis can be used in a similar way. The coach can point out to the team that they are making errors in a particular area of the field or court. As those of you who play or coach team sports know, players are reluctant to admit to mistakes, and it is always their team-mates' fault, never their own. Notational analysis data of all kinds can be used by the coach to point out errors and stop disagreements as to who is to blame.

Conditioning coaches often use feedback from heart rate monitors, blood lactate concentrations and oxygen uptake to provide feedback concerning the

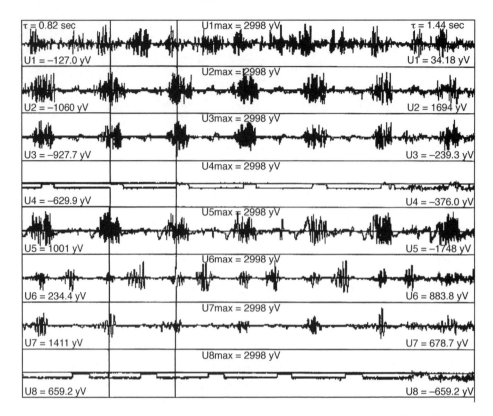

Figure 7.6   An example of a printout from an electromyograph. It is not possible for lay people to understand and needs interpretation by a sports biomechanist

fitness levels of performers. Figure 7.7 shows a table tennis player using a Cosmed K4b^2 portable monitor, which provides feedback on, among other things, heart rate, oxygen uptake and energy expenditure. This information can be used to determine the intensity of the exercise. By using a digital video analysis system, I have been able to point out to players what runs they did not make that they should have. Discussing with the player the reasons for not making these runs often results in the athlete admitting to being too fatigued. By looking at laboratory results of fitness tests we can motivate the athlete to improve fitness, especially when they know that this will result in them being more effective in the game.

Biomechanical modelling

A fairly recent development in biomechanics has been the development of models of the correct technique for any given task. These can be given to

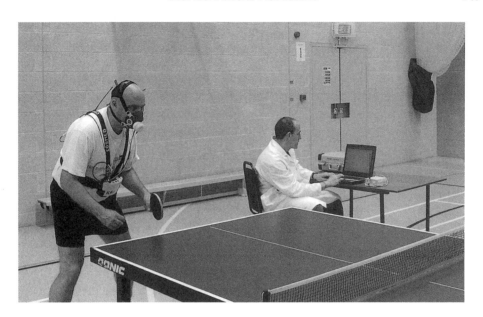

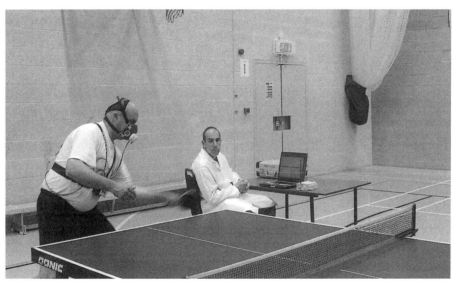

Figure 7.7 A table tennis player wearing a CosMed K4b², which allows oxygen uptake to be measured in an actual game situation

athletes as prescriptive feedback. However, one must be careful with this. These models are developed based on the assumption that the athlete is totally 'normal', i.e. they do not have any physical or neurological idiosyncrasies. It is well known that very few, if any of us, are totally 'normal'. This can particularly be seen by the fact that the vast majority of people are not 100 per cent symmetrical. Therefore, it may not be possible for a particular athlete to perform in the same way as the model.

Key points

- observation requires good perception, particularly selective attention

- observation is a process of working memory

- working memory consists of
  - short-term memory
  - information recalled from long-term memory
  - decision making

- mechanical aids to observation include
  - video analysis
  - eye-mark recorders
  - digitization
  - force platforms
  - electromyographs (EMGs)
  - heart rate monitors
  - measures of oxygen consumption

- notational analysis can provide information concerning work rate and tactical performance

- feedback is all information resulting from an action

- feedback can be intrinsic (from within the person themselves) or extrinsic (from an outside body)

- feedback can be knowledge of results (KR) (information concerning the outcome of the action) or knowledge of performance (KP) (information concerning the nature of the movement)

- the feedback delay (the time between performing the skill and receiving feedback) can be negatively affected by interpolated activity (activity taking place during the delay)

- the post-feedback delay (the time between receiving feedback and having another try) can be negatively affected by interpolated activity
  - if the post-feedback delay is too short, the learner does not have time to reconstruct his or her action plan

- too much feedback can lead to the learner becoming coach dependent
  - beginners need a lot of feedback; this should be slowly reduced as the person learns the skill – this is called the fading technique

- feedback needs to be meaningful to the learners
  - very detailed, precise feedback can be too difficult for the learner to understand
  - very limited, imprecise feedback can mean nothing to the learner
  - beginners need prescriptive feedback (they need to be told what they did wrong and how to put it right)
  - experienced performers need descriptive feedback (they need to be told the outcome)

- the use of bandwidth feedback can aid learning
  - feedback is only given if the response falls outside parameters (the bandwidth) set by the coach

- feedback can be used to aid motivation

- for feedback to work, the learner must use the feedback to generate a new response

- the use of checklists aids observation

- coaches must position themselves where they can best see the action

- feedback should aid bootstrapping, i.e. progressing to more advanced levels of performance.

III

Physiological Factors

Introduction

Coaching science, particularly at the elite level, requires the application of appropriate physiological knowledge to individuals performing specific sports. The key to successful coaching lies in two things. The first is the recognition that some guiding principles have been discovered, initially by the largely unaided trial-and-error approach adopted by the early coaches, but more recently through applied research driven by partnerships between athlete, coach and sports scientist, while the second is that these guiding principles need to be intelligently adapted to the *specific* needs of individual sportsmen and sportswomen undertaking *particular* activities.

That second element brings with it its own difficulties. We need to understand the fundamental physiological knowledge arising from human responses to various forms of strenuous exercise. Put simply, the question that needs addressing is 'How much, and what sort, of physical effort is required?'. We need to know whether the intensity of the effort, expressed as a percentage of a measured maximum ($\%_{max}$), is high or low – e.g. rowing versus snooker. Is the duration of the effort long or short – 100 m versus the marathon? Is the effort continuous or intermittent – track athletics versus football?

> **Task 1** *Using appropriate adjectives, categorize the following activities: cricket; tennis; Olympic weightlifting; 100 m, 400 m, 1500 m and 10 000 m track events; game of football; four 2 min rounds of boxing; single-handed dinghy sailing.*

Each of the above activities taxes physiological mechanisms in different ways. Thus, we need to understand the inter-play between various body systems, and, more importantly, to detect the areas of weakness in our physiological make-up. For example, all of the events listed in Task 1 require knowledge about the primary energy sources.

Task 2 *How would you describe the energy sources?*

Energy sources, critical though they are to all actions, form only part of a complex picture of the range of physiological attributes needed for different sports. Some obvious attributes that spring immediately to mind are general endurance, local endurance, speed, strength, power, flexibility, stability and body size and shape.

Task 3 *Think of examples of activities that depend essentially on one of each of these attributes. Now think of activities requiring more than one of these attributes.*

Over the next three chapters, we cover three key areas of the physiology of the coaching process. First, we explore the mechanisms by which we meet the energy requirements of particular activities. Then we explore the ways in which physiological factors limit performance in those activities, and the probable uniqueness of individual athletes' responses. Finally, we consider the physiological principles underpinning sport specific training, touch on the consequences of over-training, and examine the problems associated with assessing performance through fieldwork and laboratory simulations.

Additional reading

Hale, T. (2003). *Exercise physiology – a thematic approach*. Wiley, Chichester.
    Wilmore, J. H. and Costill, D. L. (2004). *Physiology of sport and exercise*, 3rd
    edn. Human Kinetics, Champaign, IL.

8

Physiological Demands of Track Athletics

Learning objectives

By the end of this chapter you should be able to

- recognize the importance of sport-specific movement analysis as the precursor to all coaching and training programmes
- define speed, velocity, acceleration and deceleration
- distinguish between aerobic and anaerobic metabolism, and substrate and oxidative phosphorylation
- describe the relative energy densities of the primary fuel sources, and link them to different activities
- outline the processes involved in the phosphagen cycle, glycogenolysis, the Krebs cycle and the electron transfer chain in the resynthesis of adenosine triphosphate (ATP) from adenosine diphosphate (ADP)
- explain the process involved in the production of lactic acid
- describe the main features of the structure and function of skeletal muscle
- explain the effect of excess hydrogen ions on skeletal muscle contraction.

Coaching Science   Terry McMorris and Tudor Hale
© 2006 John Wiley & Sons, Ltd

In this chapter, we explore the energy systems that underpin all of our activities. We examine a sample of running events as a source of useful basic information on the systems that drive muscle actions. We begin where all good coaches begin by analysing running performance, and then look at the physiological mechanisms supporting that performance. In this way, we introduce some important links between practice and theory.

The physiology of elite sprinting

At the elite level, the 100 m takes less than 10 s from gun to finishing line. You may think that an event lasting such a short time cannot contain a great deal of information that needs to be uncovered. After all, only two attributes are required – a fast start, and the maximum effort possible. However, detailed analysis suggests that 100 m running is not so simple.

A fast start depends on

(a) a well prepared athlete who is confident, committed, relaxed and focussed on the task in hand; this is the province of the sports psychologist;
(b) a short reaction time; this is the province of the psychologist interested in motor control and the way athletes respond to their environment;
(c) a powerful thrust off the starting blocks; to examine the starting technique requires force platforms in the starting blocks, and is more properly the province of the sport biomechanist.

The maximum effort possible requires good technique through

(a) a balance between leg-speed, stride length and arm co-ordination;
(b) relaxation of the upper body to maintain the athlete's stability.

These are the provinces of the technical coach, who needs to combine all three forms of scientific analysis, with the aid of a video recording of the entire 100 m. For the physiologist, this timed video recording provides important pointers on the physiology of muscle contraction.

> **Task 1** *Think about your own 100 m efforts. Draw a graph of speed against distance of what you imagine your performance would be like e.g. slow start–fast finish, the reverse of this, steady effort throughout. Now try drawing the graph of an elite sprinter.*

If we look at six world class 100 m runners in action, we find that at the finishing tape the winner is a mere 0.1 s – equivalent to a distance of about one metre – ahead of the sixth placed runner. The raw data appear in Table 8.1.

Table 8.1 Athlete reaction times, split times and average velocities of the 100 m finalists in the 1991 Tokyo World Championships (Hyman R. (2003) IAAF World Records with permission of the IAAF)

Athlete	1		2		3	
Reaction time (s)	0.140		0.120		0.090	
Distance (m)	Time t (s)	Velocity v(m/s)	Time t (s)	Velocity v(m/s)	Time t (s)	Velocity v(m/s)
10	1.88	5.32	1.83	5.46	1.80	5.56
20	2.96	9.26	2.89	9.43	2.87	9.35
30	3.88	10.87	3.80	10.99	3.80	10.75
40	4.77	11.24	4.68	11.36	4.68	11.36
50	5.61	11.91	5.55	11.49	5.55	11.49
60	6.46	11.77	6.41	11.63	6.42	11.49
70	7.30	11.91	7.28	11.49	7.28	11.63
80	8.13	12.05	8.12	11.91	8.14	11.63
90	9.00	11.49	9.01	11.24	9.02	11.36
100	9.86	11.63	9.88	11.49	9.91	11.24
Average velocity(m/s)	10.14		10.12		10.0	

Athlete	4		5		6	
Reaction time (s)	0.126		0.151		0.114	
Distance (m)	Time t (s)	Velocity v(m/s)	Time t (s)	Velocity v(m/s)	Time t (s)	Velocity v(m/s)
10	1.85	5.41	1.86	5.38	1.81	5.53
20	2.91	9.43	2.92	9.43	2.88	9.35
30	3.83	10.87	3.84	10.87	3.79	10.99
40	4.72	11.24	4.73	11.24	4.68	11.24
50	5.57	11.77	5.60	11.49	5.54	11.63
60	6.43	11.63	6.47	11.49	6.41	11.49
70	7.29	11.63	7.33	11.63	7.29	11.36
80	8.14	11.77	8.18	11.77	8.16	11.49
90	9.04	11.11	9.07	11.24	9.06	11.11
100	9.92	11.36	9.95	11.36	9.96	11.11
Average velocity(m/s)	10.08		10.05		10.04	

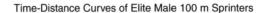

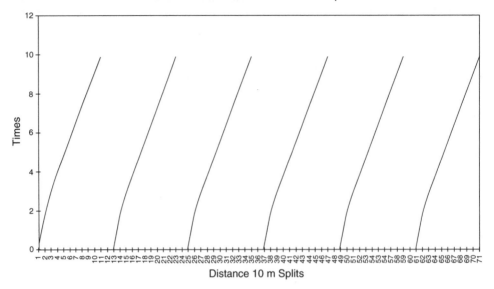

Figure 8.1   Time–distance curves of elite male 100 m sprinters (published with permission from IAAF)

Task 2 *Using Table 8.1, (a) say who had the fastest and slowest reaction times and (b), (c) put the athletes in order from fastest to slowest (b)over the first 10 m and (c) over the last 10 m.*

Now, if we simply plot time taken against serial 10 m blocks for this group of sprinters (see Figure 8.1) we find it difficult, if not impossible, to distinguish between the runners on anything except time taken. We get little more information from this graph than if we simply calculate the individual's average speed – i.e. distance in metres divided by time in seconds ($m\,s^{-1}$).

Task 3 *Do this calculation for the first and last athletes and compare speeds (10.14 m s^{-1} for the winner compared with 10.04 m s^{-1} for the sixth).*

This merely confirms what we already know – that the winner is always faster than the last placed runner! However, if we examine the time taken for *each* 10 m split, we can calculate speed – or to use the precise term 'velocity' in metres per second ($m\,s^{-1}$) – and see where *changes* in velocity – i.e. 'acceleration/deceleration' in metres per second per second ($m\,s^{-2}$) – occur during the race. A typical graph of 100 m performance shows three basic phases (Figure 8.2). There is an increase in speed over the first 30–40 metres, followed

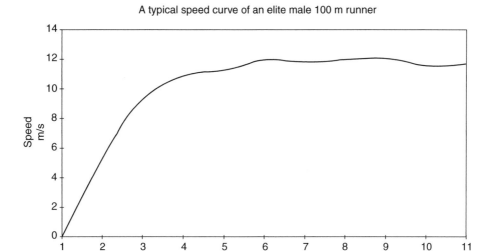

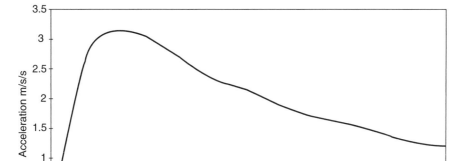

Figure 8.2 (a) A typical speed curve of an elite male 100 m runner and (b) a typical acceleration curve (published with permission from IAAF)

by a plateau over the next 40–70 m, and speed is at its lowest over the final 20–30 m. In terms of acceleration, the initial 10 m always gives the greatest change in velocity, because the athlete is starting from zero, but after that the overall picture is one of gradual, but progressive deceleration.

However, if we examine each individual's graph two obvious features stand out. First, each sprinter produces an individual profile, and second, no profile is

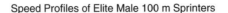

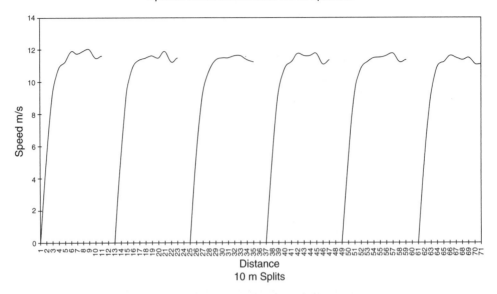

Figure 8.3 Speed profiles of elite 100 m male sprinters (published with permission from IAAF)

smooth (Figure 8.3). We can see other interesting features on the graphs. For example, the gradients of different 10 m segments show not just the fact that average velocity changes throughout the race, but that there are segments where actual deceleration occurs. We also see that athletes reached peak velocity at different points during the race.

> **Task 4** *From the graphs, can you detect (a) the instances of deceleration in each run and (b) the approximate distance at which each athlete reached peak velocity? Speculate on the possible causes of deceleration.*

Sources of energy for muscle contraction

All of our energy comes initially from the sun, packaged in the form of proteins, carbohydrates and fats in the food we eat. We can ignore proteins as a major source of energy except for particular circumstances (high protein intake immediately before exercise, or long-term starvation). Fats provide a very valuable source of energy; they are high in calorific content but their metabolic breakdown – catabolism – is too slow and uses too much oxygen to be useful to the 100 m runner. This leaves carbohydrate; this is stored in the muscles in long chains of glucose molecules

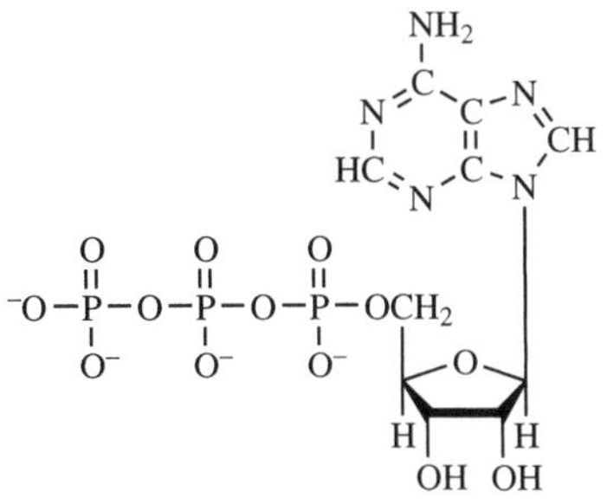

ATP consists of a base, in this case adenine (red), a ribose (magenta) and a phosphate chain (blue).

Figure 8.4 The ATP molecule is composed of three components. At the centre is a sugar molecule, *ribose* (the same sugar that forms the basis of DNA). Attached to one side of this is a *base* (a group consisting of linked rings of carbon and nitrogen atoms); in this case the base is *adenine*. The other side of the sugar is attached to a string of *phosphate* groups. These phosphates are key to the activity of ATP

called glycogen. This is the preferred fuel for all events lasting less than ~90 min.

The fuel that drives *all* cellular activity, including muscle contraction, is a compound – adenosine triphosphate – usually shortened to ATP. Without it, muscle fibres cannot contract and relax (the stiffening of the body after death – *rigor mortis* – is due to gradual but progressive reduction in adenosine triphosphate stores). The adenosine triphosphate molecule is made up of three components: first, a sugar – ribose; second, linked rings of carbon and nitrogen atoms attached to this core – adenine; finally, a string of three phosphate bonds – triphosphate (Figure 8.4). The energy for muscle contraction derives from a chemical reaction that splits off the final phosphate bond, producing adenosine *di*phosphate.

Oddly, in view of its importance, there is relatively little adenosine triphosphate stored in muscle cells – about $25\,\text{mmol}\cdot\text{kg}^{-1}$ in dried type II muscle. Thus, we need physiological mechanisms that enable us to continually replenish these stores so that contraction can take place. There are two main mechanisms involved – one requires access to adequate supplies of oxygen; the other can do without it.

Task 5 Do you know the technical names for these two processes? Which process do you think predominates in the 100 m?

Although oxygen is present within the muscles, carried in the blood and stored in myoglobin, the rate at which it can be used to convert glycogen to adenosine triphosphate is much too slow for the task of running the 100 m as fast as possible. Thus, *aerobic* processes, which are covered in detail later in the chapter, contribute only ~10 per cent of the energy needed. The remaining 90 per cent of the energy requirements come from two *anaerobic* processes – the phosphagen cycle, and glycogenolysis (the breakdown of glycogen) – working in combination.

The phosphagen cycle

We have seen that muscle cells contain three essential materials needed for contraction: two high-energy compounds – adenosine triphosphate (ATP) and phosphocreatine (PCr) – and glycogen. When the muscle fibres are stimulated to contract by impulses from the motor neurons reacting to the starter's pistol, adenosine triphosphate molecules interact with water, a process called hydrolysis. This results in the terminal phosphate bond being split off from the adenosine *tri*phosphate molecule, under the influence of the enzyme *actinomyosinATPase*. This splitting releases energy for contraction and leaves adenosine *di*phosphate (ADP) and inorganic phosphate (P$_i$).

$$\text{ATP}\text{—}actinomyosinATPase \rightarrow \text{ADP} + \text{P}_i + \text{energy} \qquad (8.1)$$

The ADP molecule is immediately restored to ATP (called phosphorylation) by attaching the phosphate that splits from the phosphocreatine (PCr) –aided by another enzyme, *creatine kinase* – to the just formed adenosine diphosphate.

$$\text{ADP} + \text{PCr}\text{—}creatine\ kinase \rightarrow \text{ATP} + \text{Cr} \qquad (8.2)$$

The process is cyclical:

$$\text{ATP}\text{—}actinomyosinATPase \rightarrow \text{ADP} + \text{P}_i + \text{energy}$$
$$\downarrow$$
$$\text{ADP} + \text{PCr}\text{—}creatine\ kinase \rightarrow \text{ATP} + \text{Cr} \qquad (8.3)$$

There is no similar mechanism for an *immediate* phosphorylation of creatine. Thus, the continued phosphorylation of adenosine diphosphate depends almost exclusively on the relatively large amount of phosphocreatine (about 3.5 times that of adenosine triphosphate) stored in the muscle. This store is readily available, but also used very quickly. At a typical rate of about 5 mmol·kg^{-1} dm s^{-1}, most of it disappears over the first 60 m of the 100 m race, and only ~20 per cent remains at the finish. The replenishment of phosphocreatine stores from the breakdown of foodstuffs has to wait until the recovery period at the end of the race.

Glycogenolysis

To make up for the declining level of phosphocreatine activity, another anaerobic process – glycogenolysis (the breakdown of the glycogen molecules) – is necessary for the phosphorylation of adenosine diphosphate to adenosine triphosphate. The reason why this process is relatively slow becomes obvious when we consider necessary reactions contained in the biochemical pathway described below.

The breakdown of glycogen needs two preliminary reactions before it can join the main glycolytic, or Embden–Meyerhof pathway (see Equation (8.4)), consisting of a series of chemical reactions that result in the re-synthesis of adenosine triphosphate. The reactions making up the pathway can take place without adequate supplies of oxygen and enabled our ancestors to maintain a high speed for up to $\sim$90 s. All of the reactions take place within the cytoplasm of the cell. Cytoplasm, known as sarcoplasm in muscle cells, is a watery, gel-like substance bounded by the cell membrane, the sarcolemma. This gel consists mainly of water, proteins, ions (charged particles) and various intra-cellular organelles such as mitochondria and ribosomes.

Steps 1 and 2

Before glycogen can enter the glycolytic pathway, the chemical bonds holding the glucose molecules together need to be broken; the enzymes that drive these reactions are *phosphorylase* and *phosphoglucomutase*.

$$\text{glycogen} + \text{P}_i\text{---}phosphorylase \rightarrow \text{glucose-1-phosphate} \qquad (8.4a)$$

$$\text{glucose-1-phosphate---}phosphoglucomutase \rightarrow \text{glucose-6-phosphate} \qquad (8.4b)$$

Step 3

The glucose-6-phosphate is converted into fructose-6-phosphate

$$\text{glucose-6-phosphate---}phosphoglucoisomerase \rightarrow \text{fructose-6-phosphate} \qquad (8.5)$$

Step 4

Paradoxically, the next reaction, rather than *producing* adenosine triphosphate, actually *uses* the compound to convert fructose-6-phosphate to fructose-1, 6-diphosphate. We now appear, temporarily at least, to be worse off in terms of adenosine triphosphate production:

$$\text{fructose-6-phosphate} + ATP—\textit{phosphofructokinase}$$
$$\rightarrow \text{fructose-1, 6-diphosphate} + ADP \tag{8.6}$$

Steps 4 and 5

The fourth step is a critical reaction for adenosine triphosphate production. Fructose-1, 6-diphosphate splits into two compounds each containing three carbon atoms.

$$\text{fructose1, 6-diphosphate}—\textit{aldolase} \rightarrow \begin{cases} \text{dihydroxyacetone phosphate} \\ \text{glyceraldehyde3-phosphate} \end{cases} \tag{8.7a}$$

The two compounds – dihydroxyacetone phosphate and glyceraldehyde-3-phosphate – are isomers. This means that the number of carbon, hydrogen and oxygen atoms is the same – $C_3H_5O_3$ – but their structures are different. However, only glyceraldehyde-3-phosphate takes part in the future reactions within the muscle cell, so *triose phosphate isomerase* rearranges the dihydroxyacetone phosphate to give a second molecule of glyceraldehyde-3-phosphate

$$\text{dihydroxyacetone phosphate}—\textit{triose phosphate isomerase}$$
$$\rightarrow \text{glyceraldehyde-3-phosphate} \tag{8.7b}$$

The last two sets of reactions have important implications for adenosine triphosphate production. The critical issue is that, from the original *one* molecule of glycogen, we now have *two* sets of reactions going on in parallel. We shall follow only one set of reactions in detail here, but record the consequences for adenosine triphosphate production from both sets of reactions.

Step 6

At the next stage, the glyceraldehyde-3-phosphate (G-3-P) interacts with a hydrogen carrier – nicotinamide adenine dinucleotide (NAD) – and organic phosphate (P_i) to form 1, 3-diphosphoglycerate, and reduced nicotinamide adenine dinucleotide (NADH) and hydrogen ions (H^+)

$$\text{G-3-P} + NAD + P_i—\textit{G-3-P dehydrogenase}$$
$$\rightarrow \textit{1, 3-diphosphoglycerate} + NADH + H^+ \tag{8.8}$$

Step 7

The following reaction sees the appearance of two molecules of re-synthesized adenosine triphosphate as 1, 3-diphosphoglycerate interacts with adenosine diphosphate and inorganic phosphate.

$$1, 3\text{-diphosphoglycerate} + \text{ADP} + \text{P}_i\text{---}\textit{phosphoglycerate kinase}$$
$$\rightarrow 3\text{-phosphoglycerate} + 2ATP \tag{8.9}$$

Task 6 What is the current state of ATP production – still in deficit, even or in surplus?

Step 8

This stage entails the re-organization of 3-phosphoglycerate by moving the phosphate to a different position within the molecule to give 2-phosphoglycerate:

$$3\text{-phosphoglycerate---}\textit{phosphoglyceromutase} \rightarrow 2\text{-phosphoglycerate} \tag{8.10}$$

Step 9

This reaction removes water (dehydration) from 2-phosphoglycerate to give phosphoenolpyruvate

$$2\text{-phosphoglycerate---}\textit{enolase} \rightarrow \text{phosphoenolpyruvate} + \text{H}_2\text{O} \tag{8.11}$$

Step 10

In the final act of glycolysis, the phosphate bond attached to phosphoenolpyruvate transfers to adenosine diphosphate to produce more adenosine triphosphate:

$$\text{phosphoenolpyruvate} + \text{ADP---}\textit{pyruvate phosphokinase}$$
$$\rightarrow \text{pyruvate} + 2ATP \tag{8.12}$$

Task 7 What is the cumulative effect of glycogenolysis/glycolysis on ATP production?

Figure 8.5 is a schematic picture of the relative contributions of the phosphagen cycle and glycogenolysis to adenosine triphosphate re-synthesis during 30 s of intermittent high intensity muscle action.

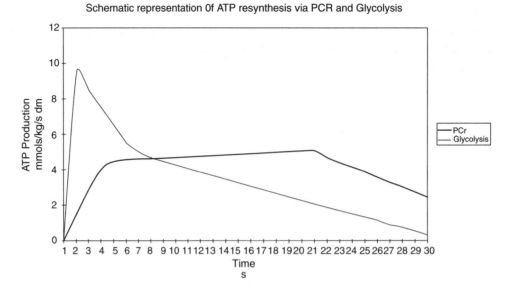

Figure 8.5   Schematic representation of ATP resynthesis via PCR and glycolysis

Figure 8.6 provides a clearer picture of the processes at work during the actual 100 m race itself.

Task 8 *What feature in Figure 10.2 seems to coincide with the PCr depletion?*

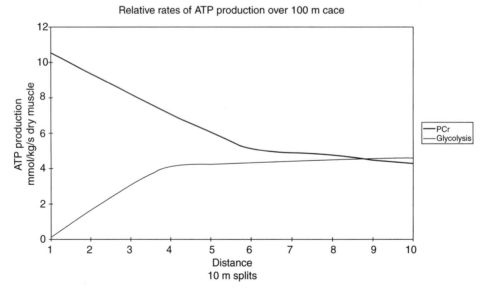

Figure 8.6   Relative rates of ATP production over 100 m race

The virtually instantaneous reactions between adenosine diphosphate and phosphocreatine are dominant, particularly in the early stages of the race. Nevertheless, by the halfway stage the glycolytic pathway is producing almost half of the required adenosine triphosphate, and by the end of the race the pathway is producing the majority. The key problem with glycolysis is that although it provides adenosine triphosphate the time taken is too slow to keep up with the muscles' demands; force generation declines as a result. We shall see similar effects, but for different reasons, when we consider our next event – the 400 m.

The physiology of the 400 m

For this event, we have access to the split times for each 100 m stage only. However, even these limited bits of information allow us to see some interesting features (Figure 8.7(a), (b)).

The first is that this event is not an all-out effort for the entire distance – individual athletes have specific strategies. In the example chosen, although the male and female athletes show similar overall profiles, the latter produces slower speeds throughout. The male covers the first 100 m in 11.3 s and the female in 12 s, at average speeds of 8.93 and 8.33 m s^{-1} respectively. The second 100 m was the fastest – 10.2 s and 10.8 (9.80 and 9.26 m s^{-1}) respectively. The last half of the race shows that, even though both are producing a maximum effort, the times inexorably increase. The third quarter took 10.8 and 12 s, with a drop in speeds to 9.26 and 8.33 m s^{-1} respectively. The final quarter was run in 11.1 and 13.4 s (9.01 and 7.46 m s^{-1}) respectively, the slowest stage for the female runner. The athletes reach peak acceleration at ~80 m and plateau until ~140 m; deceleration takes over during the final 200 m. The fuel used is still glycogen. Aerobic metabolism now provides about 30 per cent of the adenosine triphosphate needed, but anaerobic metabolism fuels the remaining 70 per cent and the 400 m taxes the athlete's anaerobic capacity to its limit.

Figure 8.5 suggests that the phosphagen cycle predominates during the first 80 m, but by 300 m adenosine triphosphate re-synthesis from the phosphocreatine–adenosine diphosphate mechanism has virtually ended, indicating that phosphocreatine stores are exhausted. In addition, the glycolytic mechanism is also showing signs of declining production. The following question arises: 'How does the athlete complete the last 100 m of this event?'. The final 260 m of gradual deceleration is linked to three main events: first, a reduced rate of adenosine triphosphate production; second, a growing level of adenosine

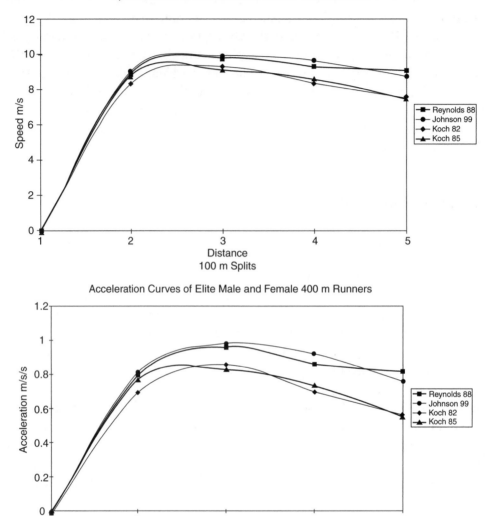

Figure 8.7 (a) Speed profiles of elite male and female 400 m runners and (b) the acceleration curves of sprinters (published with permission from IAAF)

diphosphate; third, an increased concentration of acid. All of these factors contribute to a reduced force generated by the skeletal muscle and the inevitable decline in power output.

The presence of acid in the muscle cell brings pain, which is a psychological barrier to further exertion, although with training we can learn to ignore it. What we cannot ignore is the fact that acid interferes with the mechanics of muscle contraction. The most obvious sign occurs in the last 50 m when athletes cannot maintain their running technique. Occasionally there is a complete loss of controlled muscle function. Athletes who are in the lead with 5 m to the finishing line stumble, even fall, and finish out of the medal places. The next section describes how this acid arises.

Lactic acid

We left the glycolytic pathway with a reaction that produced pyruvic acid and adenosine triphosphate (Equation (8.13)). If oxygen is available, the pyruvate (a salt of pyruvic acid) enters an *aerobic* pathway – the Krebs cycle – that produces very large quantities of adenosine triphosphate. However, in the 400 m we are not in this position – we are still dependent largely ($\sim$70 per cent) on anaerobic metabolism for most of our adenosine triphosphate.

We need to go back to a critical reaction (Equation (8.9)) between glyceraldehyde-3-phosphate (G-3-P) and the hydrogen carrier nicotinamide adenine dinucleotide (NAD^+) and inorganic phosphate (P_i) that formed 1, 3-diphosphoglycerate, reduced nicotinamide adenine dinucleotide (NADH) and hydrogen ions (H^+):

$$\text{G-3-P} + NAD^+ + P_i - G\text{-}3\text{-}P \; dehydrogenase$$
$$\rightarrow 1, 3\text{-diphosphoglycerate} + NADH + H^+ \tag{8.13}$$

This reaction is critical. Without nicotinamide adenine dinucleotide, glycolysis, and therefore adenosine triphosphate re-synthesis, ceases. Unfortunately, NAD^+ stores are limited, and the usual process for restoring them makes use of aerobic metabolism. As the 400 m runner is dealing essentially with anaerobic metabolism, and molecular oxygen is not available in sufficient quantities a short-term solution is available.

Instead of *adding* oxygen to nicotinamide adenine dinucleotide, we can achieve the same effect by *removing* hydrogen from it. The reduced nicotinamide adenine dinucleotide, driven by the enzyme *lactate dehydrogenase*, reacts with pyruvate to restore nicotinamide adenine dinucleotide levels. This permits continued adenosine triphosphate resynthesis.

$$\text{G-3-P} + NAD^+ + P_i - G\text{-}3\text{-}P dehydrogenase$$
$$\rightarrow 1, 3\text{-diphosphoglycerate} + NADH + H^+ \tag{8.14}$$

$$\text{pyruvate} + NADH + H^+ - lactate \; dehydrogenase \rightarrow \text{lactate} + NAD^+ \tag{8.15}$$

$$1, 3\text{-diphosphoglycerate} + ADP + P_i - phosphoglycerate \; kinase$$
$$\rightarrow 3\text{-phosphoglycerate} + 2ATP \tag{8.16}$$

The benefit of these reactions is important as it allows the athlete to continue to perform; the penalty, as we have already mentioned, is increasing acidity. Acids break down temporarily (dissociate) into protons – also known as hydrogen ions (H^+) – and salts. Increasing hydrogen ion concentration ($[H^+]$) results in acidosis, and adversely affects the contractile process in skeletal muscles. What we are seeing at the end of the 400 m are the consequences of that interference. To understand how that occurs we need to look at issue of acids and bases in the body, and the way skeletal muscles contract.

Acids and bases

A substance that *donates* a proton/hydrogen ion (H^+) – e.g. lactic acid – is an acid; one that *accepts* a hydrogen ion – e.g. bicarbonate (HCO_3^-) – is a base The measure of acidity and alkalinity of a solution is the negative logarithm of its hydrogen ion concentration – its pH:

$$pH = -\log_{10}[H^+] \qquad (8.17)$$

The pH scale ranges between 0 and 14; pure water at 25 °C is neither acid nor alkaline: it is neutral with a pH of 7. Increasing the hydrogen ion concentration of a solution increases acidity; adding bicarbonate ions increases alkalinity. Solutions with a pH below 7 are acids; those above 7 are alkaline. Body fluids are all slightly alkaline – arterial blood for example is 7.4, whilst intra-cellular fluid is 7.0. However, because pH is temperature sensitive, at body temperature the neutral pH is slightly lower at 6.8.

Acids in the body arise from several sources: the breakdown of food into amino, fatty, and pyruvic acids; the combination of water and carbon dioxide – carbonic acid (H_2CO_3) and, as we have seen earlier in this chapter, the production of lactic acid during short-term high-intensity exercise. Indeed, the intra-muscular pH of the 400 m runner can get as low as 6.5 as the result of the acids generated by the need to maintain levels of nicotinamide adenine dinucleotide and adenosine triphosphate in muscle cells.

Task 9 Any theories on what you might do to minimize the drastic effects of lactic acid?

Let us look at the effect of this intra-muscular change in pH on skeletal muscle contraction. To do this we must begin by looking at the nature of skeletal muscle.

Structure and function of skeletal muscle

Skeletal muscle consists of overlapping thick (myosin) and thin (actin) protein filaments, giving fibres their striated (striped) appearance, embedded in sarcoplasm and constrained by a membrane called the sarcolemma. The entire unit is a sarcomere. Many sarcomeres linked together form myofibrils; these in turn go to make individual muscle fibres attached to bones via tendons.

Motor nerves are attached to muscle fibres by motor end-plates that allow nerve impulses, originating in the brain, to induce the voluntary muscle contractions needed to complete the 400 m. The nerve impulse, known as an action potential, disturbs the electro-chemical balance between intra- and extra-cellular fluids surrounding the muscle–nerve unit.

The impulse triggers the release of calcium from storage vessels (cisternae) in an enveloping sleeve of tubules called the sarcoplasmic reticulum. The calcium interacts with actin filaments to reveal binding sites. The protruding heads of the myosin filaments engage with the actin filaments and drag them rather like oars drag a boat through water. The actin filaments slide between the myosin filaments, thus shortening the sarcomere.

The hydrogen ions produced from the dissociation of lactic and other acids increase the acid environment of the muscle cell. Increased acidity adversely affects the functions of both key glycolytic enzymes and the proteins that make up the actin and myosin filaments. In addition, the hydrogen ions compete for the myosin binding sites on the actin filament, thereby inhibiting the ability of the myosin heads to deliver the power stroke that leads to contraction. Thus,

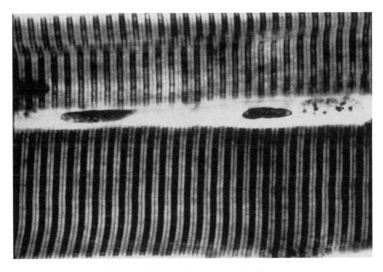

Figure 8.8 Striated muscle fibres

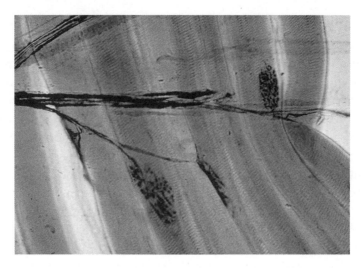

Figure 8.9   Section of a muscle fibre showing striations and multiple nuclei

the deceleration seen towards the end of the 400 m is a combination of a lack of cellular phosphocreatine, an excess of hydrogen ions and increasing levels of adenosine *di*phosphate. This combination results in the inability of some muscle fibres to deliver maximal force and leads inevitably to a loss of form and declining performance.

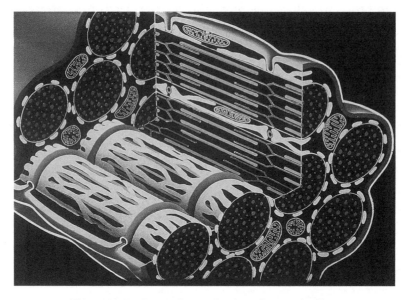

Figure 8.10   Internal organization of a muscle fibre

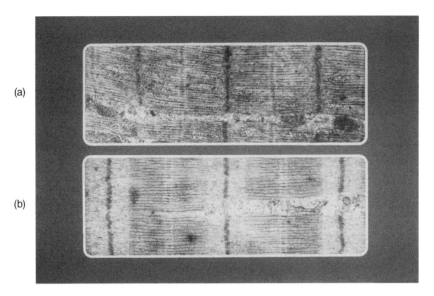

Figure 8.11 Sarcomere of a myofibril (a) contracted and (b) relaxed

The physiology of the 10 000 m

Thus far, we have concentrated on the anaerobic end of the track spectrum. As we move through the 800 m, 1500 m up to the 10 000 m and beyond, the ratio of anaerobic:aerobic metabolism changes from 9 : 1 for the shortest track event to about 0.3 : 9.7 for the longest track event, the 10 000 m. In the marathon (42 195 m), the ratio is 0.1 : 99.9. Each of these long distance events has different requirements. We rely on a preponderance of type I slow-twitch fibres, and slightly different energy providing mechanisms producing sufficient adenosine triphosphate to cope with average speeds of 6.3 m s^{-1} and 5.63 m s^{-1} for over 26 min and 2 h respectively.

> **Task 10** Draw a speed/distance graph of the typical 10 000 m event. Compare it with Figure 8.12.

Aerobic metabolism

Although the aerobic metabolic process is similar in 10 000 m and marathon, there is a significant difference in glycogen needs for the two races. Thus, although there is a considerable overlap we will deal with each event separately.

Men's 10 000 m Speed Profiles

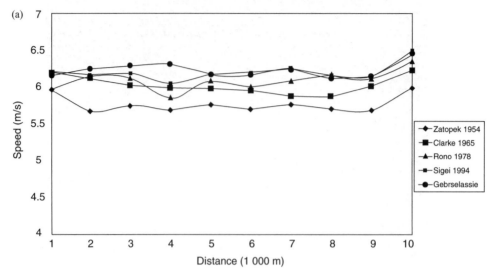

Women's 10 000 m Speed Profiles

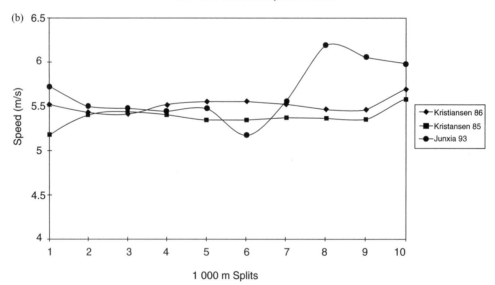

Figure 8.12 (a) Men's and (b) women's 10 000 m speed profiles (published with permission from IAAF)

We can use data (Table 8.2 and Figure 8.12) from 10 000 m performances by five men – Emile Zatopek (1954), Ron Clarke (1965), Henry Rono (1978), William Sigei (1994) and Haile Gebrselassie (1995) – and two women – Ingrid Kristiansen and Wang Junxia – to illustrate some underlying physiological mechanisms.

Table 8.2 1000 m split times for five 10 000 m world record holders from four decades and three continents (Hyman R. (2003) IAAF World Records with permission of the IAAF)

Distance (m)	1954 Zatopek (s)	1965 Clarke (s)	1978 Rono (s)	1994 Sigei (s)	1995 Gebrselassie (s)
1 000	167.8	161.5	167.5	161.34	162.3
2 000	176.4	163.5	162.7	162.40	160.0
3 000	174.0	166.0	163.4	161.67	158.9
4 000	175.8	167.0	171.0	165.15	158.2
5 000	173.6	167.0	164.4	162.15	162.0
6 000	175.4	168.0	166.7	161.37	161.9
7 000	173.4	170.0	164.3	159.68	159.9
8 000	175.2	170.0	162.1	162.19	163.0
9 000	175.8	166.0	163.4	162.51	162.6
10 000	166.8	160.4	156.9	153.77	154.8

In the case of Zatopek, Clarke and Kristiansen, we see a phenomenon known as 'steady-state running'. The strategy adopted is maintenance of an optimum running speed that was determined during training. Apart from the first and last kilometres, there is very little variation in the 1000 m (2½ lap) split times – 3 and 5 s km^{-1} for Kristiansen, 3 s km^{-1} for Zatopek and 4 s km^{-1} for Clark – for the majority of the race. There is a difference in tactics however. Figure 8.12(a) reveals Zatopek's famous surges, when he would inject a faster lap to test the resolve as well as the physiology of his rivals. Clark, on the other hand, conserves his energy during the middle of the run, and leaves his major surge until the last three kilometres, when he increases speed inexorably. His times fall by a full 10 s over the last 3 000 m. Kristiansen adopts slightly different tactics for her 1985 and 1986 record runs, but the faster speed over the majority of the run led to a lowering of her own world record by 45.68 s.

The three African runners, however, use much more disruptive tactics. Rono's opening kilometre – 167.5 s – is almost his slowest; but his second kilometre – 162.7 s – is his second fastest. Sowing confusion in the minds of his rivals, his 4000 m split of 171 s is the slowest kilometre, before injecting pace in progressive surges over the final 6 000 m. Sigei, who like Rono is a Kenyan, follows a similar pattern. Gebrselassie, the Ethiopian, sets out to destroy his rivals in the first 4000 m as his kilometre times fall progressively from 162.3 s to 158.2 s; a second surge occurs at 5000 m, with a final kilometre run in 154.8 s. However, Junxia produces a run that undermines the steady-state theory. Kilometre times over the run vary by 31.5 s. After a brisk start, kilometre times for the next 4000 m follow a typical steady-state approach. She runs the sixth stage in the slowest time, but follows this with two kilometres during which speed increases by an average of $1.1\,\mathrm{m\,s^{-1}}$, and lowers the previous record by 42 s.

Aerobic metabolism and steady-state running

To fuel steady-state running at this level the most important requirement is a plentiful supply of adenosine triphosphate. The mechanism responsible for such fuel production is a process known as aerobic metabolism. This process consists of three distinct phases – glycogenolysis, the Krebs cycle and the electron transfer chain.

Aerobic glycogenolysis

We have already dealt with the fundamentals of *anaerobic* glycogenolysis via the glycolytic pathway (Equations (8.4)–(8.13)). The start of the *aerobic* process follows the same pathway, but with two additional reactions that are essential for the long-term production of adenosine triphosphate. The two reactions occur because an adequate supply of oxygen is available – hence the term 'aerobic' (literally 'with air').

Task 11 Can you remember how many molecules of adenosine triphosphate have been produced via anaerobic glycogenolysis?

   The increased oxygen supply available for aerobic glycogenolysis is the result of several inter-connected physiological mechanisms. These include the following.

(a) Secretion of the hormone adrenaline that dilates airways in the lungs to assist in the ventilation of the blood; it also raises cardiac output via increased heart rate and stroke volume.
(b) Adrenaline, together with nor-adrenaline, the other sympathetic hormone, redistributes the total blood volume of the body – about 5 litres – *away* from resting tissues, by constricting their blood vessels, and *towards* the working muscles by dilating their blood vessels.
(c) This results in better perfusion of the muscle bed as more capillary blood vessels open.

(d) Changing conditions within the muscle cells brought about by exercise – increases in acidity, carbon dioxide production and temperature – release more oxygen from the blood that diffuses into the muscle cell.

We need to return now to the key reactions of Equation (8.9) above and the critical position of nicotinamide adenine dinucleotide (NAD^+) stores in the muscle cell.

$$G\text{-}3\text{-}P + NAD^+ + P_i \text{---} G\text{-}3\text{-}P \; dehydrogenase$$
$$\rightarrow 1, 3\text{-diphosphoglycerate} + NADH + H^+ \tag{8.18}$$

Task 12 Can you recall how NAD^+ stores are maintained during anaerobic exercise?

The Krebs or tricarboxylic acid (TCA) cycle

You will recall that if nicotinamide adenine dinucleotide levels fall too far, glycogenolysis ceases. Under aerobic conditions, the $NADH + H^+$ is oxidized through the removal of protons (H^+), via a process known as the electron transfer chain, that restores NAD^+ levels so that glycogenolysis can continue. The last reaction in the electron transfer chain requires an oxygen atom; this combines with two hydrogen atoms to give water. Without the presence of oxygen, this final combination cannot take place and nicotinamide adenine dinucleotide reverts to the anaerobic process described earlier. More importantly, the oxidation of reduced nicotinamide adenine dinucleotide via the electron transfer chain results in the production of *three* molecules of adenosine triphosphate to add to those already generated by the earlier reactions that have taken place.

Task 13 How many molecules of ATP have been generated by aerobic glycogenolysis?

The second reaction in the aerobic metabolic process deals with the fate of the pyruvate produced by glycolysis in the original Equation (13) above.

$$\text{phosphoenolpyruvate} + ADP \text{---} \textit{pyruvate phosphokinase} \rightarrow \text{pyruvate} + 2ATP \tag{8.19}$$

With adequate oxygen available, the pyruvate enters a cyclical process, known as the Krebs cycle in recognition of its discoverer Hans Krebs (also known as the citric acid or tricarboxylic acid (TCA) cycle). The pyruvate is broken down to carbon dioxide and water with the production of large amounts of adenosine triphosphate.

Step 1

The first step in the process is the removal of carbon dioxide (decarboxylation) from pyruvate together with its oxidation by the removal of hydrogen from nicotinamide adenine dinucleotide through a compound called *coenzyme A* (CoA).

$$\text{pyruvate} + \text{CoA} + \text{NAD}^+ \text{—}pyruvate\ dehydrogenase$$
$$\rightarrow \text{CO}_2 + \text{acetyl CoA} + \text{NADH} + \text{H}^+ \tag{8.20}$$

The removal of hydrogen takes place via the electron transfer chain and results in the production of *three* molecules of adenosine triphosphate from a single molecule of glycogen broken down during glycogenolysis.

Step 2

We now jump onto the Krebs roundabout. The acetyl CoA produced combines with the acid oxaloacetate to form citric acid.

$$\text{acetyl CoA} + \text{oxaloacetate} \text{—}citrate\ synthase \rightarrow \text{citrate} + \text{CoA} \tag{8.21}$$

The CoA is available to take part in continuous removal of carbon dioxide from pyruvate, whilst the citric acid is decarboxylated to α-ketoglutaric acid and carbon dioxide. During this reaction, hydrogen is again removed from nicotinamide adenine dinucleotide via the electron transfer chain, resulting in a *further* three molecules of adenosine triphosphate.

$$\text{citrate} + \text{NAD}^+ \text{—}aconitase \rightarrow \text{α-ketoglutarate} + \text{CO}_2 + \text{NADH} + \text{H}^+ \tag{8.22}$$

Step 4

A similar oxidative decarboxylation process takes α-ketoglutarate, coenzyme A and nicotinamide adenine dinucleotide to give succinyl CoA, carbon dioxide and three *more* molecules of adenosine triphosphate.

$$\text{α-ketoglutarate} + \text{CoA} + \text{NAD}^+ \text{—}\alpha\text{-}ketoglutarate\ dehydrogenase$$
$$\rightarrow \text{succinyl CoA} + \text{CO}_2 + \text{NADH} + \text{H}^+ \tag{8.23}$$

Task 14 *How many molecules of ATP have been produced by the TCA cycle up to this point?*

Step 5

The next step sees *one* further molecule of adenosine triphosphate produced by splitting succinyl CoA to give succinic acid. The energy released fires a reaction in which a compound found in the sarcoplasm of the muscle cell – guanosine diphosphate (GDP) – is phosporylated to guanosine triphosphate (GTP). The guanosine triphosphate interacts with adenosine diphosphate (ADP) to give adenosine triphosphate.

succinyl CoA + guanosine triphosphate + ADP—*succinyl CoA synthetase*

   → succinate + ATP   (8.24)

Step 6

Two *more* ATP molecules are provided at the next reaction, where succinate reacts with another adenine nucleotide – flavin – to produce fumaric acid and reduced flavin adenine dinucleotide.

succinate + flavin adenine dinucleotide—*succinate dehydrogenase*

   → fumarate + $FADH_2$ (8.25)

Step 7

The fumaric acid is hydrated to give malic acid.

$$\text{fumarate}—\textit{fumarase} \rightarrow \text{malate} \qquad\qquad (8.26)$$

Step 8

The malic acid is converted to oxaloacetic acid and reduced nicotinamide adenine dinucleotide, producing the final three molecules of adenosine triphosphate.

$$\text{malate} + NAD^+—\textit{fumarase} \rightarrow \text{oxaloacetate} + \text{NADH} + H^+ + \text{ATP} \quad (8.27)$$

The 'roundabout' has now completed one circuit, and is back at the start of the process, where oxaloacetic acid interacts with acetyl CoA to begin further production of adenosine triphosphate.

Task 15 *What is the total number of ATP molecules produced by one turn of the TCA cycle?*

The electron transfer chain (ETC)

We have mentioned the electron transfer chain on several occasions already. This is a critical process in aerobic metabolism. It is important for understanding the mechanisms that we recognize the three ways in which oxidation of substance A takes place. The first is obvious – we simply *transfer* oxygen from substance B to A.

$$A + BO_2 \rightarrow AO_2 + B \tag{8.28}$$

The other two ways are less obvious. One entails the *removal* of hydrogen (dehydrogenation) from A.

$$AH + B \rightarrow A + BH \tag{8.29}$$

The other involves the *removal* of a negatively charged sub-atomic particle, called an electron, from A.

$$A^{2+} \rightarrow A^{3+} + e^- \tag{8.30}$$

All three methods occur during aerobic metabolism. Many of the enzymes involved in removing hydrogen are *dehydrogenases*, and are included in the earlier equations. Splitting hydrogen into a proton (H^+) and an electron (e^-) and transferring the electrons during a reaction is the work of the electron transfer chain. Oxygen, acting as the final electron acceptor, is the final step in the aerobic process (Figure 8.13).

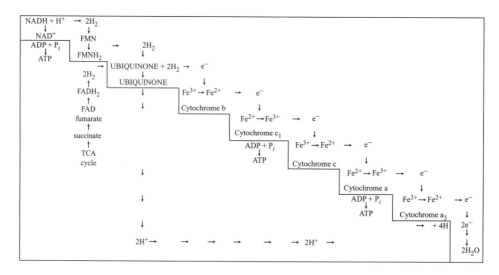

Figure 8.13   Energy source contribution for maximal work

Now we can calculate the total amount of adenosine triphosphate derived from the aerobic breakdown of glycogen. You will recall that, unless adequate oxygen is available, there is a net gain of only three molecules arising from the reactions leading to pyruvic acid. We *consume* adenosine triphosphate in Equation (8.6), but in Equations (8.7a) and (8.7b) one molecule of glucose-6-phosphate is split into two parallel pathways, each *producing* two molecules of adenosine triphosphate at Equations (8.10) and (8.13). The net gain, therefore, is three molecules. We describe this rapid process as *substrate* phosphorylation.

However, in Equation (8.9), the two parallel pathways produce two molecules of nicotinamide adenine dinucleotide. Both are oxidized by the three-stage process of removing hydrogen, transferring electrons and adding oxygen. Each NAD^+ molecule provides *three* molecules of adenosine triphosphate. The total for aerobic *glycogenolysis* therefore is *nine* molecules of adenosine triphosphate per molecule of glycogen. We call this much slower process *oxidative* phosphorylation. The total produced by each turn of the Krebs roundabout, or tricarboxylic acid cycle is *15* molecules of adenosine triphosphate; because of the parallel pathways, there are two simultaneous turns of the cycle, giving *30* molecules. Adding the products of aerobic *glycogenolysis* and the TCA cycle gives us *39* molecules of adenosine triphosphate for each molecule of glycogen.

However, it is worth noting that there is some debate about the actual number of adenosine triphosphate molecules generated via aerobic metabolism. Experimental investigations have only produced 30 molecules, not the 39 calculated from the glycogenolytic pathway and the Krebs cycle. This debate should not detract from the major point, which is that aerobic metabolism provides much greater quantities of the essential fuel for muscle contraction, and without the TCA cycle and electron transfer chain 10 000 m running would look very different from the data we saw earlier.

The physiology of the marathon

The men's current best – 2 h 4 min 55 s – was set by the Kenyan Paul Tergat in 2003, at an average speed of $5.63 \, m \, s^{-1}$. The current women's best, set also in 2003 by Paula Radcliffe, is 2 h 15 min 25 s – an average speed of $5.39 \, m \, s^{-1}$. Typical oxygen uptakes (V_{O2}) throughout the race are ~ 4.5 and $4.0 \, L \, min^{-1}$ respectively.

Figure 8.14 is a typical time profile for elite male and female marathon athletes showing the 5 km split times. The most notable difference between the

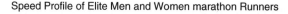

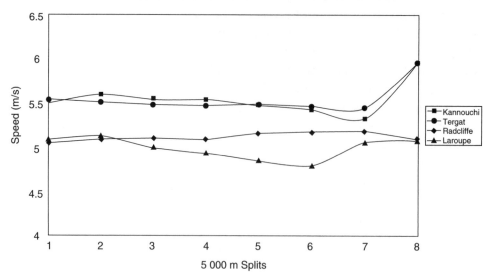

Figure 8.14 Speed profiles of elite men and women marathon runners (published with permission from IAAF)

two is the range between the fastest and slowest 5 km times. For the male athlete it is only 11 s (14 min 58 s–15 min 9 s); this is a good example of steady-state running, even though there are still indications of small but regular surges in running speed. The range of the female athlete is 22 s (16 min 5 s–16 min 27 s).

The intensity of the exercise determines the fuel used. The phosphagen and lactate mechanisms will certainly have made some contribution at the very earliest stages of the race – the first lap around the stadium, or the dash to secure a good position in the massed-start events – but aerobic metabolism is the predominant mechanism in this race. Thus, all of the physiological mechanisms described for the 10 000 m runner apply to the marathon runner, but there are two additional, equally important, physiological demands arising from competing over a total distance of 42 195 m. First, there is a question about the fuel source used to produce adenosine triphosphate – i.e. is it carbohydrate or fat? Second, there are the inter-linked problems of temperature regulation and dehydration. The former problem is ever present, but the latter is environment dependent. Running the London Marathon on a cool, dry spring morning is less environmentally stressful than the same distance in hot, humid conditions.

Sources of fuel

The total energy requirement of steady-state marathon running amounts to ~12 000 kJ (almost 3000 kcal). At the intensities seen in an event such as marathon running – i.e. ~80 per cent of maximal oxygen uptake, carbohydrate, in the form of glycogen and glucose, is the *preferred* fuel. Although less energy dense than fat, carbohydrates are more readily available to the exercising muscle.

> **Task 16** *What do you think might happen when muscle glycogen stores are virtually exhausted?*

The major storage areas for glycogen are the liver – about 75–100 g – and skeletal muscle – 300–400 g. The blood holds about 10 g of glucose. We have known for over 70 years that in untrained individuals typical muscle glycogen stores can only support ~70 ± 10 min of continuous strenuous exercise, and that such demanding exercise is accompanied by progressive depletion of muscle glycogen stores. When glycogen is no longer available, we have to switch to fat (lipids) as the main source of fuel for adenosine triphosphate production. Recreational runners often reach this switching-point about three quarters of the way (~30 km/18 miles) around the course; they call it 'hitting the wall'. The speed drops to a slow jog, and the last quarter of the race can take as long, if not longer, than the previous three quarters.

Fat is an efficient means of storing energy, and provides the life support mechanism for over-wintering hibernating animals. We store lipids in the plasma, skeletal muscle and fat cells. The lower the exercise intensity and the longer its duration the more we depend on the oxidation of free fatty acids to deliver adenosine triphosphate to support whatever activity we are undertaking. It is the fuel used for everyday activities such as housework, gardening, walking and jogging.

Lipids have a much higher calorific value (39 kJ – 9.3 kcal g^{-1}) than carbohydrates (17 kJ – 4.1 kcal g^{-1}). The total energy of stored fat is roughly equivalent to 314 000 kJ (75 000 kcal) compared to the 8 300 kJ (2 000 kcal) available from stored glycogen. Lipid breakdown also produces more than three times the amount of adenosine triphosphate per molecule of fatty acid –130 molecules compared to the 39 molecules derived from a molecule of glycogen; we can see how in the following equations for glycogen and palmitic acid:

$$C_6H_{12}O_6 + 6O_2 + 39ADP + 39P_i = 6CO_2 + 6H_2O + 39\underline{ATP} \tag{8.31}$$

$$C_{16}H_{32}O_2 + 23O_2 + 130ADP + 130P_i = 16CO_2 + 16H_2O + 130\underline{ATP} \tag{8.32}$$

Task 17 *Can you see in these two equations why recreational runners 'hit the wall' during their marathon run?*

The kind of lipid that provides the energy – triacylglycerol – consists of three free fatty acid molecules attached to one of glycerol. The oxidation of free fatty acids is a three-stage process. The first is lipolysis – the breakdown of triacylglycerol into free fatty acids and glycerol assisted by enzymes called *lipases*. The second stage – β-oxidation – is the breakdown of free fatty acids in the mitochondria of the muscle cells. This entails the stripping of pairs of carbon atoms from fatty acids – palmitic (seen in Equation (8.32) above), stearic or oleic acids are the most common types – and attaching the carbon to coenzyme A to give acetyl coenzyme A (acetyl CoA). The third stage involves acetyl CoA entering the Krebs cycle and the electron transfer chain and the production of the substantial number of adenosine triphosphate molecules shown in Equation (8.32).

Task 18 *Where have we met acetyl CoA before?*

Although fat provides the major source of energy for low intensity activities, it has considerable disadvantages for the marathon runner. Two things are clear from the above equations. First, free fatty acids are more complicated compounds than glycogen. They contain more carbon (16–18), hydrogen (32–36) and fewer oxygen (2) atoms than the 6 carbon, 12 hydrogen and 6 oxygen atoms found in glycogen, and require more reactions to produce adenosine triphosphate. Second, we need considerably more oxygen to break down free fatty acids than we do to break down glycogen. Herein lies the problem.

At elite level, we are running at our maximum steady state lactate level (MSSL) – i.e. about 80 per cent of our maximal oxygen uptake. Any increase in adenosine triphosphate demand is likely to push us over the threshold into non-steady-state lactate production, and thus hydrogen ion accumulation, with the inevitable consequence of impaired performance. 'Hitting the wall' is a clear sign of glycogen depletion; slower running speed is the only option if we are to complete the race. This strategy reduces adenosine triphosphate requirements, and allows oxygen supply to match the increased demands of fat metabolism. It also loses you the race!

Non-running sports

The processes outlined for the four track events provide the key concepts that underpin the energy requirements for many sports and cardio-vascular fitness programmes. Some sports, however, require no running at all – e.g. canoeing, cycling, rowing and swimming. Most of these sports are directly comparable to the track events just described for two reasons. First, they have similar competitive structures to athletics, namely a range of distances from the phosphagen/anaerobic driven sprints, through the aerobic/anaerobic middle- and long-distance events, to the 24 h Devizes to London canoe race, and the 21 day Tour de France. Second, the physical effort demanded is largely steady-state energy production. Thus, as far as energy sources are concerned, the nature and relative contribution of those sources to events of varying durations, can be one of the starting points for the preparation of general physical conditioning programmes in many sports.

Activities other than steady-state running

However, few sports require uncomplicated, 'steady-state' running. Think about the demands of middle-distance running compared with repeated-effort sports such as boxing, gymnastics, judo and table tennis. Do the same for the marathon and sports lasting between one and three hours – e.g. basketball, football, hockey, tennis, baseball, cricket and single-handed dinghy sailing. What are the requirements for events that last for most of the day – e.g. cricket and rock climbing, or even weeks – e.g. round the world sailing and the Tour de France? Finally, we come to the sports where strenuous physical activity is negligible – e.g. darts, golf and snooker, but where, for the elite player, the crucial attributes are very precise skills and sustained concentration over several days.

***Task 19** Using the following headings, make a guess at the relative contributions of each energy source to all of the sports listed in the previous paragraph, e.g.*

Sport	Phosphagen cycle	Anaerobic glycogenesis	Aerobic glyco-genolysis	Lipolysis
Outfield football	40%	20%	37.5%	2.5%
Amateur boxing				
Judo				
Gymnastics				
Basketball				
Dinghy sailing				
Field hockey				
Rugby				
Cricket – bowling				
Cricket – fielding				
Cricket – batting				
Tour de France				
Snooker				
Darts				

Training programmes need to reflect the physiological demands of particular sports. However, our inherited physiological make-up varies between individuals. Each of us will have strengths and weaknesses. We can modify some of these by appropriate training, but this is not always the case. The next chapter explores some physiological factors that limit performance.

Practical implications

Just as in Part III we demonstrated the need to analyse skill, so the evidence of the theory and research covered in this chapter shows that we must also examine the nature of the physiological factors involved in performance in some detail. It is not good enough to say that an athlete runs 200 m or 400 m or 1500 m; we need to know the energy systems that he/she will be using. This is fairly simple for the 100 m runners, who use the phosphagen system. However, even for them we must not forget the need for a quick responses at the start and the differing biomechanical principles for running over the first few metres compared with those needed in the rest of the race. Once we step up from 100 m, however, the problems become more complex. Running the 400 m requires the use of the phosphagen system early in the race but soon it depends on anaerobic glycolysis. The 800 m and 1500 m require the use of the aerobic system as well as the anaerobic glycolytic system. Moreover, each athlete differs in the way he/she runs these races. When exactly do they make a burst that results in their changing from the aerobic pathway into the anaerobic glycolytic? So we must examine what *our* athlete does, not what we generalize from exercise physiology texts.

The problem of which energy systems are used, and when, is difficult enough in track athletics, but in team games it becomes very difficult indeed. As we saw in Part III, time and motion analysis is very useful. We can make certain generalizations with regard to the speed and length of run to decide whether it will draw mostly on the phosphagen, anaerobic or aerobic systems. However, one must be careful with this. If someone makes several short sprints, each of which would draw on the phosphagen system, but there is little time for recovery in between sprints, they will begin to use the anaerobic glycolytic pathway. Moreover, the need in team games to recover quickly in between short bursts requires oxygen, hence the aerobic system is important for repeated short high intensity sprinting.

Task 20 Which energy systems do you think that most midfield players in hockey or football would use?

I have asked the question in Task 20 because it highlights the danger of coaches generalizing from data given in exercise physiology texts and coaching manuals. Most people would probably say the aerobic system and in general they are correct. However, I recently watched a ladies hockey game in which the midfield players played very different types of game. One of them played a defensive role and made only short sprints (phosphagen system) and a lot of low intensity running (aerobic glycolysis). Another player made many comparatively long runs into the opposition D and equally many high intensity recovery runs. These runs would have taxed her anaerobic glycolytic system as well as her aerobic system. So do we train both of these ladies in the same way? The answer is, of course, no, but how many teams do you know that differentiate between player types and training schedules? It is only fairly recent that football goal-keepers have received separate training from the outfield players.

Once we have decided which energy system our athletes need to work on we must then devise the training schedules. Schedules are covered in Chapter 10, but here we will look at ways of training each system in a single training session.

Task 21 *How do you think we would train each system?*

The phosphagen system lasts for only a very small time period, between 10 and 30 s, although the latter probably only applies to well trained athletes. Therefore, training this system requires short, sharp, high intensity bursts of activity. For track athletes, say 100 m runners, the gaps in between trials would be fairly long. The actual time would depend on how far they had run. We would be looking for full replenishment of ATP by phosphorylation. However, for team game players we might have less of a gap as they will not always have the luxury of comparatively long inactive periods between sprints. A common practice for team game players is to run 30 s sprints followed by 30 s rest. In fact, it cold be argued that this is actually training the role of the aerobic system in aiding recovery more than the phosphagen system itself. Nevertheless, there is some evidence to say that such training lengthens the time for which the individual can draw on the phosphagen system.

The anaerobic glycolytic system can maintain high intensity work for ~90 s. Therefore, training should be based around runs of that time period. Again the rest period in between runs will depend on the type of activity in which the person is involved. 400 m runners can have long rest periods while team game players need less time, although it should be remembered that most team game players rarely use 90 +s high intensity runs in a game. In games such as basketball, this will almost never happen, so the amount of time spent on such training needs to be carefully scheduled. Our attack minded midfield hockey player, above, may well need far more anaerobic training than her more defensive team-mate.

All activities require an aerobic base, so training the aerobic system is important. Steady-state running for fairly long periods >30 min appears to be best for track athletes. Indeed, we would expect them to be running for >1 hour. For middle and long distance runners 1 hour would be insufficient. For many team game players, however, this is tantamount to punishment that would be more in place in the middle ages. Imagine the rugby prop going on a 1 hour cross-country run. This problem can be overcome by the use of *interval training*. Although the most common form of interval training is the 30 s sprint followed by 30 s rest, repeated several times, which works the phosphagen and aerobic systems (see above), it can be used for aerobic training. Runs of ≥5 min (preferably longer) at a steady, sub-maximal intensity can be interspersed with rests of about the same time length. As we will see in Part VI, these can be part of technical training and so sugar the pill of long distance running even more.

Nutrition

The fact that we use glycogen and fat as the fuel bases of our energy systems means that we must be careful with our diets. This is, of course, more the case with athletes. The need to 're-fuel' properly is very important. As we have seen, for most athletic performances carbohydrate is more important than fat. Possibly very long distance low intensity swims, such as across the Channel, will draw more heavily on lipolysis, but otherwise carbohydrate is the main food source, so athletes' diets need to be high in carbohydrate. We must not forget proteins, however, as these are needed to help repair the wear and tear of training. Muscle damage requires proteins if it is to recover.

Although most professional athletes know the importance of a good diet, they do not always follow it. Even some athletes in sports such as boxing and wrestling, which require meeting weight demands, eat the wrong kinds of food. The eating of diets high in fat should be avoided. However, athletes under-taking heavy training can probably eat more fat than the average person. It is, however, more important to eat food high in carbohydrates, as this is what has been depleted in training and competition. The sub-cultures of many sports cause problems for coaches trying to get athletes to eat a healthy diet. Until very recently many football mangers had their players eat beef about 2 hours before a game. Beef cannot be fully digested in this time. They would be far better eating pasta. Immediately after a game, we need not only to re-fuel but to re-hydrate. In rugby and other team games a few (well several) beers after a game is the norm. While beer is high in carbohydrate it can make dehydration worse rather than better. The sports nutritionist Ron Maughan told me that he tells Rugby players to drink a few shandies (half lemonade and half beer) before starting on the beer. The lemonade guards against dehydration while the beer provides the carbohydrates. He also advises that they have a meal high in carbohydrate as well. Ron admits, however, that some rugby players will not drink shandy because 'it is not a man's drink'. These attitudes are gradually changing but coaches should be aware of them.

Key points

- carbohydrates are the main source of energy for sprinters

- carbohydrates are stored in long chains of glucose molecules called glycogen

- adenosine triphosphate (ATP) drives all cellular activity

- ATP is made up of ribose (a sugar), adenosine (linked rings of carbon and nitrogen atoms), triphosphate (three phosphate bonds)

- energy is produced when one of the phosphate bonds splits off, producing adenosine diphosphate (ADP)
- energy in sprinting is supplied by two anaerobic systems – the phosphagen system and glycogenolysis

- the phosphagen cycle involves the interaction between ATP, phosphocreatine (PCr) and water
  - ♦ this process is termed hydrolysis
  - ♦ hydrolysis results in the formation of ADP and inorganic phosphate (P_i) and requires the presence of actinomysinATPase (see Equation (8.1))

- the restoration of ATP is by the process of phosphorylation
  - ♦ this requires the presence of the enzyme creatine kinase (see Equations (8.2) and (8.3))

- when PCr stores breakdown energy is produced by glycogenolysis
  - ♦ glycogenolysis does not require oxygen

♦ it can operate for ~90 s

- this takes place in the cytoplasm of the cell (called sarcoplasm in muscle cells)
  ♦ it is a watery, gel-like substance bound by the cell membrane (or sarcoplasm)

- the glycolytic pathway can be broken down into 10 steps and requires the presence of several enzymes (see Equations (8.4)–(8.16))
  ♦ this process results in increased acidity in the muscle
  ♦ the acids break down into hydrogen ions (H^+) and salts
  ♦ increased H+ results in acidosis, which negatively affects muscle contraction
  ♦ a substance that donates a H^+ is an acid
  ♦ a substance that accepts a H^+ is a base
  ♦ the measures of acidity and alkalinity are shown in Equation (8.17)
  ♦ hydrogen ion concentration is measured by pH

- acids in the body come from several sources
  ♦ breakdown of food into amino, fatty and pyruvic acids
  ♦ the combination of water and carbon dioxide (carbonic acid [H_2CO_3])

- production of lactic acid in the glycolytic pathway (see Equation (8.15))

- skeletal muscle consists of overlapping thick (myosin) and thin (actin) protein filaments
  ♦ the fibres are said to be striated (striped)
  ♦ they are embedded in the sarcoplasm and constrained by the sarcolemma
  ♦ together these are called sarcomeres
  ♦ many sarcomeres form myofibrils
  ♦ many myofibrils form muscle fibres

- motor nerves are attached to fibres by motor endplates
  ♦ neural messages from the brain via the motor nerves energize the muscle
  ♦ nerve impulses are called action potentials (see Figures 8.9, 8.10 and 8.11)

- steady-state running is fuelled by the aerobic system
  ♦ the aerobic system consist of three stages – glycogenolysis, the Krebs cycle and the electron transfer chain

- increased oxygen supply is available due to

♦ the action of adrenaline (dilates airways and increases cardiac output)
♦ adrenaline and nor-adrenaline redistributing blood away from resting tissue to working muscles
♦ increased acidity, carbon dioxide production and temperature in muscle cells releases more oxygen into the blood

- the beginning stages of the aerobic system are as for the glycolytic pathway up to Equation (8.9), but with oxygen available
  ♦ nicotinamide adenine dinucleotide (NADH) $+ H^+$ is oxidized by the removal of H^+ protons – known as the electron transfer chain (see Equations (8.28)–(8.30) and Figure 8.13)
  ♦ NAD^+ is restored so glycogenolysis can continue
  ♦ pyruvic acid enters the Krebs cycle (see Equation (8.19))

- there are eight steps to the Krebs cycle (see Equations (8.20)–(8.27))

- aerobic metabolism produces much more ATP than the other systems

Sources of fuel

- carbohydrate, in the form of glycogen and glucose, is the main source during exercise
  ♦ glycogen is stored in the liver and skeletal muscle

- when glycogen is no longer available we use fat (lipids)
  ♦ fat is stored in plasma, skeletal muscle and fat cells
  ♦ fat produces more energy than carbohydrate but the mechanism is slow (see Equations (8.31)–(8.32))

- triacylglycerol is the main fat providing energy
  ♦ it consists of three molecules of free fatty acid and one of glycerol
  ♦ it is broken down in three stages:
  ♦ breakdown of triacylglycerol into free fatty acids and glycerol assisted by the enzyme lipase – the process is called lipolysis
  ♦ breakdown of free fatty acids in the mitochondria, called β-oxidation (see Equation (8.28))
  ♦ this produces acetyl coenzyme A (acetyl CoA)
  ♦ acetyl CoA enters the Krebs cycle.

9

Factors that Limit Performance

Learning objectives

By the end of this chapter you should be able to

- describe a range of key factors that limit human sporting performance
- name the three muscle fibre types and list their structural and physiological characteristics
- link these characteristics to sports performances and discuss the effects of training on each type
- outline the physiological mechanisms underpinning maximal oxygen uptake, and indicate the physiological characteristics that distinguish elite athletes from untrained subjects
- explain the relationship between glycogen and long-term sports performance and the strategy of carbohydrate loading
- outline the effects of heat stress, explain the conflict between oxygen delivery to skeletal muscle and temperature regulation and discuss strategies that reduce the chances of temperature regulation failure
- describe the factors limiting anaerobic performance, and discuss the pros and cons of creatine supplementation and bicarbonate loading
- outline the links between strength, power and flexibility
- define the 'all-or-none' law, and discuss the mechanisms by which skeletal muscles produce force

---

Coaching Science   Terry McMorris and Tudor Hale
© 2006 John Wiley & Sons, Ltd

- explain the relationship between force and velocity of muscle fibre contraction
- discuss the importance of neuro-muscular facilitation to maximal strength production
- explain the role and mechanisms of proprioception in force production
- define flexibility, summarize the morphological factors limiting joint flexibility and discuss the merits of various stretching methods.

The factors that limit human performance encompass biochemistry, biomechanics, meteorology and the physical environment, physiology, psychology, social environment, strategy and tactics, and travel. Even physiological factors cover a substantial list of subjects – genetics, aerobic and anaerobic power and capacity, speed, strength and mechanical power, flexibility, diet, dehydration and heat stress. In dealing with these topics, it seems sensible to follow the pattern laid down in the previous chapter in using selected athletic track events to link physiological theory to sporting practice.

Given the variability of performances shown in the velocity–time graphs of all the events, the first, and probably most important, limiting factor, and the one we can legally affect least, is our genetic make-up. Coaching and training can refine and enhance what is already there, but the genes we inherit from our ancestors play a large part in the kinds of activity at which we excel, and in elite level track events determine whether we are going to be a sprinter, middle distance or marathon runner.

A major attribute passed down from our evolutionary past is the composition of the muscle fibres we inherit. In environments more hostile than those that exist now, the ability to out-sprint our main predator was a key factor in our survival. If we survived, we passed the appropriate genes to our offspring, which helped them and their descendants to survive. In this instance, it was a case of the survival of the *fastest*.

Another survival attribute was endurance. Primitive hunters shot their prey with curare tipped arrows, and jogged after the beast until progressive muscle paralysis, induced by the curare, finally allowed the hunter to catch up with and kill the prey. In this instance, it was a case of the survival of the most *durable* (and possibly skilful) cross-country archer.

Muscle fibre types

The two kinds of muscle fibres we inherit – fast-twitch and slow-twitch fibres – reflect the two running attributes seen in the two previous paragraphs.

We can divide the fast-twitch type into two sub-groups – fast glycolytic (type IIb) and fast oxidative (type IIa). We all have both the slow-twitch and the two kinds of fast-twitch type in our make up, but the proportions of each vary between individuals. All three types of fibre contain very important organelles called mitochondria (singular – mitochondrion); these act as the power stations for all of our cellular activity including the muscle cells. Although all three types are activated during an all-out effort such as the 100 m, the type we are especially interested in here is fast-twitch glycolytic fibres.

100 m

These fast-twitch glycolytic fibres, usually abbreviated to (FG), are the palest of the three types because they lack myoglobin (Mgb), an important oxygen-binding molecule that gives muscle its red colour. They are also the thickest fibres and generate the highest power output – about three times that produced by the slow-twitch type – an important factor in a 100 m sprint. Large motor nerves (neurons) innervate the fibres, inducing contraction and relaxation roughly twice as fast as slow-twitch fibres.

The muscle cells contain important materials that are more plentiful than in the slow-twitch type. Among these are the substrates fuelling the contractions – adenosine triphosphate, glycogen and, crucially, phosphocreatine. The major glycolytic enzymes that drive the chemical changes – phosphofructokinase and phosphorylase – are also more plentiful and active in fast-twitch muscle. Endurance capacity is low, so the fast-twitch fibre type fatigues quickly, an effect detectable in the speed profiles seen earlier in Chapter 8 (Figures 8.3, 8.7, 8.12(a) and (b) and 8.14).

400 m

The 400 m runners, like the short-sprint athletes, have a high proportion of type IIb FG-fibres. However, the longer event introduces the other type II muscle fibre – type IIa or fast oxidative glycolytic type (FOG). This muscle fibre type is capable of using both anaerobic and aerobic mechanisms to produce adenosine triphosphate. The two major characteristics of this form of fast-twitch fibre are their resistance to fatigue and their high power output. They share large motor neurons, high glycogen and phosphocreatine content and increased glycolytic enzyme activity with their fast glycolytic fibre cousins, but are red, reflecting increased myoglobin, and therefore muscle oxygen content, and are capable of both high glycolytic and high oxidative enzyme activity.

Long-distance events

The typical long-distance runner's major muscle fibre type – type I, slow oxidative (SO) – is the complete opposite of the type II fibres seen in 100 m and 400 m runners. Both type II fibres will be present, but the overwhelming characteristic of 10 000 m and marathon runners is the proportion – approaching 80 per cent - of type I fibres. Their red colour arises from the presence of large quantities of stored myoglobin. These are the thinnest of the three types, contract relatively slowly, generate relatively low forces and hold the lowest glycogen but highest fat (triglyceride) content of all of the fibre types. The capillary density and mitochondrial content are high; these ensure a plentiful blood – and therefore oxygen – supply, and greater oxidative enzyme activity. The outcome is a fibre type that has a high oxidative capacity and is highly resistant to fatigue.

Maximal oxygen uptake and long-distance running

Without oxygen, human life as we know it would not exist. The gas is the essential requirement for all of our cellular activity. Although we use little of it during the 100 m, we use it post-race to re-synthesize phosphocreatine. In the 400 m, we use it not only during the race but also to convert lactic acid to glycogen in post-race recovery. For the 10 000 m and the marathon, oxygen is vital for releasing the large amounts of energy needed to complete these events. We now turn to consider the factors that limit maximal oxygen uptake.

   The maximal rate at which we can consume oxygen ($V_{O2 max}$) is the outcome of a chain of physiological mechanisms linking the delivery of atmospheric oxygen to skeletal muscle contraction. The oxygen transport chain consists of four main elements – lung ventilation, oxygen carriage by the blood, oxygen delivery by the heart and oxygen uptake by the tissues. Within these, there are sub-divisions. Lung ventilation entails transport of inspired air down the airways to the respiratory bronchioles and diffusion down the alveolus and across the alveolar–capillary membrane into the blood. Oxygen carriage in the blood depends on the number of oxygen carrying red blood cells available, and the speed of these cells through the pulmonary circulation. Oxygen delivery – i.e. cardiac output – is the outcome of the strength of the heart muscle and the rate at which it beats. Oxygen uptake by the skeletal muscle is a function of the number of open capillaries, the speed of the red cells through the capillary bed, the number of mitochondria and the rate at which biochemical reactions occur within the sarcoplasm and mitochondria of individual muscle fibres.

A chain is only as strong as its weakest link, and the issue of which physiological mechanism is the weakest continues to exercise the minds of sport and exercise scientists. Healthy people easily meet the resting oxygen demands. The difference between trained and untrained adults occurs when we undertake more than two to three minutes of strenuous aerobic exercise.

In most athletes, each link is much stronger than that of the untrained individual. This is especially true of endurance athletes – e.g. 800–42 190 m runners, all cyclists save the sprinters, invasion and net game players, swimmers and rowers. We can see this when comparing the Fick equation for oxygen in two groups – trained endurance athletes and untrained individuals of similar age and size. The equation is

$$V_{O2\,max} = Q_{C\,max} \cdot C_{a-v\,O2\,max}$$

It says that maximal oxygen uptake ($V_{O2\,max}$, L min^{-1}) is the product of maximum cardiac output ($Q_{C\,max}$, L min^{-1}) – itself the product of heart rate ($f_{C\,max}$, beats min^{-1}) and stroke volume ($V_{S\,max}$, mL beat^{-1}) – and the maximum difference in the oxygen content (C_{O2}) of arterial (a) and mixed venous (v) blood ($C_{a-v\,O2\,max}$, mL L^{-1}). Typical data for the two groups look like this:

$$V_{O2\,max}\,(\text{L min}^{-1}) = Q_{C\,max}\,(\text{L min}^{-1}) \times C_{a-v\,O2\,max}\,(\text{mL L}^{-1})$$

Untrained

$$3.50 = 25 \times 14$$

$$(200\ \text{beat min}^{-1} \times 125\,\text{mL L}^{-1})$$

Trained

$$6.40 = 40 \times 16$$

$$(200\ \text{beat min}^{-1} \times 200\,\text{mL L}^{-1})$$

In the healthy untrained individual, the major difference is a significantly lower cardiac output, resulting from a 37 per cent reduction in stroke volume; a secondary feature is a 5 per cent lower oxygen extraction by the muscles. This is the model currently favoured by many in the sports science community.

However, Table 9.1 reveals that, even within a small group of elite endurance athletes, the ways in which individuals reach their maximal oxygen

Table 9.1   Maximal values of oxygen uptake, cardiac output and peripheral oxygen extraction of eight Swedish elite endurance athletes, showing the varying relationships between the three factors (adapted from Ekblom and Hermansen, 1968)

Subject	$V_{O_2\,max}$ $L\,min^{-1}$	Q_{max} $L\,min^{-1}$	$C_{a-v\,O_2}$ $mL\,L^{-1}$
1	5.122	31.5	163
2	5.776	37.8	153
3	4.661	27.8	168
4	5.604	34.4	163
5	5.503	36.2	152
6	5.645	38.1	148
7	6.007	39.8	151
8	6.248	42.3	148

uptake levels differ. Some have very high cardiac output with relatively low peripheral oxygen extraction, some have the opposite, whilst a third group lies somewhere in between. Thus, the actual picture is rather more complex – too complex to cover in detail here (for a more detailed review of this topic see Hale, 2003).

However, we can highlight the potential weaknesses at each stage of the oxygen cascade from atmosphere to muscle cell as follows: maximal oxygen uptake will be impaired if there is any impediment to

(a) gas transport through the lungs – e.g. asthma, longer diffusing time across the alveolar–capillary membrane – e.g. pulmonary oedema,

(b) oxygen uptake by the pulmonary blood – e.g. low red cell count, low haemoglobin levels, too fast red cell transit time through the pulmonary capillaries,

(c) oxygen delivery via the heart and circulatory system – e.g. low blood volume, low cardiac output – via low maximum heart rate and low stroke volume, singularly or in combination, poor blood perfusion of the skeletal muscle capillary bed, inadequate venous return or

(d) oxygen extraction by skeletal muscle – e.g. low capillary density, too rapid red cell transit time through the capillaries, low mitochondrial content, low oxidative enzyme activity, low 2,3-diphosphoglycerate content of red blood cells.

Endurance training focuses on legally maximizing the effectiveness of each of these links in the oxygen uptake chain. Methods that increase the oxygen carrying capacity of the blood, such as blood doping and the use of synthetic erythropoietin (EPO), are illegal. However, there is some evidence that *moderate* caffeine ingestion, which is legal, 60 min prior to exercise increases endurance. Field trials are scarce, and the proposed mechanism underpinning the greater endurance – i.e. increased free fatty-acid mobilization leading to glycogen sparing – has not been confirmed.

Glycogen depletion

Any event involving continuous strenuous exercise for more than 75–90 min – the marathon, invasion games such as football, rugby and hockey – may run into limitations in glycogen availability. Fortunately, we can manipulate glycogen stores before, during and after exercise by various dietary and supplemental strategies. A high carbohydrate diet ingested for the 2–3 days *before* an event – carbohydrate loading – optimizes liver and muscle glycogen stores and leads to improved endurance performance. Carbohydrate drinks taken *during* an event maintain blood glucose levels and reduce demands on muscle glycogen stores. High carbohydrate intakes immediately *after* an exhausting event or training schedule not only restore muscle glycogen to their original levels but can double or triple them. These strategies are essential for marathon runners and commonplace among endurance athletes of all kinds, including repeated-effort sports such as football and rugby. It is important for successful coaching that we understand the physiological basis for these strategies.

Figure 8.12 suggests that 'hitting the wall' is not the pattern seen in elite marathon runners, and the explanation lies in the combination of dietary manipulation and the training they undertake. Aerobic training increases endurance capacity through changes in muscle anatomy and biochemistry. Type I (slow-twitch oxidative) fibres may hypertrophy (become thicker); but more importantly, the size and number of mitochondria found in the fibres – the organelle where the key reactions of the Krebs cycle and electron transfer chain take place – increase, thereby enhancing oxidative phosphorylation. Some type IIa (fast-twitch oxidative) fibres seem to take on more of the attributes of type I muscle fibres and enhance oxidative phosphorylation without losing their ability to generate force quickly. The blood supply to the muscle fibre improves through increases in the capillary density of the fibres, thus enhancing oxygen delivery. Oxy-myoglobin ($MgbO_2$) stores increase, providing a useful additional oxygen reservoir. Glycogen stores, accompanied by appropriate dietary regimes, also increase. Intra-muscular free fatty acid stores also develop; this leads to enhanced utilization of fat as a fuel source, and to the sparing of glycogen catabolism. With these attributes, the elite marathon runner is capable of maintaining an average speed of more than $5 \, \text{m} \, \text{s}^{-1}$ for the entire race.

Heat stress and dehydration

The marathon, however, imposes demands other than simply the availability of appropriate fuel sources. The linked problems of body temperature control and dehydration can provide the final straw that impairs some marathon runners' performances. The exercising human does not transfer energy into actual work very efficiently; most of the work done by exercising muscle (70–80 per cent) merely produces heat. Because we only function optimally within a relatively narrow core temperature band – $37 \pm 1 \, ^\circ\text{C}$ – we have developed survival mechanisms to deal with conditions lying outside this range. At rest, providing we are not suffering from a fever or hypothermia, we maintain core temperature at about $37 \, ^\circ\text{C}$. Marathon running results in increased heat production of about $60 \, \text{kJ} \cdot \text{min}^{-1}$ ($14.5 \, \text{kcal} \cdot \text{min}^{-1}$), which, if left unchecked, is sufficient to raise core temperature by about $1 \, ^\circ\text{C}$ every 10 min. Increases beyond $41.5 \, ^\circ\text{C}$ are regarded as life threatening and need immediate medical attention. Long distance runners often sustain core temperatures of $40 \, ^\circ\text{C}$ without any obvious ill-effect, so some regulatory mechanisms must come into play.

The main mechanisms for heat loss from the body are radiation, conduction, convection and, most importantly for the marathon runner, evaporation of sweat; the last named accounts for about 80 per cent of heat loss during exercise. The difference in body core and ambient temperatures, together with the area of the body in contact with the outside air and the running speed, determines the effectiveness of radiation, conduction and convection. The smaller the temperature gradient between athlete and the ambient air, and the more the athlete is covered up, the less effective the heat loss by these mechanisms. Indeed, our body *gains* heat if ambient temperatures exceed that of the body; this is particularly so when skies are clear and solar radiation is at its maximum – just think of the perspiration that results from just lying on the beach.

In cool, dry environmental conditions, our normal temperature regulatory mechanisms are usually adequate to deal with the added heat production of marathon running. Problems arise during hot, humid conditions. The effectiveness of sweat evaporation depends on the relative humidity of the ambient air. Low humidity means that sweat evaporates readily from the surface of the

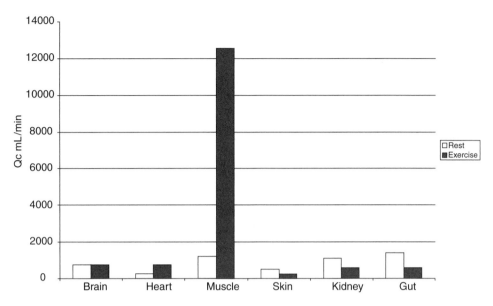

Figure 9.1 Distribution of blood at rest and during exercise

skin, thereby cooling the surface blood; high humidity leads to the sweat dripping from the body rather than evaporating from it, thus losing the benefits of evaporative heat loss.

We know that oxygen supply to working skeletal muscle is critical to marathon performance. Figure 9.1 shows the distribution of blood, and therefore oxygen, at rest and during exercise. To ensure sufficient oxygen is available to support the increased adenosine triphosphate needed when exercising, we shunt blood *away* from areas such as the skin and guts *towards* the working skeletal muscles.

Temperature regulation, however, requires the shunting of blood *away* from the body's core to its outer shell, where blood-cooling mechanisms can be more effective. Thus, we have a conflict between adenosine triphosphate production and control of body temperature. Diverting blood to the periphery is of minimal help unless accompanied by sweat secretion from eccrine glands found all over the body's surface. They secrete a weak (99 per cent water) solution containing sodium and chloride ions (Na^+ and Cl^-, i.e. salt), along with urea, uric acid, ammonia and lactic acid. The evaporation of the water from the skin is the major mechanism in cooling the venous blood returning to the body's core. Evaporation – changing water to water vapour – requires heat; this is the latent heat of vaporization. Vaporizing a litre of water leads to a loss of almost 2 500 kJ (580 kcal) of heat from the body.

Sweat production is a double-edged sword, however. Although during competition elite marathon runners *produce* about 500 mL of water via aerobic metabolism, they *lose* up to 5000 mL of water via sweating and increased ventilation. Total body water accounts for ~60 per cent of whole body mass. A loss of 2–4 per cent leads to impaired performance in endurance events; losses of 10–12 per cent are usually fatal.

There is another problem associated with the sweating mechanism. Sweat contains electrolytes – mainly sodium and chloride, albeit at much lower concentrations than those found in blood plasma. Insufficient water intake during the race can lead to increased electrolyte concentrations in the blood that upset the balance between intra- and extra-cellular fluids. Higher than normal sodium levels in the plasma – hypernatraemia – induces water to move from the intra-cellular fluid compartment, resulting in cellular dehydration and impaired performance. Dehydration triggers secretion by the adrenal glands of the hormone aldosterone, which minimizes sodium excretion in the sweat. Even so, if there is no water replacement the athlete becomes increasingly dehydrated, and suffers heat exhaustion, and possibly life-threatening heat stroke. On the other hand, excessive water intake without added sodium can lead to below normal sodium levels – hyponatraemia. The result is movement of water from the plasma into the tissues leading to muscle weakness, and dizziness and confusion as the brain does not tolerate the swelling produced by the influx of water.

There are considerable individual differences in sweat production and electrolyte content; too much sodium to combat hyponatraemia may make the drink unpalatable; too little is ineffective. Adequate pre-competition hydration, combined with fluid intake at feeding stations, is prudent. A mutually beneficial combination of a flavoured drink containing carbohydrate and sodium is common practice. The former assists in glycogen sparing, the latter combats sodium difficulties. However, we must take considerable care to establish the precise combination for individual athletes, and a process of 'trial and error' during training sessions is necessary if we are to optimize the potential benefits.

Factors limiting anaerobic performance

There are psychological, physiological and metabolic processes at work that limit an athlete's ability to maintain maximum anaerobic activities. Psychologically, the untrained individual is disinclined to ignore pain, and lacks the desensitization to the presence of hydrogen ions that results from prolonged anaerobic training. Physiologically, a below average first-line defence mechanism – i.e. the blood buffers in the intra- and extra-cellular fluids, principally, hydrogen carbonate (often described as bicarbonate), phosphate and haemoglobin – would be unhelpful. Metabolically, depletion of glycogen stores results in a switch in the primary fuel for contraction from carbohydrate to the much slower process of lipid breakdown.

For the sprint athletes, the limiting factor is the phosphocreatine content of the major muscles involved. Research suggests two things: first, the maximum creatine content of muscle is $\sim 5\,\mathrm{g\,kg_{muscle}}^{-1}$; second, about half of this is used per day by elite athletes undergoing strenuous training and must be replaced. There are three ways in which this replacement can occur: synthesis during glycolysis, dietary intake and direct supplementation.

Creatine supplementation

The main sources of naturally occurring creatine are dietary meat and fish. The body also manufactures creatine from the amino acids methionine, glycine and arginine. The first of these is an essential amino acid – i.e. it cannot be synthesized in humans and so must arise from the dietary intake. We generate the remaining two amino acids during anaerobic and aerobic catabolism of glucose. 3-phosphoglycerate (Equation (8.10)) is a precursor to glycine synthesis, and arginine is made from intermediaries released during aerobic metabolism. However, supplemental creatine is available in powder, tablet and sports drink form as creatine monohydrate.

Research shows significant benefits following creatine supplementation for some power athletes, particularly when accompanied by strenuous training – e.g. weight training, short sprints and plyometric exercises, all of which feature in the preparation of 100 and 400 m athletes. There are also potential benefits for middle distance athletes, and those involved in repeated effort sports such as American football, rugby and football.

As with most supplements, there are some concerns. These centre on the quality control of some creatine supplement production, and on exaggerated claims by some producers. Not all athletes respond positively to creatine supplementation and it is impossible to screen for such athletes. The individual most likely to benefit is a previously sedentary vegetarian; such a person may have chronically low creatine levels and a greater potential for improving physical performance, but hardly fits the profile of an elite 100 m runner.

Creatine attracts water, and therefore increases body mass; this is counter-productive in weight-controlled sports such as boxing. The optimal supplementation strategy is uncertain; dosages vary from $20\,\mathrm{g\,day^{-1}}$ for 5 days to $10\,\mathrm{g\,day^{-1}}$ for 51 days to $3\,\mathrm{g\,day^{-1}}$ for 30 days. However, the body cannot absorb all of the creatine provided. In response, the liver and kidneys work overtime to metabolize the material and excrete the surplus, leading to possible damage to both organs. There have also been reports of muscle cramps, nausea and gastro-intestinal problems. In spite of these caveats, however, creatine is not an illegal ergogenic aid, and there is evidence that some athletes will benefit from an appropriate, athlete-specific supplementation strategy.

For the 400 m group there are two additional factors. First is the burden of increasing pain; second, and more important, is the growing interference from higher hydrogen ion concentration of the excitation-coupling action of actin and myosin that destroys running technique. The problem facing the coach is 'What else, can be done to enhance performance by the smallest of percentages apart from the anaerobic training strategies designed to develop tolerance to hydrogen ions, enhance the ability of the blood and muscle to buffer the acid and increase the activity of essential anaerobic metabolic enzymes?'. Improvements of less than 1 per cent represent a huge difference at the elite level; in 1999, an improvement of 0.25 per cent (0.11 s) was sufficient for Michael Johnson to beat Butch Reynolds's eight-year-old world record.

Logically, increasing the intake of an alkaline compound – ordinary kitchen bicarbonate of soda for example – ought to increase the power of the body's buffering mechanisms. Buffers are compounds that transport hydrogen ions in ways that do not lower pH. Amongst the most powerful are phosphates, haemoglobin and hydrogen carbonate – previously described simply as bicarbonate. Ingesting bicarbonate of soda before an anaerobic event ought to raise blood pH. Such an increase facilitates the efflux of hydrogen ions from the muscle into the blood, thereby raising the intra-cellular pH and removing some of the inhibiting mechanisms to muscle fibre contraction.

Bicarbonate loading

Research evidence points to some beneficial effects of bicarbonate loading. These effects are primarily delaying the onset of fatigue rather than any actual improvement in work capacity or power output. In 1988, one study reported the effect of a bicarbonate dose of $400\,\mathrm{g\,kg^{-1}_{body\,mass}}$ on trained 400 m runners in simulated competition. The experimental group improved by 2 per cent compared with control and placebo groups. The fact that a similar effect at world class level would see the present 400 m record fall to 42.32 s suggests that the choice of subjects has some influence over the results. Highly trained elite 400 m runners may not be as susceptible to such interventions as club or county athletes.

The evidence also points to considerable variability in responses between subjects; this also applies to the range of side effects experienced. The most common approach is $300–400\,g\,kg^{-1}$ with more than $500\,mL$ of water, 60–90 min before the event. However, this needs testing by an individual trial-and-error approach during the training stage. Side-effects can include nausea, vomiting, diarrhoea, cardiac arrhythmias and muscle spasm. It is not clear whether any further benefits accrue by combining bicarbonate ingestion to raise pH with creatine supplementation to enhance phosphocreatine stores.

Factors limiting strength, power and flexibility

Many sports require additional physical attributes for success at elite level. Consider the 110 and 400 m hurdle events. The basic energy requirements are similar to the 100 and 400 m flat events, but there is the additional need for flexibility to attain the necessary hurdling technique. Now turn your attention to the field events and compare the additional demands for jumps to the throws. In both elements, explosive power is the crucial feature, and the type II FOG muscle fibres and the phosphagen cycle will dominate power and energy production. However, each event has its own special technical requirement. In the jumps, power, flexibility and precision are necessary; in the throws, power needs matching with shoulder flexibility in the javelin, with body mass in the shot and hammer, and with body mass and long levers in the discus. We look first at the fundamentals of strength and power.

Strength is the ability of muscle to generate force. Muscles generate force through three muscle actions – concentric, eccentric and isometric. Concentric action – force production during muscle fibre *shortening* – occurs during the lifting stage of a biceps curl. Eccentric action – force production during muscle fibre *lengthening* – occurs during the lowering phase of a biceps curl. Isometric action – force production where fibres *neither* lengthen *nor* shorten – occurs when attempting a biceps curl with a weight that is too heavy to lift.

Motor units and gradation of force

Muscles actions occur when motor units are stimulated. A motor unit consists of an incoming motor nerve, a group of skeletal muscle fibres and a myoneural junction linking the two. A nerve impulse from the motor cortex or the spinal cord travels down the nerve to the myoneural junction. Here, a neuro-transmitter, acetylcholine, is released from the nerve ending, allowing the impulse to cross the gap between nerve and muscle fibre and stimulate the muscle to contract. The motor units responsible for fine movements trigger very few – two to five – individual muscle fibres, whereas those responsible for the gross movements seen in most athletic events trigger 2000–3000 muscle fibres.

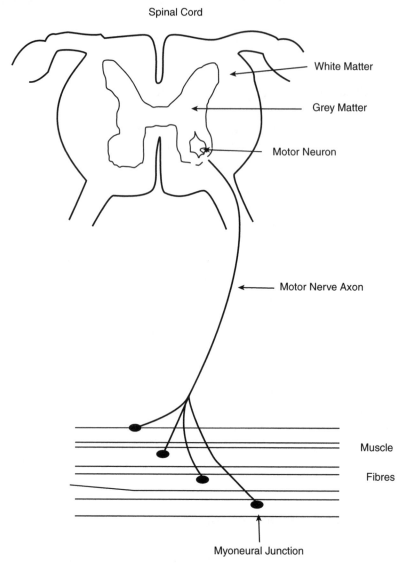

Figure 9.2   Motor unit

The muscle contracts *only* when a stimulus exceeds a threshold, and then it contracts *fully* – this is the 'all-or-none' law; thus, a stronger stimulus does not lead to a stronger contraction. The simplest contraction, responding to a single stimulus, is the muscle twitch seen only in the laboratory. It consists of a stimulus, a short latent period, contraction and relaxation; an increased frequency of stimulation leads to twitch summation, un-fused and fused tetany.

A maximum voluntary isometric contraction of the quadriceps muscle for example needs to develop fused tetany in *all* motor units. However, *untrained* individuals are unable to engage all of the available motor units in such a manoeuvre. Researchers have compared voluntary maximal efforts against external stimulation of the femoral nerve of the quadriceps and found greater force generation through artificial stimulation.

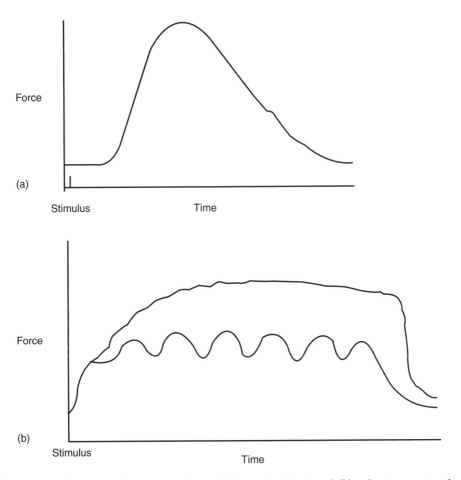

Figure 9.3 Diagrammatic representation of (a) muscle twitch and (b) voluntary contraction

This practice is not without risk; over-stimulation may lead, and indeed in a few cases has led, to rupture of the patella tendon. The important point, however, is that strength training, particularly in the early stages, has more to do with improving neuro-muscular facilitation than with any structural changes – i.e. increased muscle fibre girth, known as hypertrophy – in the muscle fibre itself. The smooth controlled muscle actions seen during sport appear to be the result of un-fused tetany of different motor units working independently of each other. The factor that enables us to perform skills as widely different as picking up a pen and sprinting is the engagement of the appropriate number of motor units exhibiting asynchronous un-fused tetany.

Strength is important in many sports. However, the major requirement for a range of dynamic sporting activities is power – i.e. the velocity at which the muscle generates force. The two key elements involved in power production are work and time, and power is work divided by time. Work is force multiplied by distance and the equation for power (P) is force (f) times distance (d) divided by time (t):

$$P = \frac{f \cdot d}{t}$$

but distance over time is velocity (v). Thus

$$P = f \cdot v$$

The relationship between force and velocity is inverse and curvilinear. This means that we cannot generate maximum force and velocity at the same time.

The maximum power output generated is the product of optimal force – about $50\%_{max}$ – and optimal velocity – about $30\%_{max}$. This represents only about 15 per cent of the theoretical maximum output. It takes almost half a second to generate maximum force. Different sports require different actions, and most take less than half a second; this requires two kinds of training. One is where a *high* force production – i.e. maximum *strength* – is vital; the other is where the *rate* of force production – i.e. maximum *velocity* – is crucial. Any inadequacies in strength or speed of movement will limit anaerobic power output. Skilled movement depends on the optimum force over appropriate time scale, and requires integrated activity within the neuromuscular system. This involves the motor cortex, the spinal cord, nerve axons, neuromuscular junctions and peripheral sense organs known as proprioceptors.

Neuromuscular facilitation

Proprioception

Muscle actions, whether arising from conscious acts or reflex arcs, require stimulation of motor neurons in the brain's motor cortex and the spinal cord. The impulses created travel to neuro-muscular junctions that link (synapse) directly with individual muscle fibres producing force. The peripheral limbs contain sense organs – the proprioceptors – in the form of stretch receptors in muscle spindles, tendons and joints. The receptors provide feedback on the length and tension of muscle fibres, and on limb position and movement. These organs control the forces generated during any muscle action via sensory (afferent) nerves and alpha and gamma (efferent) motor nerves linked to the central nervous system.

Muscle spindles are modified muscle cells, known as intra-fusal fibres, lying parallel to the normal muscle cells. The spindle contains two kinds of fibre. The first – nuclear *bag* – responds to dynamic stretching. The second – nuclear *chain* fibres – responds to static stretching (for a more thorough coverage of this topic see Åstrand and Rodahl, 1986). The main body of the spindle cannot contract but does respond to stretching. It does this in two ways. The first is via the encircling annulospiral sensory nerve fibres that interface with alpha motor neurons in the spinal cord. Stretching the spindle generates afferent nerve impulses – i.e. signals travelling from the periphery to the central nervous system; these signals stimulate efferent – i.e. from the centre to the periphery – alpha motor neurons, to produce contraction in skeletal muscle cells. The second is via gamma motor neurons found in contractile fibres at the ends of the spindle. The motor cortex of the brain stimulates these gamma neurons directly. The fibres contract; the spindle stretches producing muscle contraction via the alpha motor neurons. The higher the force required, the greater the degree of stretching, leading to the engagement of more motor units stimulating muscle fibres to contract.

The stretch receptors found in the tendons of muscles – the Golgi organs – provide a safety mechanism against excessive forces that could damage both types of tissue. Unlike the muscle spindles, which respond to muscle *length* by facilitating muscle contraction, the Golgi organs respond to muscle *tension* by inhibiting contraction. The sensory nerve from the Golgi organ feeds directly into the spinal cord. Golgi organ impulses synapse with an inhibitory neuron in the spine reducing the stimulation of the alpha motor neurons; this leads to muscle relaxation and a release of tension. The activation of the tendon organ is responsible for the failures seen in weight lifters trying to exceed their maximal effort.

Joint receptors are responsible for passing information on joint position, movement and tendon tension. Ruffini receptors respond to pressure within the joint capsule. Pacinian corpuscles respond to pressure in connective tissues around joints resulting from joint acceleration and deceleration. The tendon organs in the joint capsule provide an inhibitory function on active muscles when joint stability is threatened.

Factors limiting flexibility

Flexibility is the greatest range of voluntary movement around a joint. We divide the range of movement (ROM) into inner, mid- and outer sectors. The most effective work done during any action occurs in the mid-sector of the movement.

Strength and flexibility exercises are mutually beneficial; focusing on either strength or flexibility at the expense of the other does not lead to maximizing power. Great strength with limited flexibility results in force generation over a short distance; great flexibility with limited strength results in lower force, albeit over a long distance. In either case, we may compromise power output. The combination of stretching exercises to increase the entire range of movement alongside strength training optimizes force generation over the longest distance in the shortest time.

The joint structure is the main limitation to flexibility. The bones and connective tissues, such as the joint capsule and supportive ligaments, account for about 50 per cent of a joint's resistance to movement. Another 10 per cent lies in the tendons crossing the joint. We cannot reduce this resistance without compromising joint safety. The least flexible joints are the hinge joints; movement is restricted largely to flexion and extension. Hyperextension of the elbow is resisted by the bony structures of the olecranon fossa of the humerus and olecranon process of the ulna. No such structure exists in the other major hinge joint, the knee. Here, the major protective features are the joint capsule and ligaments, principally the patellar, the medio-lateral and anterior–posterior cruciate.

The most flexible joints are the multi-axial, or ball-and-socket, joints of the hip and shoulder allowing fullest range of movement – abduction, adduction, circumduction, flexion, extension, rotation. The head of the femur is located in the acetabulum; this is a deep socket of the pelvic hipbone surrounded by a strong capsule and ligaments. The head of the humerus is located in the much shallower glenoid fossa of the scapula, has a greater range of movement than the hip joint, and is more easily dislocated.

The connective tissues of muscle groups are made of 'visco-elastic' materials – collagen and elastin. These can account for a further 40 per cent of the resistance to movement. When we stretch viscous material – 'Plasticine' for example – it retains its stretched shape. When we stretch an elastic band, it returns immediately to its original state when released. The combination of these two materials means that when stretched, muscle will stay stretched for a time before regaining its original position. These features are the key to flexibility training.

Ligaments and tendons have limited elasticity; attempting to increase flexibility by stretching these tissues leads to joint weakness and an increased risk of injury. The majority of the elastic material lies in the muscle fascia, of which there are three kinds. The deepest is the endomysium – the tissue surrounding individual muscle fibres. Next is the perimysium – the structure that binds bundles of muscle fibres to form a fasciculus. Finally, there is the epimysium – the outermost tissue that binds fasciculi into discernable muscle groups such as biceps and quadriceps.

Flexibility training uses the visco-elastic nature of the muscle and fascia, and works on two areas. The first is stretching the individual sarcomere of each muscle fibre to its maximal resting length. When this point is reached, any further stretching rearranges the fibres of the muscle fascia, adding further movement. The second is desensitizing the muscle spindles – and therefore the stretch reflex – and enhancing the Golgi tendon organs' response, through *controlled* stretching. A good time to engage in stretching is immediately following a weight-training session.

There are four basic stretching methods – ballistic, dynamic, proprioceptive neuromuscular facilitation and static stretching. There is considerable overlap between the methods, however. Ballistic stretching – e.g. the vigorous use of upper body movement to try to touch one's toes – is not recommended, as it reinforces the stretch response thus not allowing the muscle time to adapt to a stretched position; it can lead to injury. Dynamic stretching is a controlled movement – e.g. arm swings taken to the limit of the present range of motion. Static stretching takes three forms: static active, e.g. leg raise to 90° and hold that position for 10–15 s; passive stretching, e.g. the splits; isometric stretching, adopt a passive stretch and then try to contract and hold the tensed muscle for 10–15 s. Proprioceptive neuromuscular facilitation – e.g. hamstring: this starts with a held passive stretch followed by an isometric contraction of the hamstring for 10–15 s; finally, there is a brief relaxation before a final 10–15 s passive stretch beyond the initial passive stretch position.

The purpose behind physical training is the reduction of the outcomes of these factors that limit performance. The next chapter outlines the key principles underpinning *all* training programmes, warns of the dangers of over-training/over-reaching, and considers the limitations of assessing performance in the laboratory and in the field.

Practical implications

Perhaps the first implication concerning the factors affecting performance is that an athlete should choose his/her parents carefully. Of course, this does not happen so the athlete and coach have to make do with what they have. Testing athletes to find out genetic factors, such as the ratio of muscle fibre types, is possible at top level but not at lower levels. Even in top class sport, where money is no problem, athletes tend to shy away from muscle biopsies. They are nowhere near as painful as they look but few people want to have one. Observation of your athletes can give a good idea of what their fibre type is. If they excel at long duration steady-state running, they are probably high in SO fibres. If they are good sprinters and jumpers they will be high in FG and/or FOG fibres. In Chapter 10, we examine some of the sports-specific tests that are used and these can give us some vital clues as to not only fibre type but also cardiorespiratory make-up.

> *Task 1* What ratio of muscle fibre types do you think you have? What are your reasons for thinking this?

Whether we can change a person's muscle fibre type is a controversial question in exercise physiology. Suffice it to say here that even if we can there are severe limitations as to how much of a difference we can make, so we will have to adapt what we ask of the athlete. For some track athletes changing the distance run has made a huge difference. Using different styles of play can have large advantages for many team game players. When Brian Clough took over as manager at Nottingham Forest, he told his reserve left-winger, John Robertson, to accept that he was slow and alter his game accordingly. Robertson did so and became first choice not only at Forest but also for Scotland. Although we may not be able to change muscle fibre type we can develop what we have. Weight training can ensure that the athletes develop their strength and power fully.

Power is essential in almost all sports. The best way to develop power is to first work on strength. This is best done using weight training (problems of weight training with children and adolescents are covered in Part IV). Heavy weights with very low, fewer than three, repetitions should be used. Once strength has been established lighter weights, but nevertheless still difficult to lift, should then be used. The lifting should be as dynamic as possible. The range and type should also be as near to the actual activity as possible. Modern multi-gyms make this more possible than it used to be. If the number of repetitions in the sport itself is low, e.g. high jump, then only a few repetitions are necessary, fewer than five. If the sport requires the athlete to not only possess power but also to be able to repeat it over and over again, e.g. volleyball, then slightly lower weights should be used but more repetitions.

Although it is difficult to affect muscle fibre type, $V_{O2\ max}$ can be greatly increased by good aerobic training. The types of aerobic training that we mentioned in the last chapter have beneficial effects on the whole of the aerobic system. Lung ventilation, cardiac output and blood transport are all improved. Sometimes improvements can be dramatic. Obviously, once a certain level has been achieved, improvement becomes more difficult and genetic factors will decide which athletes are going to the top. Lung size and heart size can probably be improved but if you start at an advantage *and train* you will keep that advantage.

While these problems are genetic, factors such as dehydration can be guarded against. The importance of drinks during marathons is well known but is perhaps ignored to some extent in team games. Water and preferably carbohydrate drinks should be available throughout a game and players encouraged to drink. This is especially so in hot climates or even in temperate climates on hot days. The use of drinks containing bicarbonate of soda, e.g. lemonade, can help limit increases in pH.

Another area that can be improved is flexibility. Stretching, particularly proprioceptive neuromuscular stretching, can increase the range of movement around joints. Flexibility is the basis of agility. While flexibility requires a range of movement, agility requires that range but in a dynamic movement. The power cannot be added until the range has been established. Genetic factors, however, play a large role in flexibility. Improvements tend to be in the way the brain reacts to the movement more than in the movement itself. The anatomical changes that are possible appear to be limited.

Key points

- genetics is the first factor affecting performance
  - muscle fibre type is genetically inherited

- there are two types of muscle fibre, fast twitch (type II) and slow twitch (type 1)
  - fast-twitch fibres are divided into fast glycolytic (type IIb) and fast oxidative (type IIa)
  - proportions of these vary between individuals

- muscle fibres contain mitochondria
  - these supply the power for all muscle cell activity

- fast-twitch glycolytic (FG) fibres generate the highest power output
  - motor neurons in these fibres work three times faster than in slow-twitch fibres

- fast-twitch oxidative glycolytic (FOG) fibres can use both anaerobic and aerobic mechanisms to produce ATP
  - they contain myoglobin (Mgb) – an oxygen binding molecule

- slow-twitch oxidative (SO) fibres contain more Mgb than FOG
  - SO are highly resistant to fatigue

- in short duration fast activity oxygen is used after the event to re-synthesize phosphocreatine
  - in long-duration events oxygen is the main source and is used during competition

- the maximal rate at which we can used oxygen is called $V_{O2 \, max}$

- $V_{O2 \, max}$ is the outcome of a chain of physiological mechanisms delivering oxygen to skeletal muscle (see Fick equation)
  - the chain consists of lung ventilation, oxygen carriage by the blood, oxygen delivery by the heart and oxygen uptake by tissues

- lung ventilation involves
  - transport of inspired air down airways to the respiratory bronchioles
  - diffusion down the alveolus and across the alveolar–capillary membrane into the blood

- oxygen carriage in blood depends on
  - number of oxygen carrying red blood cells available
  - speed of those cells through the pulmonary circulation

- oxygen delivery (cardiac output) is the result of
  - strength of heart muscle
  - rate at which the heart beats (heart rate)

- oxygen uptake by the skeletal muscle is a function of
  - number of open capillaries
  - speed of red cells through the capillary bed
  - number of mitochondria
  - rate of biochemical reactions within the sarcoplasm and mitochondria of individual muscle fibres

- glycogen depletion is a major factor limiting performance
  - a high carbohydrate diet 2-3 days prior to performance optimizes liver and muscle glycogen stores
  - carbohydrate drinks during performance maintain blood glucose levels
  - high carbohydrates immediately after an event restore muscle glycogen and can increase it

- heat stress and dehydration limit performance
  - humans only function optimally within a core temperature band of $37 \pm 1\,°C$
  - increases above $41.5\,°C$ are life threatening

- radiation, conduction, convection and evaporation of sweat help keep core temperature low during exercise and in heat
  - sweat is responsible for 80 per cent heat loss during exercise
  - the efficiency of radiation, conduction, convection to aid heat loss depends on the difference between core temperature and ambient temperature
  - the smaller the gap the less heat is lost
  - if ambient temperature is greater than core temperature heat will be gained

- humidity adds another problem
  - high humidity makes it difficult for the air to evaporate the sweat

- loss of water through sweating can lead to increased electrolyte concentration in the blood
  - which causes dehydration
  - extremes of dehydration can be fatal

- water helps against dehydration BUT
  - excessive water intake without added sodium causes hyponatraemia
  - this causes water to move from plasma into muscle leading to muscle weakness

- the limiting factor for anaerobically produced energy is the phosphocreatine stored in muscle
  - this can be replaced by synthesis during glycolysis, dietary intake and creatine supplementation

- a limiting factor for the anaerobic glycolytic system is increased muscle pH
  - bicarbonate of soda helps limit increases in pH

- strength is the ability of muscles to generate force

- there are three muscle actions – concentric, eccentric and isometric
  - concentric force is when muscle fibres shorten
  - eccentric is when muscle fibres lengthen
  - in isometric force fibres neither shorten nor lengthen

- muscle action occurs when motor units are stimulated

- a motor unit consist of a motor nerve, a group of skeletal muscle fibres and a myoneural junction linking the two
  - the neurotransmitter acetylcholine allows the impulse to cross the myoneural junction and contraction occurs
  - the stimulus must exceed a threshold before the motor unit will respond
  - response is 100 per cent – the 'all-or-none law'

- power is the velocity at which muscles generate force

- work is force × distance
  - power is force × distance divided by time
  - we cannot generate maximum force and velocity at the same time

- proprioceptors are sensory organs
  - muscle spindles are intra-fusal fibres within the muscle
  - the nuclear bag responds to dynamic stretching
  - the nuclear chains respond to static stretching
  - stretching generates nerve impulse which stimulate the alpha motor neurons to produce contraction

◆ the brain directly stimulates gamma motor neurons which also stimulates the alpha motor neurons following stretching

• Golgi tendon organs are stretch receptors in tendons
  ◆ they respond to tension and inhibit contraction

• joint receptors provide information about joint position, movement and tendon tension

• flexibility is the greatest range of voluntary movement around a joint

• joint structure is the main limiting factor in flexibility

• flexibility can be enhanced by stretching exercise

• there are four stretching methods – ballistic, dynamic, proprioceptive neuromuscular facilitation and static stretching
  ◆ ballistic stretching is not recommended as it can lead to injury
  ◆ dynamic stretching is a controlled movement – e.g. arm swings taken to the limit of the present range of motion
  ◆ static stretching takes three forms: static active, e.g. leg raise to 90° and hold that position for 10–15 s; passive stretching, e.g. the splits; isometric stretching, adopt a passive stretch and then try to contract and hold the tensed muscle for 10–15 s
  ◆ proprioceptive neuromuscular facilitation – e.g. hamstring: this starts with a held passive stretch followed by an isometric contraction of the hamstring for 10–15 s; finally, there is a brief relaxation before a final 10–15 s passive stretch beyond the initial passive stretch position.

10

Principles of Physical Training

Learning objectives

By the end of this chapter you should be able to

- list the principles of training
- discuss the relationships between the overload principle and its component parts – volume, frequency, duration and intensity of training programmes
- outline the importance of specificity to successful training outcomes
- recognize the importance of athlete uniqueness, and give examples of how such uniqueness may manifest itself
- discuss the values of sport specific ergometry, and the problems associated with laboratory simulations
- recognize the difficulties of field tests and the possibility of errors arising from predictive tests
- outline the causes of over-training and how it may be prevented
- discuss the relationship between recovery, rest and reversibility.

The most important survival attribute of the human body is its plasticity. This attribute takes many forms. Initially designed for life in tropical temperatures at sea level, humans now live and work at high altitudes and sub-zero

Coaching Science   Terry McMorris and Tudor Hale
© 2006 John Wiley & Sons, Ltd

temperatures and have undergone adaptive physiological and morphological characteristics. Altitude dwellers have more red blood cells than those living at sea level. SCUBA-divers extract more oxygen from a litre of inspired air than untrained individuals of similar size. Elite tennis players often have thicker racket-arms. Body-builders have extensive muscle development. Coaches use the body's plasticity to enhance sports performance in the same way that physiotherapists use exercise to restore quadriceps' strength to limbs immobilized through injury.

The over-arching characteristic of any training programme is that it is *goal oriented*. As we saw in Part I, the process of goal setting involves collaboration on an equal footing between coach and athlete, and entails consideration of age, previous experience and performance, present level of fitness, the future competitive framework and the aspirations of the individual athlete. This is the most important process. Done well, some/most of the goals may be achieved; done badly, disappointment and possible long-term injury await. Crucially, the athlete must be fully committed to the goals set.

In addition to goal orientation, there are four key principles underpinning all forms of physical training, whether for elite athletes or fitness and health seekers. These are *progressive overload*, *specificity*, *recovery* and *reversibility*.

Progressive overload

All individuals start from an existing exercise tolerance baseline. Working below that baseline does not result in overload or improved performance. The aim is to find a training *threshold* that stresses our existing biological mechanisms. The training programme ensures there is an adaptive response and a higher threshold is achieved. This is how the *overload* principle works.

There are several ways of establishing thresholds. A popular approach aimed at improving aerobic endurance for fitness and health goals as well as elite athletes is calculating a *training heart rate*, e.g.

$$[(\text{maximum heart rate} - \text{resting heart rate}) \times 0.70]$$
$$+ \text{ resting heart rate} = \text{training heart rate}$$

Other methods use relationships between heart rate and oxygen uptake, heart rate and blood lactate levels, heart rate and power output, power output and blood lactate levels and a simple percentage of maximal oxygen uptake.

Developing strength uses weight training as the stimulus. A threshold is calculated as a percentage of the maximal weight lifted – i.e. a one-repetition maximum (1RM) – e.g 60 per cent 1RM. The percentage chosen depends on the time in the competitive season, the age and experience of the athlete and the goals set by athlete and coach.

Whatever the threshold happens to be, it needs to be sufficiently strenuous to disturb the body's primary goal of a physiological steady state (homeostasis). In response, the body adjusts its physiological mechanisms to deal with the added stress and restore homeostatic balance. Repeated bouts of a stressor – i.e. training – result in an enhanced homeostatic response. Our physiological mechanisms adapt to cope with this stress. Thus, over time, a cycling load that elicited a pre-training heart rate of 175 beats min^{-1}, or an initial bench press of 60 kg, progressively result in less stress. The result of such adaptive responses is a fall in post-training heart rates – both exercising and resting – or an increase in our 1RM load. However, if we are to improve performance even further, we must create an even greater level of stress.

This is *progression*, a critical feature of the *overload* principle. We can increase the cycling load by maintaining the same distance but reducing the target time, or maintaining the same time but increasing the distance to be covered. In the case of weight training, we can increase the number of repetitions at the same 1RM, or establish a new 1RM and maintain the same percentage. Both are examples of *progressive* overload.

The progressive overload principle revolves around a balance between the building blocks of *volume*, *frequency*, *duration* and *intensity* of training. Volume is a function of distance covered, number of repetitions in a set of exercises or number of sets per session. Frequency is the number of sessions per day/week/cycle. Duration is the length of time of each session. Intensity governs the strenuousness of the exercise. Clearly, there is interaction between these training building blocks. Volume can increase through greater frequency or longer duration of a session, singly or in combination. The intensity of a session governs the frequency and duration of a session, particularly in terms of the work–recovery patterns, and takes account of the competitive calendar. The art of coaching requires a specifically constructed balance between these particular elements for individual athletes.

Specificity

Sport specificity

Specificity takes various forms. The most obvious is the athlete's particular sport or event – different sports need different training approaches. Track athletes offer the clearest example, readily falling into sprints, middle- and long-distance, marathon and ultra-marathon categories. Whilst there is some overlap across each category, sprinters do not train by running 10 km intervals, and 10 000 m runners do not practise fast starts from starting-blocks. Specific training is necessary to produce *appropriate* adaptations.

This does not always seem to be the case, and within some sports, the training undertaken seems far from specific. Here are some examples. 100 m free-style swimmers – elite times <60 s – spend hours ploughing up and down the pool at sub-competition pace. A typical training programme for 5000 m elite pursuit cyclists may include routine three-hour squad rides where average heart rates lie between 120 and 140 beats min^{-1}. This is in spite of evidence showing heart rates of riders reach 180–190 beats min^{-1} within 45 s of starting an event, and blood lactate levels reach 14 mmol L^{-1} by the end. Research shows outfield football players spend about a third of a match standing or walking, a third jogging and the final third in short bursts of sprinting over distances ranging between 5 and 25 yards accompanied by a power action such as a jump, shot or tackle. Time spent in excessive cross-country running seems to be a waste of time and energy, when repeated shuttle runs of 5, 10, 15, 20 and 25 yards reflect the actual running patterns of the game. Single-handed dinghy sailors need to 'hike' – i.e. lean out over the side of the dinghy to prevent the boat from capsizing. Traditional training insists on static isometric muscle action in the hiking position. Performance analysis shows that modern elite sailors spend most of their time in dynamic hiking. This entails repeated trunk flexion, extension and rotation, as well as fore and aft body movements to maintain the greatest speeds. Prolonged static isometric hiking is not going to deliver the appropriate level of fitness for elite sailors.

Training specificity

A simple example of specific training occurs in the sport of Olympic weight lifting. Here athletes in several different weight categories undertake two lifts – the snatch, and the clean and jerk. Biomechanical analyses of each lift reveal the key stages of each lift, allowing coaches to break down the complete action into its component parts. Training focuses on these components specifically, thereby ensuring maximum benefit.

Many sports use weight training as part of an overall programme. A crucial characteristic of Olympic lifters' training is their use of 'free weights'. This enables them to use specific movements that mimic the precise actions of the actual lifts. The difficulty with weight training for other sports is that there is a greater risk of injury through poor technique when using free weights. The development of weight training machines with pre-set movement patterns is safer than free weights, but these restrict the trainee to a particular movement pattern, often from one body position. For anyone undertaking a general weight training routine for fitness and health reasons, this restriction is probably unimportant. However, the restriction becomes very important for the elite athlete looking for specific movement patterns at specific speeds. If the set *movement* pattern and/or body position practised does not feature in the actual movement pattern of a particular sport, no benefit accrues to post-training sports performance – i.e. there is no *crossover* training effect. Furthermore, training for *speed* must mimic the real-time speed at which an event occurs. These features inevitably require the use of free weights. Thus, shot putters, discus and javelin throwers and golfers, for example, would look to combine lower body – e.g. high resistance isometric squat or leg-press action – and core strength to provide the stability needed to sustain powerful upper body action and fast trunk rotation.

However, the issue of power training is rather more complicated. For example, discus throwing requires strength *and* fast explosive movements. We saw in the previous chapter that a trade-off exists between the force and the velocity of movements – the greater the velocity the less force generated. To maximize *strength* – i.e. force development – we need to engage as many of the available motor units in a muscle group as possible. The most effective way to achieve this is through *slow* actions. This provides a sound initial level of *strength* fitness. This enables coaches to maximize power – i.e. work divided by time – through increasingly specific *velocity* training activities. Thus, the specificity of the weight training element of the overall programme demands a combination of both actions, with strength development taking precedence during the early stages of the training programme.

Herein lies a possible dilemma for the coaches. Specific training requires a foundation of general fitness. The greater this foundation, the more specific the training can become. Runners and swimmers use the off-season to develop their foundational fitness before introducing the crucial element of specific training as the competitive season approaches. The problem lies in deciding how much general training should precede specific work to achieve the optimum return.

Athlete specificity

All coaches recognize that the most important element in the specificity of training is the individuality of each athlete. Our inherited DNA (deoxyribo-nucleic acid) provides the essential blueprint for who we are and what we could become. There is no way of knowing whether each one of us is unique, but sufficient evidence exists to say that we are unique enough to use our DNA as the critical marker in criminal cases.

The interaction of our environment and our DNA produces, for example, individuals who fall into distinct groups – sprinters, discus throwers and high jumpers. All of these athletes share common characteristics – an abundance of type II fast twitch muscle fibres is one example. Conversely, marathon runners have an abundance of type I slow twitch fibres. Often, we regard this difference in muscle fibre types as sufficient to group athletes, and that the training needs of each athlete in a particular group are the same. Here are some examples involving endurance athletes that show that this is not always the case.

Maximal oxygen uptake

A study by Ekblom and his colleagues published in 1968 followed eight male students over a 4 month mixed running training programme entailing 30–60 s sprints, interval running, times varying between 3 and 7 min, and 45–75 min continuous running. The average post-training improvements were as follows. Maximal oxygen uptake rose by 17 per cent (3.13–3.68 L min^{-1}); cardiac output increased by 8 per cent (22.4–24.2 L min^{-1}); maximum heart rate fell by 4.5 per cent (199–190 beat min^{-1}); stroke volume grew by 13.4 per cent (112–127 mL beat^{-1}) and peripheral oxygen extraction improved by 3.6 per cent (138–148 mL L^{-1}). These are impressive gains and at first sight indicate the value of this general approach to endurance training.

However, if we look at how each *individual* reacted to this common training programme we get a very different picture, as seen in Table 10.1.

Table 10.1 Percentage changes in key mechanisms producing maximal oxygen uptakes following a four-month mixed running training programme. (Based on data originally published in Ekblom B, Å strand PO, Saltin B & Wallstrom B (1968) Effect of training on circulatory response to exercise. *J Appl Physiol* **24**: 518–528)

Subject	$V_{O_2\,max}$ L min^{-1}	Q_{max} L min^{-1}	$f_{c\,max}$ beat min^{-1}	V_S mL beat^{-1}	$C_{a-v\,O_2}$ mL L^{-1}
1	+16%	+6%	−8%	+15%	+10%
2	+11	+10	−5	+15	+1
3	+18	+27	−2	+30	−8
4	+10	+14	−1	+15	−4
5	+13	+10	−1	+10	+4
6	+1	−8	−11	+3	+9
7	+15	+2	−7	+10	+13
8	+7	+5	−3	+8	+1

Subject 6 had minimal improvement in maximal oxygen uptake and stroke volume, and compensated for a fall in cardiac output by increasing peripheral oxygen extraction. Subject 3 had the greatest increase in maximal oxygen uptake and cardiac output, but the greatest fall in oxygen extraction. Four subjects (2, 3, 4 and 8) increased their maximal oxygen uptake largely through increased cardiac output. Two subjects (6 and 7) improved maximal oxygen uptake mainly through better oxygen extraction by the working muscles. Only subjects 1 and 5 showed improvements in both cardiac output and oxygen extraction. The programme clearly suited some individuals better than others, but the important feature is the individuality of responses. The subjects in this research were students. The obvious question is 'Does it happen with elite athletes?'. The answer appears in Table 10.2.

This second 1968 study by Ekblom and Hermansen examined the maximal oxygen uptake of elite Swedish endurance athletes. The obvious features here are firstly the very high maximal oxygen uptakes, and secondly the different mechanisms used to deliver that high level of oxygen to the working muscle. Subjects 6 and 8 are cardiac output dependent, 1 and 3 are peripheral extraction dependent, whilst 2, 4, 5 and 7 rely on a combination of both mechanisms.

The key question facing the coaches of these individuals is whether different training strategies might have produced higher maximal oxygen uptakes by improving the weaker links in the oxygen uptake chain whilst retaining the very strong ones.

Unfortunately, we are unlikely to test this hypothesis because the method used – i.e. cardiac catheterization – is invasive and is a process that is not routinely available to coach or athlete, even if the latter were willing. However, the principle is clear; a rigid approach to training is not going to benefit every athlete.

Table 10.2 The Fick equation for maximal oxygen uptake, showing differences between elite endurance athletes. (Based on data originally published in Ekblom B & Hermansen L (1968) Cardiac output in athletes. *J Appl Physiol* **25**: 619–625)

Subject	$V_{O_2\,max}$ L min^{-1}	Q_{max} L min^{-1}	$C_{a-v\,O_2}$ mL L^{-1}
1	5.122	31.5	163
2	5.776	37.8	153
3	4.661	27.8	168
4	5.604	34.4	163
5	5.503	36.2	152
6	5.645	38.1	148
7	6.007	39.8	151
8	6.248	42.3	148

The anaerobic threshold

A physiological assessment of all of the middle and long distance world record holders reveals highly developed aerobic systems – i.e. maximal oxygen uptake ($V_{O_2 max}$). All are capable of steady-state running at more than 80 per cent of their maximum uptake. However, African runners seem to demonstrate something extra – the ability to inject increased speed at different points during the race as well as over the last kilometre (see Chapter 10). This ability suggests a number of attributes other than just a high aerobic capacity. First, they are well endowed with type I (SO) fibres. Second, they also have sufficient type IIa (FO) fibres to sustain bursts of increased speed. Third, they have good running economy (RE) – i.e. the oxygen cost of the individual's running style is relatively low. Finally, and probably most importantly, they have a relatively high anaerobic threshold (An_{Thresh}) – the running speed at which hydrogen ions begin to accumulate in the blood and diminish performance.

The term anaerobic threshold arose from a 1964 investigation into the exercise tolerance of patients recovering from a heart attack. The threshold indicates the increasing involvement of anaerobic metabolism as a source of energy, and locates the point during an exercise bout at which lactic acid – or more precisely hydrogen ions – begins to accumulate in the blood. The acronym used is OBLA – the onset of blood lactate accumulation. Research in the 1980s found that a particular value of OBLA – $\sim$4 mmol L_{bl}^{-1} – was critical for endurance performance. Below the critical figure, performance was maintainable; a value above the critical figure led to a rapid and often catastrophic loss of performance.

The whole purpose of injecting pace into an event is to induce the production of hydrogen ions in competitors whose anaerobic threshold is comparatively low. A successful outcome of such tactics is obvious. The less gifted runners who choose to respond to the change in speed find themselves exceeding their threshold and slipping into non-steady-state running and hydrogen ion accumulation. The outcome is the inability to maintain their *chosen* race pace because of falling intra-muscular pH and the consequent interference with force generation of the running muscles. There is also perhaps the realization of imminent and inevitable defeat and accompanying mental fatigue. As we saw in Chapter 8 (Figure 8.12), Emile Zatopek successfully inflicted this strategy on his opponents in the 1950s with an almost rhythmical change of pace in the middle of the race, but the African runners adopt various physiologically disruptive strategies that make a mockery of the theoretically sound steady-state running strategy in middle and long-distance running.

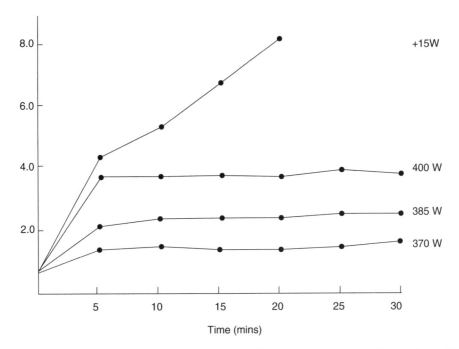

Figure 10.1 Blood lactate concentrations of a cyclist exercising at four different intensities

An illustration of the fine line between triumph and disaster comes in evidence from cycling shown in Figure 10.1, but studies on runners show similar patterns. Here an elite cyclist performs four 30 min sessions at power outputs ranging from 370 to 415 W, whilst having blood lactate (La_{bl}) levels recorded at 5 min intervals. Each increase in power results in an initial sharp rise in blood lactate in the first 5 min. At the three lower power outputs, the raised lactate levels remain constant for the rest of the 30 min task. However, at the fourth level, the increase in power output of less than 4 per cent – i.e. a mere 15 W – is sufficient to tip the athlete into a state where lactate accumulates in the blood and rapidly reaches a level at which the athlete is unable to complete the 30 min task. In actual competition, the only strategy to prevent this happening is to reduce the demand by cycling/running slower.

It is important to note a number of things here.

1. It is the hydrogen ion released from the lactic acid that is creating the problem, not the lactate itself. However, as there is a close relationship between blood lactate levels and intra-muscular pH, blood lactate levels provide a reasonable marker for the pH of skeletal muscle.

2. *Specific* training can improve aerobic capacity and running economy and move the anaerobic threshold to a more advantageous position in the work–lactate relationship.

3. However, the most important is that there is no *standard threshold* of $4 \, mmol \, L_{bl}^{-1}$. Research shows that the point at which the lactate begins to accumulate in the blood varies considerably between individuals, ranging from 3 to $7 \, mmol \, L_{bl}^{-1}$. Each athlete is unique, and the individual threshold needs to be determined, a process that *is* routinely available in good sports science laboratories.

Ergometer specificity

Regular monitoring of athlete progress, particularly during the non-competitive part of the year, plays an important part in the training process. Coaches and scientists recognized the need for sport specific ergometry, and in most sports science laboratories treadmills and cycle ergometers are the major tools of physiological monitoring. These offer a reasonably valid test environment for sports involving these two activities. However, even within running and cycling, ergometer specificity is vital. Monitoring a runner's maximal oxygen uptake on a cycle, and a cyclist's anaerobic threshold on the treadmill, would be perverse. Cycling has gone a step further in developing the King cycle, a device that allows cyclists to use their own bicycles rather than the 'one size fits all' laboratory cycle ergometer.

This need for specificity applies to sports where running is not involved, such as rowing and swimming. The development of the rowing ergometer and swimming flume responded to these particular needs. Research into the physiological demands of boxing, single-handed dinghy sailing and sail-boarding include details of sport specific ergometers (see Figure 10.2 for an example of a boxing specific ergometer). These innovations have accompanied developments in miniaturized heart rate monitors, eight-channel EMG radio-telemetry and the portable CosMed (see Figure 7.8) device that analyses expired air, allowing more valid laboratory simulations, and even in-competition monitoring of physiological performance.

Test specificity

The measurement of the aerobic power and capacity, and anaerobic threshold, is relatively simple. However, in the case of short-term events that rely very

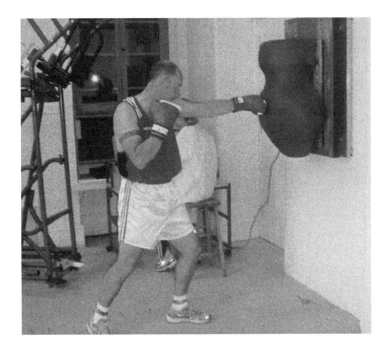

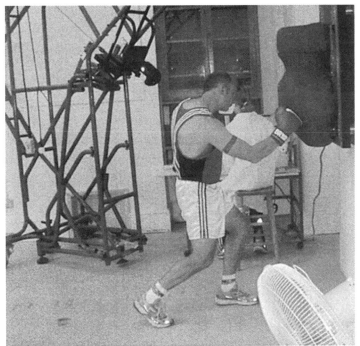

Figure 10.2   A boxing specific ergometer, which measures the power of the punch

heavily on anaerobic metabolism the practical application of our knowledge is less well developed. Several tests claim to measure anaerobic power or capacity, but all produce indirect measures and none possess the validity of the maximal oxygen uptake and anaerobic threshold tests.

The two most frequently used – the Margaria step and the Wingate 30 s – are indirect measures of anaerobic power introduced in the 1960s. The former, involving a timed run up a short set of steps, calculates power by multiplying the mass of the subject by the vertical distance of the steps, divided by the time taken, i.e.

$$\text{power} = \frac{\text{mass (kg)} \times \text{vertical distance (m)}}{\text{time (s)}}$$

and gives the product in kilogram metres per second – $kg\,m\,s^{-1}$. This needs to be converted into the SI unit of power – the watt (W) – where $1\,W = 6.12\,kg\,m\,min^{-1}$. Thus, a subject with a body mass of 70 kg, who completes the vertical distance of 1 m in 0.5 s, generates a power output of $140\,kg\,m\,s^{-1}$, or 1372 W $((140 \times 60)/6.12)$. Clearly, body mass is a significant factor in this equation; a heavier subject completing the run in the same time as a lighter one does more external work, but whether this translates into greater anaerobic power is not clear. Thus, this test may be a useful indicator in a longitudinal training study, but of dubious value in cross-sectional studies.

The Wingate test is a computer-monitored 30 s all-out cycling test to assess both anaerobic power and capacity. Figure 10.3 is a typical power output profile from the test.

The time taken to reach maximum wheel revolutions gives an idea of anaerobic power; the total amount of work done gives an idea of anaerobic capacity. The computer programme captures wheel revolutions and calculates power (W) from the work done over time. However, this calculation is of questionable validity, as the simple work/time equation does not take into account acceleration and deceleration. On the other hand, the computer captures wheel revolutions very precisely and these data give the same profile as those derived from the invalid calculations. The intra-subject variability on tests repeated over several days is low, so the test is a useful tool in assessing anaerobic capabilities before and after training.

The attempts to transpose the principles behind the Wingate test from cycling to running resulted in mixed outcomes. The method involved a non-motorized treadmill with the runner attached to a strain gauge by an inelastic harness. The natural forward lean adopted during sprinting imposed a load on the gauge and movement of the treadmill bed. A maximal 30 s sprinting effort was recorded on a computer, and the combined distance and forces generated

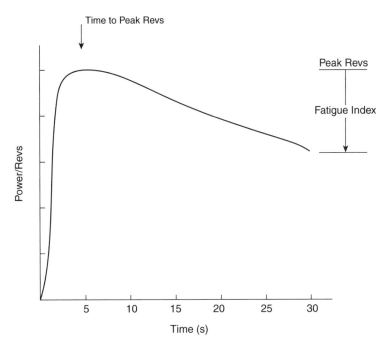

Figure 10.3 A typical power output (fly-wheel revolution) profile from a 30 s Wingate test. Note the sharp rise in the first few seconds, to peak power, and the gradual decline in power output over the remainder of the time

used to calculate power. The validity of the method and the resulting calculations has been questioned, however.

The principles underpinning the 30 s test have been applied to repeated-effort sports such as invasion games. The new test entails several short all-out efforts on the cycle ergometer interspersed with short recovery periods – e.g. 10 sprints of 6 s, with 10 s recovery between each sprint. The decline in peak revolutions provides a baseline against which we can measure post-training efforts. There are two major inter-linked problems for the coach. The first is whether the results from the exercise mode adopted – cycling – validly reflect running performance. The second is whether results from cycling or running are transferable to sports such as rowing and swimming.

The most recent attempt to assess anaerobic capacity is the maximal accumulated oxygen deficit (MAOD) devised in 1988. The procedure takes the linear relationship between sub-maximal running speed and oxygen consumption and estimates (by extrapolation) the oxygen consumption at supra-maximal exercise (Figure 10.4).

The test requires two stages. First, the progressive sub-maximal running test provides the speed/V_{O_2} relationship that we use to predict the supra-$V_{O_2 \, max}$.

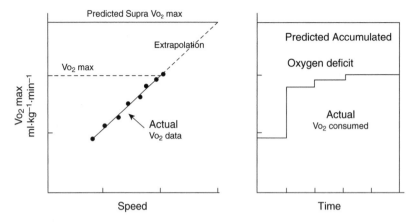

Figure 10.4   Calculating maximal accumulative oxygen deficit

Second, the athlete performs a maximal 2 min run, during which we record the actual oxygen consumption. The difference between the *actual* and the *predicted* oxygen consumptions gives us the maximal accumulated oxygen deficit; the greater the deficit, the greater the anaerobic capacity.

This approach is ingenious and offers an alternative to the simple measurement of excess post-exercise oxygen consumption (EPOC) used in the past to assess the extent of anaerobic metabolism during strenuous exercise. However, we have no sound evidence regarding the precise relationship between running speed and oxygen consumption whilst running at supra-maximal speeds.

Specificity of field tests

Most coaches want robust but uncomplicated ways of monitoring their athletes' progress. These must be administered within the training environment, thereby avoiding the costs in time, energy and finances associated with validated laboratory tests. The key issues of any test – field or laboratory – are the twin requirements of validity and reliability. For example, a running-based maximal oxygen uptake test for cyclists and swimmers might provide *reliable* information, but its *validity* is questionable. Validity entails specificity – the test measures what it is supposed to measure. Reliability entails repeatability – i.e. a standard stimulus always produces the same result every time. A test that has high reliability but lacks validity is fatally flawed; we are repeatedly measuring the wrong thing. High validity but low reliability is equally useless; here we are measuring the right thing, but the results are inconsistent.

Most tests require a maximal effort – how many press-ups/sit-ups in a minute, the 30 s Wingate test, the $V_{O_2\,max}$ test. The problem here is whether we can be certain that the athlete is making that maximal effort. A young healthy male subject undertaking a test to volitional exhaustion who stops at a heart rate of 150 beats min^{-1}, or a blood lactate level of 2 mmol L^{-1}, may not be motivated enough to make a truly maximal effort.

There are sub-maximal tests that predict maximal performance, which are particularly useful in fitness tests for the general population. The Lewis nomogram predicts anaerobic power from the Sargent jump and reach test. The Åstrand-Rhyming nomogram predicts maximal oxygen uptake from heart rates ranging from 120 to 170 beats min^{-1}. There are questions regarding the validity of the predictive processes used that, whilst not seriously affecting general fitness assessment and monitoring, make the use of these test in elite groups of questionable value.

One such test – the Cooper 12 minute run – predicts $V_{O_2\,max}$ from the distance completed in 12 minutes, was designed for general fitness testing and is highly motivation dependent. A minimum 3000 m completed within the time limit gives a rating of 'excellent' for a 20-year-old man and a predicted $V_{O_2\,max}$ of 56 mL kg$_{bm}$$^{-1}$ min^{-1}. For a woman of the same age, the distance required for the 'excellent' rating is 2300 m; this equates to a $V_{O_2\,max}$ of 40 mL kg$_{bm}$$^{-1}$ min^{-1}. For experienced athletes, the minimum distances for men and women are 3700 m and 3000 m, leading to predicted $V_{O_2\,max}$ of 71 and 56 mL kg$_{bm}$$^{-1}$ min^{-1} respectively.

We can apply this procedure to elite athletes. The men's record holder at 3 000 m is Daniel Komen of Kenya. If he were capable of maintaining his record pace for Cooper's 12 minutes, he would cover 4896 m; his predicted $V_{O_2\,max}$ would be 98 mL kg$_{bm}$$^{-1}$ min^{-1}. Haile Gebreselassie, the world 5000 m record holder, completed his run in 12 min 39.35 s. This pace over a 12 min run results in 4745 m and a $V_{O_2\,max}$ of 101 mL kg$_{bm}$$^{-1}$ min^{-1}. Taking the women's records we see a $V_{O_2\,max}$ of 88 mL kg$_{bm}$$^{-1}$ min^{-1} for the 3000m holder Wang Junxia, and $V_{O_2\,max}$ of 81 mL kg$_{bm}$$^{-1}$ min^{-1} for 5 00 m holder Jiang Bo. These predicted $V_{O_2\,max}$ values may be an over-estimate, and serve to illustrate the problems of valid predictions with elite athletes.

Recent advances in electronics – e.g. polar heart rate monitors and portable lactate analysers – have offered coaches additional useful information during training and even competitive events. However, these devices are more likely to be available in a laboratory rather than a field setting. The type of test favoured by many coaches requires not much more than a tape measure, a stopwatch and perhaps some cones.

The multi-stage fitness test is a well-known test used by many coaches, particularly those associated with sharp changes of direction such as football, rugby, hockey and tennis, and predicts an athlete's aerobic power. Repeated 20 m shuttle runs at increasing speed form the basis of the test. Audible signals, generated from a compact disc through an amplifier, dictate precisely the times for each 20 m shuttle and each level. A single audible signal controls the time allowed for a shuttle; three audible signals indicate an increase in speed of the next level. The duration of a level is $\sim$60 s, and there is a maximum of 23 levels. The starting speed at level 1 is $\sim$2.36 m s^{-1}, increasing by $\sim$0.14 m s^{-1} per level. The aim is to complete as many levels as possible in time with the set time frames. The more levels completed, the higher the predicted $V_{O_2\,max}$ derived from normative tables; the oxygen costs increase by $\sim$3 mL kg^{-1} min^{-1} for each level. A high degree of motivation is required for this test.

A simpler version, used by football coaches since the early 1960s, requires a 25 m course divided into 5 m sections. The athlete sprints to the first 5 m mark and touches the ground with the hand before returning to the start line, which must also be touched before progressing to the 10 m line, continuing until the full 25 m have been covered. The time for completing one shuttle is 30 s; recovery time between shuttles is 30 s. Note the number of shuttles completed within these time frames; the aim, based on match analysis, is 17 shuttles.

A running version of the Wingate 30 s cycle test of anaerobic power exists. It entails accurate timing of six all-out 35 m sprints with 10 s recovery between sprints. The derived SI unit for power (P) is joules per second ($J s^{-1}$), or the watt (W) – which is equal to 60 J s^{-1}. Power is the product of mass (M), length squared (L^2) and the reciprocal of time cubed (T^{-3}).

$$P = \frac{ML^2 J s^{-1}}{T^3}$$

To obtain an estimate of the power generated for each 35 m sprint, we require the mass of the athlete in kilograms and the time taken as the length is a standard 35 m. From these we can easily obtain peak and mean power, and the rate of power decay over the six sprints.

Recovery and rest

Rest and recovery are essential for all training programmes, but athletes often ignore these features. This can lead to over-training, loss of form and ultimately recurrent injury. The signs of over-training are present in three areas – physical, mental and technical. The physical indicators include weight loss; loss of appetite; increased resting heart rate; muscle and joint pain; listlessness; insomnia; headaches; gastro-intestinal problems; dehydration – small urine volume, dark yellow/brown in colour; repeated upper respiratory tract infections; raised levels of cortisol; reduced strength and endurance; slower recovery times; recurrent injuries. The mental signs are poor motivation; work avoidance; anxiety; depression; lack of concentration; uncooperativeness; giving up; melancholy; neuroticism. Technical signs include recurrence of bad habits; poor technique, particularly at key times; poor tactical and strategic decision making.

One of the key values of regular laboratory and field-testing lies in their ability to detect the onset of over-training through changes in various physiological markers including the following: changes in the balance between the twin stress hormones cortisol and dehydroepiandrosterone (DHEA) – i.e. raised cortisol and lower DHEA values; impaired immune function; increased white cell count; lowered lymphocyte count; reduced blood volume; increased ventilation, heart rate and blood lactate at standard work; slower recovery heart rates; lower maximal power output and maximal oxygen uptake.

A routinely taken waking heart rate is the most readily available predictor of over-training. Any persistent increase over several days is a cause for concern. A follow-up standardized sub-maximal exercise test recording heart rate, blood lactate and oxygen cost, is advisable; increases in each measure confirms the initial diagnosis.

The major cause of over-training lies in an inappropriate increase in the level of physical *demand*, such that the body's adaptive response fails; or incomplete *recovery* from the demand, or both. The inappropriate demand may result, singly or in combination, from an imbalance between the principles of volume, frequency, intensity and duration of sessions; inadequate recovery times within a training session; insufficient rest periods between training sessions and an excessive number of competitive events (e.g. successful football players – the Premier League, Champion's League, Carling Cup, FA Cup, international matches). The source of these imbalances may lie in an athlete with an addictive behaviour syndrome, an over-zealous coach or financial considerations for the sport's governing body.

It is difficult to prescribe a standard treatment to cover the many situations that may arise. The best approach is to prevent it happening in the first place. This requires a balance between sessions of low, moderate and high intensity sessions, a variety of training tasks, and careful attention to dietary regimes because of the danger of creeping glycogen depletion. Depending on the severity and duration of the symptoms, prolonged rest may be the only course open to athlete and coach; if injury or illness accompanies the diagnosis of over-training, this is often the case. In less severe cases, however, a short period – e.g. 3–5 days – of complete rest is advisable, followed by a gradual return, consisting primarily of low-intensity exercise, to a full training load. This controlled return is necessary to avoid the possibility of detraining – a feature of the final principle of reversibility.

Detraining

This principle, also known as reversibility, requires a grasp of the fact that what we can gain we can readily lose. An experiment conducted in 1968 examined the cardiovascular responses of young men to sub-maximal and maximal exercise following three weeks complete bed-rest. This extreme example of detraining may not be directly applicable to the over-trained athlete, but there are some useful pointers for athletes and coaches. For example, maximal oxygen uptake fell by an average of $\sim$27 per cent; the major contributory factor was a reduction of similar magnitude in maximal cardiac output through smaller stroke volume. Sub-maximal heart rate at a standard workload also rose markedly.

The interesting feature of the study relating directly to aerobic athletes is the finding that those with the highest $V_{O_2\,max}$ values at the start of the experiment not only lost a greater proportion of their aerobic power but also took longer to return to their original value during the recovery training programme. Sub-sequent research has confirmed that aerobic power and muscular endurance diminish following as little as 14 days of inactivity. Absolute strength and power appear to be less vulnerable to periods of reduced training; but even here, the research evidence points to an impaired power output during *technical* performance; this suggests that inconsistent practice leads quickly to a loss of precision in skills performance.

Practical implications

Just as with practice, training needs to be goal oriented. Not only does the coach need to know what they are doing but why; and this needs to be passed on to the athletes. One way in which this can be done is to carry out some formal testing of fitness. For coaches of professional athletes this may mean going to a laboratory and measuring a whole variety of performance indicators. It is best if the exercise physiologists explain to the athletes what each test means. For most coaches, however, simple tests such as the bleep test will have to suffice. It may simply be measuring how many press-ups or pull-ups in minute or how heavy one maximal lift is with the weights. No matter what test is used, it lets the athletes know where they stand. It helps set goals, so that the athlete has something to aim for.

Once the goals have been set the coach needs to work out the training schedule. In doing this he/she must take into account the four principles of training – progressive overload, specificity, recovery and reversibility. Progressive overload itself can be obtained by increasing intensity, duration and/or frequency. So you can increase the number of training sessions per week or make the sessions longer.

A very common way of developing the phosphagen system, which is commonly used for team game players, is to use interval training. The long-term goal is to have the players run for ~30 s, have 30 s rest and repeat this a chosen number of times. The actual number of times will depend on the nature of the game. We expect the players to run at ~90 per cent of their maximum speed. Most trained athletes can cover ~230 m (250 yards) in this time. Therefore, the maximum distance you wish to cover should be equivalent to that which time and motion studies have shown that players in your game run at speed. This is not easy and it is best to start with rest periods of about 1 min between runs. Some coaches start with the players covering ~50 per cent of the actual total distance at which they are aiming. Others split the number of runs up into sets of five, with the total running at 100 per cent of the distance run in a game. So the players cover a set of five, have a break of between 2 and 5 min, then complete another set and so on. As the players get better the rest interval between runs can be cut down until it reaches 30 s. Also, the number of runs per set can be increased until there is only one set.

A similar method can be used to train the anaerobic glycolytic system, although the runs will have to take more than 60 s to complete. The goal would be to get the athletes up to 90 s runs at 90 per cent speed. The length of run could be gradually increased. Similarly, the rest interval could be shortened or the number of repetitions increased, depending on the type of activity for which you are training. If you use interval training to work the aerobic system similar increases in length of run and lowering of rest intervals can be used. The most common way of training the aerobic system is simply to undertake long distance sub-maximal runs. The distance can be lengthened or the speed increased to aid progressive overload.

Task 1 Devise a series of training sessions for your own sport, showing the use of progressive overload. Try to make them as specific to the sport as possible.

In order to develop power, a strength base needs to be established. The maximum weight for one repetition should be obtained. Training can then be 90–95 per cent resistance with one to three repetitions. Re-testing should take place often and the maximum gradually increased. For power, the resistance would come down but more repetitions used and the movement be dynamic. The amount by which the resistance is lowered will depend on the end goal, as will the number of repetitions. Similarly, for the development of agility, flexibility must first be worked on. The range of movement can be gradually increased. When you move to agility work, the range may not be 100 per cent but the movement will be dynamic.

Task 2 *Do the same as for Task 1 except for sessions that develop power and agility.*

So far we have assumed that the athletes will be enthusiastic and enjoy the training; this is not always the case, especially with team game players. In Chapter 17, we show some ways of 'sugaring the pill' for game players. These are based on the principle of specificity. There are other ways however, such as making sessions competitive or giving rewards and punishments. Putting results of tests on a notice board has an effect with highly competitive athletes.

We should not forget the need to rest. Over-training is a problem, especially with track and field athletes, cyclists and swimmers. Rest periods need to be included and the reason for them pointed out. This, in itself, does not always solve the problem. I have seen athletes who have just been given the results of medical tests that showed over-training syndrome still go out and continue working hard. In Chapter 15, we look at how rest periods can be included in an annual programme. Good coaches will watch their athletes carefully for the effects of over-training. Good coaches also take into account the principle of reversibility. After lay-offs for injury or at the beginning of a new season the coach must not expect the athletes to be at the same level as when they last trained. This is why testing is necessary. It also shows the need for some sort of maintenance programme during the off-season (see Chapter 13).

Key points

- training should be goal oriented

- the four key principles of training are progressive overload, specificity, recovery and reversibility

- progressive overload requires the person to find their threshold – the point where existing biological mechanisms are stretched
  - training should ensure an adaptive response and a new higher threshold

- thresholds can be calculated by training heart rate; the relationships between heart rate and oxygen uptake; heart rate and blood lactate levels; heart rate and power output; power output and blood lactate levels; a percentage of $V_{O_2 max}$
  - training heart rate is calculated by [(maximum heart rate – resting heart rate) $\times$ 0.7] + resting heart rate

- strength is improved by weight training

- the threshold is calculated by a chosen percentage of maximum strength (the most lifted in one repetition)

- repeated training leads to the body adapting to the physiological stress

- overload needs to be progressive

- progressive overload is a balance between volume, frequency, duration and intensity of training
  - volume is such factors as distance covered, number of repetitions of an exercise
  - frequency is the number of sessions per day/week/cycle
  - duration is the length of time of each session
  - intensity represents the amount of physiological stress
  - intensity will determine the frequency and/or duration

- training should be specific
  - specificity is determined by analysis of the activity

- power requires training that incorporates speed and strength
  - strength requires slow actions with heavy weights
  - by increasing velocity power can be developed

- specific training requires a foundation, e.g. strength for power, aerobic base for anaerobic activity

- specificity must take account of the athlete's genetic make-up

- the anaerobic threshold refers to the point at which anaerobic metabolism begins to be used increasingly as a source of energy during exercise
  - at this point lactate is increased due to increases in muscle pH
  - this point is called the onset of blood lactate (OBLA)
  - OBLA is critical and performance after this cannot be maintained
  - OBLA occurs at different percentages of V_{O2}max in different people

- the Margaria step test and the Wingate 30 s test are used to examine anaerobic power
  - power is measured in watts (W)

- the maximum accumulated oxygen deficit (MAOD) also measures anaerobic capacity (see Figure 10.4)
  - there are two phases in the MAOD test
  - a progressive sub-maximal run from which the supra-V_{O2max} is calculated and
  - a maximal 2 min run during which oxygen consumption is calculated
  - the difference between actual and predicted oxygen consumption gives the MAOD value

- predictive tests can be used to estimate $V_{O_2 \, max}$
  - the Cooper 12 min run test is easy to administer
  - the multi-stage fitness test is commonly used in sport

- a running version of the Wingate test requires six all-out 35 m sprints
  - power is calculated by multiplying the athlete's mass by 35^2 (distance run squared) and dividing by the time taken cubed

- rest and recovery are essential for training

- over-training results if rest is not taken

- over-training results in
  - weight loss; loss of appetite; increased resting heart rate; muscle and joint pain; listlessness; headaches; gastro-intestinal problems; dehydration; respiratory infections; depression etc.
  - biochemical responses are raised cortisol and lower dehydroepiandrosterone (DHEA) levels; impaired immune function; reduced red blood volume; increased white cell count etc.

- lack of training leads to a detraining effect with the threshold falling (reversibility principle).

IV

Developmental Factors

Introduction

As we saw in Chapter 5, the developmental stage of the learner is one of the factors that the coach must take into account pre-instruction. It also affects how the coach should deal with the socio-psychological and physiological preparation of the athlete. In sports, developmental factors are more concerned with child development than with adult development or ageing. The latter should not be forgotten though, as some of you will be coaching sports such as golf or lawn bowls, which attract populations that are older than the more physically demanding sports. The bulk of this part of the book, however, is concerned with child development. Moreover, as we are interested in children of coachable age, we deal with children from 6 years onwards. It should be noted that the child has already gone through much in the way of development by this age. This is particularly so with regard to motor development and the physical and anatomical development of the brain.

Although I have divided this part into two chapters and sub-divided each chapter further, the reader should keep in mind the fact that development is holistic. Development in one area affects development in another. The behaviour of the person is the result of the interaction of all of the factors – cognitive, emotional, physiological and motor. The reader may also wish to keep in mind the fact that development is not as well researched as some of the other areas we cover in this book. A great deal more research is required.

Additional reading

Gallahue, D. L. and Ozmun, J. C. (1995). *Understanding motor development.* Brown and Benchmark: Madison, WI.

Piaget, J. (1952). *The origins of intelligence in children.* International Universities Press: New York.

11

Cognitive and Social Development

Learning objectives

At the end of this chapter, you should

- have a basic understanding of Piagetian theory
- have an understanding of mental space theory
- have an understanding of domain-specificity theory
- have an understanding of information processing theory explanations of cognitive development
- have a basic understanding of ecological psychology theories of cognitive and social devolvement
- have an understanding of selected theories of moral development.

In this chapter, we consider how the cognitive and social development of the individual, particularly that of children, affects the way in which they learn and play. We should note that social development is in many ways a sub-section of cognitive development. It is, perhaps, more affected by experience of social interaction than is cognitive development but it is, nevertheless, dependent on the person's ability to make sense of what he or she is experiencing. The main aim of this chapter is concerned with examining how theories of cognitive and social development aid our understanding of why and how individuals learn and

Coaching Science   Terry McMorris and Tudor Hale
© 2006 John Wiley & Sons, Ltd

behave. The implications for coaches are once again covered in the latter part of the chapter. We only examine the ageing process to a limited extent, as it is not so important in coaching as child development, but also because its inception and rate vary so greatly between individuals. Moreover, older individuals who engage in sport, have been shown to age more slowly than sedentary individuals. The best way of dealing with older adults is to assess each person individually rather than make general assumptions. Of course, this is also true for children but, with children, there are some fairly strong guidelines that will help.

Piagetian theory

The most widely cited cognitive developmental theorist is undoubtedly Jean Piaget. Piaget (1952, 1969) claimed that cognitive development occurred through a process that he termed 'adaptation'. Adaptation is an intellectual-ization of the individuals' need to make adjustments with respect to their interaction with the environment. It comes about through the processes of 'accommodation' and 'assimilation'. Accommodation is when the person adjusts his or her responses to meet the specific demands of a new situation, while assimilation is the incorporation of new information into previously learned cognitive structures. Changes are believed to occur in determined stages.

Piaget identified four stages of development: the sensorimotor phase (birth to 2 years), the preoperational thought phase (2 to 7 years), the concrete operations phase (7 to 11 years) and the formal operations phase (11 years onward). As we are concerned primarily with people of coachable age, we will concentrate on the last three stages. In the *preoperational thought* phase the child is interested in 'why' and 'how' things occur. The understanding of this is not through mental processes but through physically manipulating objects. In the next stage of cognitive development, the *concrete operations* stage, the child moves forward but his/her mental operations are still based on physical manipulations. The key issues are the use of rules for thinking, the ability to differentiate between appearance and reality, and the principle of reversibility, i.e. the capacity of the child to understand that changes in the environment can be reversed to their original positions. This capacity allows the child to think through a series of events or actions, and as such he/she can understand what happened and why. According to Piaget, perception, at this stage, is much better developed than at the preoperational thought stage.

Cognition at this stage, however, is still fairly simple. It consists of being able to respond to what the present environment affords. There is no attempt to manipulate the display to achieve personal goals. This does not occur until the *formal operations* stage. In this stage, the person develops a systematic approach to problem solving. Perhaps more importantly, deduction by hypothesis solving and judgment by implication allow the individual to mentally restructure the environment. This enables the performer to be innovative.

Mental space theory

The neo-Piagetian Pascual-Leone (1970) believes that, in normal children, age is the major determinant of a type of cognitive development that he calls 'structural mental capacity'. Structural mental capacity is the number of distinct schemes that are available to the person. He claims that by the age of 3 years the child has developed a basic mental capacity, which he calls '*e*'. Then every two years the child adds one more scheme to his/her initial repertoire, or *e*, until about 15 years. These changes occur during the sub-stages of Piaget's stages of development.

According to Pascual-Leone, individuals may have the same structural mental capacity but can differ in the amount of that capacity that they are able to utilize at any given time. Pascual-Leone calls the amount that can be used the 'functional mental capacity'. Therefore, cognitive development will be determined more by the interaction between the number of schemes available (structural mental capacity) and the amount that the person can utilize (functional mental capacity).

Domain-specificity theories

Theorists believing in domain-specificity theory (e.g. Roth, Slone and Dar, 2000) claim that there are probably two processes occurring as the child develops. One process they call the 'structural domain-general process', which is almost identical to the Piagetian theory of a generic stage of development. They believe that the second process is *domain specific*. Although the domain-general structure will affect the whole process of development, experience in a specific domain means that the child can be at different stages of development in different domains. It is not unusual to find children who are of average ability, or even below, in schoolwork but well above average at sports.

Task 1 Think about any children you know (or your friends during your school days): do (did) you know any whose ability in a particular domain is (was) well above their general stage of development?

Information processing theory and cognitive development

Although there is little empirical evidence to support Piagetian theory, which is based on observational and interview data, information processing theories of cognitive development are based on empirical data. Much research has been carried out that compares different age groups in the performance of tasks that measure the different factors that make up the information processing model, e.g. perception, short-term memory and reaction time. Like Piaget, information processing theorists give approximate chronological ages that correspond to when changes in information-processing capacity occur. Similar to Piaget, some accept that, if a child has considerable experience in a specific activity, a particular area could be better developed than others. Research into developmental aspects of perception has shown that static and dynamic visual acuity, depth perception and figure–ground perception (the ability to visually disembed an object from its background) all demonstrate periods of improvement from early childhood until the age of 12 years.

The proficiency of short-term memory in children has been examined by a number of researchers. Even in adults short-term memory has severe capacity limitations. While adults can handle 7 ± 2 bits of information, children's limitations are much more severe. Pascual-Leone claims that by 3 years the child can handle one bit of information. Every two years, from then on, the child adds one more bit as its structural mental capacity increases (see Table 11.1). Adults overcome the capacity problems by utilizing strategies such as chunking, i.e. joining several pieces of information together to make one bit. An example of chunking in sport would be remembering a triple jump as one movement rather than three. Chunking can be used by children as young as 5 years old, but only if the child is shown how to do so. Spontaneous chunking is thought to develop at about 9 years old. Spontaneous adult type rehearsal, also, occurs at about the age of 9 years. Rehearsal refers to physically and/or mentally practising the

Table 11.1 Pascual-Leone's stages of structural mental capacity

Age	Mental capacity	Piagetian stage
3 and 4 years	$e + 1$	pre-operational
5 and 6 years	$e + 2$	pre-operational
7 and 8 years	$e + 3$	concrete operations
9 and 10 years	$e + 4$	concrete operations
11 and 12 years	$e + 5$	formal operations
13 and 14 years	$e + 6$	formal operations
15+ years	$e + 7$	formal operations

skill. All of this has particular importance in the child's ability to develop a significant long-term memory store, because without rehearsal the information will not transfer from short-term memory to long-term memory.

It is this limited long-term memory store that causes the most problems for the child in processing information. It has particularly inhibiting effects on decision making. If decision making depends on the person's ability to compare the present situation with past experiences stored in long-term memory, then a poor long-term memory store must hamper decision making. Furthermore, the limited long-term memory store severely affects selective attention and anticipation. Due to limited past experience, the child is not able to differentiate between relevant and irrelevant stimuli and, therefore, processes much information that is irrelevant. Similarly, the child is unable to recognize patterns of movement that would allow him/her to anticipate the actions of others, as the child has no memory of similar actions observed in the past.

Ecological psychology theories and cognitive development

It could be argued that ecological psychology theories of cognitive development have their basis in the work of the Russian Lev Vygotsky (1978). Vygotsky believes that development comes about due to an interaction between the child and his/her environment. Hence the appeal to the ecological psychologists. Vygotsky argued that a child moves forward when he/she reaches the *zone of proximal development*, i.e. the child is ready physically and mentally to acquire new skills. When this is reached it is possible for significant others to stimulate the child to acquire new skills. The term *bootstrapping* was given to this process, as it is seen as a 'pulling together' of potential and actual levels of ability. The significant others could be parents, coaches, teachers or even other children. This explanation fits in with the claims of the ecological psychologist Uri Bronfenbrenner (1989; Bronfenbrenner and Ceci, 1994) that the child possesses 'actualized' and 'non-actualized genetic potential'. Actualized genetic potential is like Pascual-Leone's functional mental capacity; it is the amount of genetic potential that the individual is actually using at that given time. Non-actualized genetic potential is the amount of ability not being utilized. Actualized and non-actualized genetic potential combined is similar to Pascual-Leone's structural mental capacity, i.e. it is the limit of the individual's potential due to genetics and rate of neuropsychological growth. Bootstrapping means adding more of the non-actualized potential to the actualized.

Although the ecological psychologists believe that there is such a thing as non-actualized genetic potential, which limits the levels to which an individual can aspire at any given time, they are strong believers in domain specificity. van Geert (1993) uses the term 'species' to describe domains. Examples of species could be problem solving, vocabulary and sport. Although van Geert believes, like Bronfenbrenner and Ceci, that a species will only develop if attention is paid to it, he claims that there are capacity limitations and that attention to one species will be at the expense of another species. However, growth in one species can support growth in another related species, e.g. growth in problem solving in non-sports domains might support growth in decision making in sport.

A comparison of the different approaches to cognitive development

Although coming from different schools of psychology, the theories of cognitive development outlined in the previous section are remarkably similar. The major difference appears to be in the identification of generalizable stages of development. Both Piagetian and information processing theorists would argue that individuals go through recognizable stages. They accept that a person may be at a higher or lower stage in any given domain, at any specific time, but overall the individual will be at a recognizable stage of development. Although ecological psychology approaches place greater emphasis on specificity of stages within any given domain, or to use van Geert's word species, they do not deny that individuals go through stages within a species. Moreover, they accept that the genetic potential of the person, at any given age, will impose limitations on how far the individual can progress. Even those following a domain-specificity approach accept that there is a genetic process, which they call domain-general development.

Piagetian theory and ecological psychology theory are very similar in the way in which they explain the process of development. Both place great emphasis on the interaction between the individual and the environment. Both schools accept that an environment rich in experience can improve the likelihood of the actualization of genetic potential, but cannot overcome limited genetic potential. According to Piaget, a rich environment is likely to lead the child to attempt adaptation and hence improve the chances of development. The ecological psychologists argue that such an environment motivates the child to attend to proximal processes, resulting in developmental advances.

Task 2 Draw up a list of abilities that develop in children from 7 years old to 14 years. Write down points of agreement and disagreement between Piagetians and ecological psychologists on how these developments occur.

Social development

Piaget, Vygotsky and Bronfenbrenner all see social development as being an interaction between cognitive development and the social experiences of the individual. To Piaget, social development follows the same pattern as cognitive development and is dependent on the child's stage of cognitive development. In the preoperational thought stage, the child moves slowly from undertaking behaviour that is almost totally egocentric, concerned with self-gratification, to becoming aware that he/she must interact with others. However, the child remains shy and self-conscious. Children at this stage will, and do, play with others but their concern is with their own enjoyment not the group's. Moreover, their attention span is relatively short.

There is not a great change in social development when the child moves into the concrete operations stage. Although the child is able to play in large groups, this appears to be limited in terms of time. Attention span is still fairly short, although it increases during this stage. Conversely, however, children at this stage will spend hours on activities that interest them. Although they remain self-centred, towards the end of this stage they begin to become interested in being part of a group. Affiliation starts to become an important social factor.

The most radical changes in social development occur during the formal operations stage. However, whether this is due to changes in cognitive development or physiological and neuropsychological changes due to the onset of adolescence is a debatable point. The need for affiliation tends to become very important at this stage. Adolescents like to be part of a group and enjoy cooperating with other group members. They enjoy competing against other individuals and other groups. Gender issues become far more important at this stage. This can have major implications for sports participation and we deal with this later in this chapter.

Vygotsky and the ecological psychologists, while agreeing that cognitive development affects social development, are less concerned with stages. Vygotsky sees social development as being dependent on the child's exposure to a variety of stimuli in the form of needing to interact with someone else, and the development of appropriate responses to situations. He sees the success of these interactions as leading to the repetition of the response. Success may be in the form of the approval of significant others or in the child achieving his/her goals. For example, if the child is seeking to be part of a group and certain responses result in acceptance by the group that behaviour will be repeated. Vygotsky accepts that the child's stage of cognitive development will affect how well he/she is to be able to perceive accurately the outcome of his/her actions. Limited cognitive ability would mean that children may not be aware of the consequences of their actions, while more advanced thinking would help children perceive the results of their actions. The ecological psychologists follow an almost identical line of thought to Vygotsky. In fact, there is hardly any difference between any of the schools of thought.

Moral development

Moral development affects the way in which the individual adheres to the rules of play, and the attitude towards and treatment of officials, opponents and team-mates. Thus a knowledge of how we develop our philosophy of morality can help the coach to understand how the athlete will react in any situation. To Vygotsky and the ecological psychologists, moral development is determined by the experiences of social interaction. It is a domain of cognitive development and follows the same rules as development in other domains. To the Piagetians and neo-Piagetians, moral development is a sub-section of cognitive development. Piaget perceived the chid as going through three main stages, closely linked with the stages of cognitive development. He called his first stage the *premoral*. From birth to 4 years the child, according to Piaget, has no understanding of rules or right and wrong. From 4 to 9 or 10 years the child goes through the stage of *moral realism*. As can be expected from children in the preoperational thought and concrete operations stages of cognitive development, the child responds to factual outcomes. Rules come from people with authority and the failure to accept these rules can lead to unpleasant experiences, e.g. punishment. Rules are laid down and children cannot change them. At the age of about 10 years, when the person reaches the formal operations stage of cognitive development, he or she enters the *moral subjectivism* stage. Rules are agreed upon by people and people can agree to change the rules. Furthermore, rules and laws should by determined by moral principles.

Piaget's theory of moral development has to a large extent been superseded by that of one of his followers, Lawrence Kohlberg. Kohlberg (1976) also named three stages, but actually called them levels and sub-divided each level into two stages. The first level he called *preconventional morality*. As this is mainly concerned with children who are too young to undertake sports coaching, we will leave this and move to the *conventional morality* level. At this level, children try to follow the rules and carry out the duties that they see as being expected of them by society. Decisions of what represents morality are not theirs but are imposed upon them by significant others. In the first stage, the need for approval is the motivation for behaving morally, while at the second stage rules are adhered to in order to comply with formal customs. Kohlberg calls his final phase the *postconventional morality* level. In the first stage the person is keen not to violate the rights of others and is aware of social contracts – formal and informal. In the second stage, the emphasis is on the underlying principles of equality and social equilibrium rather than the 'letter of the law'.

Ageing

In this chapter, we have concentrated particularly on child development and largely ignored changes in cognition and social interaction in old age. This has been deliberate because it is difficult to actually pinpoint when cognition begins to deteriorate and social interactions change. Indeed, the latter are probably more affected by changes in the individual's social situation rather than anything to do with development *per se*. The person who takes up lawn bowls, after many years playing hockey or rugby, is probably doing so because his or her motivation for affiliation or competition or mastery remains the same rather than diminishing or changing. He or she would probably like to keep playing the physically more demanding game but unfortunately, because of physical development or ageing, cannot. He or she is not going through a developmental stage of moving to more genteel games but simply continuing to be competitive. Try telling the competitive bowler that this is just a 'bit of fun' for 'old men and women'.

Ageing cognitively is also difficult to gauge. There are definite physical changes in the brain that affect cognitive functioning but when this begins varies greatly from person to person. Moreover, there is substantial evidence to show that having an active lifestyle helps to slow the ageing process. Deteriorations in eyesight and hearing, however, can affect perception, and we know that the older we get the slower our reaction time becomes. This may be indicative of a slowing of cognitive functioning. It would be silly of coaches, however, to make assumptions concerning a relationship between an individual's cognitive ability and their chronological age.

Practical implications

In this section, we will examine how cognitive and social development affect factors such as performance, learning and motivation. Moreover, we will look at how they often interact to affect these processes. It must be remembered, however, that physical and motor development may also interact with the developmental changes, outlined in this chapter, to affect performance and learning.

Skilled performance

From a performance point of view, cognitive developmental factors have a major bearing on the learning of decision making. Below I give some examples of how this occurs. These are taken from a more comprehensive review (McMorris, 1999). Children in Piaget's preoperational thought stage can master fairly simple decisions. Simple 1 vs 1 type tasks provide the child with a display that is not too demanding and the type of decisions require the child to think in simple terms; e.g., in tennis, if there is a space to my opponent's left, I can hit the ball into that space. If we follow the principle of bootstrapping, the child must be introduced to new problems once the simple ones are mastered. If we move to 2 vs 2 games, the child has to deal with more perceptual information. This, in itself, should lead to advances in the domain of perception, as the environment forces the child to interact in a more sophisticated manner than in the 1 vs 1 situation. However, without intervention from the coach or teacher, advances in decision making may not occur. Without help the child may not be able to determine what is relevant and what is irrelevant information. With help, however, such tasks are within the capability of children in the preoperational thought stage.

Children in the preoperational thought stage can see that, when playing in a singles game of tennis, if you hit the ball straight to your opponent he or she is more likely to return it than if you hit it to one side or the other. Children in the concrete operations stage can go further. They understand that, if they hit the ball to one side, their opponent will have to move to that side in order to return the ball. Furthermore, they can see that, if the opponent is unable to get back into the centre of the court when the ball is returned, they can hit it into the space vacated by their opponent and win the point. Even in more complex team games, e.g. basketball and ice hockey, they are able to understand that it is better to pass the ball (or puck) to an unmarked team-mate than to one who is marked. They can also understand defensive duties such as marking an opponent when the opposition has the ball/puck. However, at this stage the child is still making decisions in a simplistic way, responding to the present display rather than thinking ahead and working on strategies to defeat the opposition. At the formal operations stage, the child should be introduced to more complex displays and decisions should require more in the way of cognitive restructuring skills, e.g. the use of decoy runs, in Rugby or basketball, to create space for others.

> **Task 3** *Choose a skill, preferably one that requires interaction with team-mates and opponents. Write down how you would expect 7-, 10- and 14-year-olds to differ in how they perform the skill.*

Optimal periods of learning

Both Piagetian and ecological psychologists believe that it is not possible to separate cognitive and socio-emotional aspects of development. Moreover, these will in turn be affected by physical and motor development. It has long been thought that there are periods in which the interaction between development in each of these areas is ideal for the person to learn. These times are known as *critical periods of learning*. The term 'critical' is based on animal studies. When animals do not learn a particular skill at the critical time, they either do not acquire it at all or acquire a very inferior version. Something similar happens with humans but not as severely, and we can learn at a time after the critical period. As a result, Robert Singer (1968) coined the phrase 'optimal periods of learning'. This is a more accurate explanation. One of the skills of coaching is being able to recognize when these periods arise. Attempting to get someone to work at acquiring a skill that he or she is not ready to attempt may not merely be fruitless but may also have a negative effect on motivation. It could even lead to the young athlete dropping out of the activity altogether. These periods are similar to Vygotsky's zones of proximal processes.

> **Task 4** *How might the interaction between physical and social development affect when it is best to introduce tackling in rugby or American football?*

Practice

In Part II of this text, we examined what the motor learning literature has to say about the nature of practice. The theories of practice found in the motor learning literature tend to come from laboratory based studies and studies with adults, particularly physical education and sports science students. While these undoubtedly have a great deal to tell us, they are limited ecologically, particularly with regard to children. Research into practice has generally been concerned primarily with the task and has shown only a limited attempt to examine socio-psychological factors. Indeed, developmental issues have been almost totally ignored, even in the physical education literature. Therefore, in this section we examine the issues that a knowledge of cognitive and social development have on the decision of what and how to practice.

As we have already seen, with regard to the learning of decision making in sport, the child's limitations in long-term memory, selective attention and anticipation must be taken into account when devising a practice. We must also take into account factors such as reaction time and figure–ground perception. It is common to see young children placed in practices that overload their cognitive and perceptual abilities. From a basic skill acquisition point of view, practices with young children need to be fairly simple, i.e. low in numbers and not demanding much in the way of selective attention and decision making. From a social psychology perspective this is also advantageous. Children under the age of 10 years can only play with small numbers of other children and even then for only short periods of time. While this may appear to be a negative point, it can be very advantageous. Children at this age are happy to work by themselves and practise basic skills. This is the time to develop technical ability.

The life stories of legendary sports performers show that most developed a wide range of techniques in this period of their lives. The great ice hockey player Wayne Gretsky leaps to mind, not to mention the football player Pelé. Another interesting issue with children of this age is a somewhat paradoxical one. Although generally their attention span is short, they will practise for long periods of time on skills that they enjoy doing. This is especially so if the practice can be subtly altered from time to time. An example of this can be seen in Figure 11.1. In (a) A passes the ball to B and runs forward to the back of the opposite line. In (b) A passes to B but this time turns and runs to the back of the line behind him. The real task, the passing, remains the same but the change in direction of movement following performance of the skill stops the individual becoming bored. This drill also helps the child develop the comparatively basic movement skill of turning.

The under 10 years old period of time is one in which we should be encouraging children to develop a wide range of technical abilities. This technical ability is the 'building block' for complex skills. Trying to get children to learn these basics later in life can be counterproductive, as we have seen with the notion of optimal periods of learning. If, however, they have sound basic skills by the age of 11 years they are ready to develop their ability to play with others in a team.

Children from 11 years onwards start to become interested in playing in teams and competing against one another. They are far less likely to enjoy

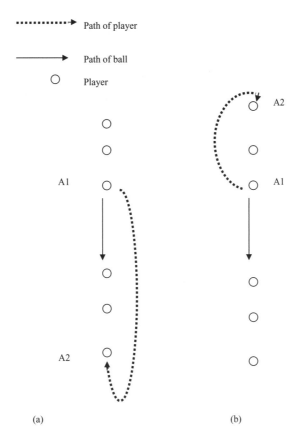

- - - - - - - - → Path of player

———————→ Path of ball

○   Player

(a)   (b)

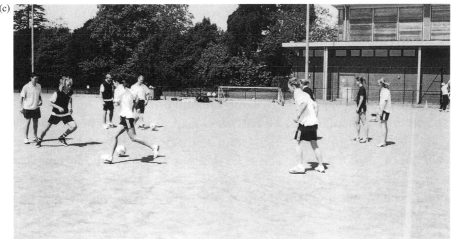

(c)

Figure 11.1 (a) and (b) show a diagrammatic representation of two simple drills, while (c) and (d) show the same drills photographically. In (a) the ball is passed from one line to the other and the passer joins the opposite line. In (b) the passing is the same but the passer runs and re-joins his own line. By changing the direction of the run, the coach can keep young children happy and motivated

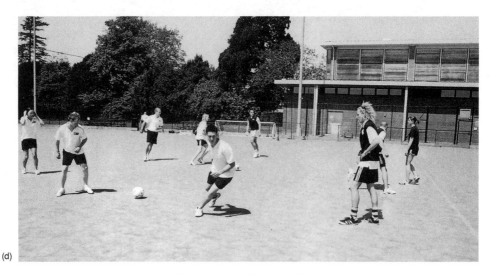

(d)

Figure 11.1   *(Continued)*

taking part in small practices and want to play a game. At 11 years they are not capable of playing games such as football, hockey and rugby in full-sided matches but are capable of handling five- and six-a-side games. Games such as netball, ice hockey and basketball can be played in the full-sided versions. If children have learned the basic skills properly then, at this stage, they are ready to develop their decision-making skills. However, if they have been poorly coached in the early years their technical skill is so poor that they are not ready to learn more complex decision-making skills or even develop more advanced skills in six-a-side games. Many years ago I had the pleasure of coaching the former England international football player Paul Gascoigne, when he was a young boy, on a number of coaching courses organized by Gateshead Borough Council in conjunction with Durham Football Association. By the age of 11 years Paul had already mastered most basic skills so he was ready to work at more advanced skills and, in particular, develop his decision making. This is a good example of the point I made at the end of the last paragraph. Paul was also a good example of someone whose development in one domain, football, was way above his development in other domains.

Task 5 Choose a skill and devise a number of practices for 7-, 10- and 14-year-olds; assuming that all are beginners. What are your reasons for choosing these particular practices and, in particular, why do they differ? (If they do not, you are doing something incorrectly.)

Motivation

Children follow similar patterns of motivation to adults and indeed achievement motivation theory developed out of the study of motivation in children.
Some researchers have claimed that children under 11 years are more concerned about participation in its own right rather than comparing themselves
with other people. This makes sense if we accept that young children are
egocentric and tend to play alone or in small groups. It has also been claimed
that young children confuse ability with effort. Very recently these claims have
been questioned and some evidence that children can differentiate between
individuals based on the quality of performance has been presented. There
appears to be little doubt that, as children approach adolescence, they are
becoming fairly stable in their self-perception. Rightly or wrongly they make
comparisons of their own and others' ability. This can have major ramifications
for the desire to continue to compete and perhaps more so for the level of
aspirations of individuals. In my years of teaching physical education, it never
ceased to amaze me how many children had 'written themselves off' as sports
performers because they had not done well at primary school. In some cases it
was not possible to get the child to realize that they were, in fact, much better
than their peers and primary school teachers had imagined.

On the other hand, many children who have some ability but little desire to
perform in sport may begin to do so at about 11 and 12 years old because they
wish to be part of a group. While this is positive, the opposite also happens,
particularly with girls. The desire to be part of the group often causes
adolescent girls to 'drop out' of sport. While adolescence may result in many
boys starting to take up physical activity to show off their masculinity, many
girls perceive sport as not being feminine, therefore they lose interest. These
girls can, and do, put great pressure on other girls to join them. The power of
such pressure groups can be very persuasive. It is sad, but true, that many girls,
even today in supposedly more enlightened times, drop out at this stage because
they do not wish to be perceived as being unfeminine.

Playing in the spirit of the game

Many coaches do not see fostering playing in the right spirit as being part of
their domain. Sport governing bodies, however, have made definite moves
towards getting coaches to develop the correct attitudes towards officials and
opponents. Moral development would appear to have an affect on how ready
and willing children are to play to the rules. If we follow Kohlberg's theory, we

would expect children at the conventional level of development to play to the rules, as they see morality as something imposed on them by important others such as adults. At the first stage of the postconventional level, children are unlikely to break the rules, particularly those they see as being mutually agreed to. This is because they see violation of the rights of others as being socially unacceptable. At the second stage, however, the child is likely to break rules that they see as being generally disregarded by most players. For example, basketball is supposed to be a non-contact sport. Few players take any notice of this and therefore the child at this stage will not perceive using contact as being unacceptable conduct. However, the child will obey the 'unwritten rules' of basketball. For example, although holding an opponent is against the rules, placing one arm across the offensive post and one behind their back, thus stopping them from sliding back into the space left by the defensive post, is considered acceptable and is rarely punished by the referee. However, hitting a player while he/she is in the air is considered totally unacceptable.

Task 6 Can you think of similar activities that are accepted and unaccepted by the 'unwritten' rules in your own sport?

There is some evidence, however, to show that children are likely to copy their favourite performers rather than follow the stages as proposed by Kohlberg. This is, of course, in line with Bandura's observational learning theory. Therefore, it is not unusual to see young football players commit the so called 'professional foul' because this is what their heroes would do. On a more positive side, children will follow the example of professionals in shaking hands at the end of a game. This is despite the fact that one would not expect this to happen until after the age of 11 years as prior to that children are very egocentric and the skills of others are of little concern to them. This is only a small gesture but can lead to children learning to win and lose graciously.

Summary

When dealing with young athletes, in particular, coaches should take into account the developmental stage of the performer. They must be careful to differentiate between chronological age and developmental age. Psychometric tests are not readily available to coaches so they have to rely on their own observational skills. A working knowledge of the 'norm' for each age is an excellent aid. Coaches should be aware that children can be very advanced in the domain of sport even if their general development is not up to the 'norm'. Coaches should also be aware of times of life that can result in major developmental changes, particularly puberty. The move into adulthood can have a major effect on child development and, in turn, on motivation and performance in sport.

An awareness that cognitive, social, physical and motor devolvement combine to define the optimal period of learning for any activity is very important. A child may be cognitively ready to learn decision-making skills in hockey, for example, but not socially ready to play in team game situations. The opposite also happens. A child who has missed out on learning the basic techniques may really need to focus on basic skills in drill type practices. However, socially they may prefer to play in game type situations. This is, in fact, a very common situation. It is best, in such cases, to make some kind of compromise. Basic skills can be learned in game situations, with just a little imagination from the coach.

Key points

Cognitive development

- according to Piaget, development occurs through the process of adaptation, i.e. the person's need to adjust with respect to their interaction with the environment

- adaptation is the result of accommodation and assimilation
  - accommodation is the adjustment of responses to new situations
  - assimilation is incorporating new information into already learned behaviours

- according to Piaget:
  - in the preoperational stage (2–7 years), the child is interested in physically exploring the environment
  - in the concrete operations phase (7–11 years), the child can react to changes in the environment but cannot consciously act upon the environment to create changes
  - in the formal operations stage (11+ years), the person can act upon the environment to create opportunities for action and has a systematic approach to problem solving

- according to Pascual-Leone, development is determined by the interaction between structural and functional mental capacity
  - structural mental capacity is the number of schemes available to the child
  - functional mental capacity is the amount of schemes the child can actually use

- the domain-specificity theorists believe that there are two processes affecting development, the structural domain general and the domain specific
  - the structural domain-general process is a generic stage of development
  - the domain-specific process refers to the child's ability in any given area or domain
  - domain-specific development can be considerably different to domain-general development but is affected by it

- according to the information processing theorists, the child's information processing capacity improves with age up to about 12 years old

- short-term memory is affected by developments in
  - capacity
  - chunking
  - rehearsal

- improvements in long-term memory aid the development of selective attention

- Vygotsky claimed that increases in developmental capacity occur when the child reaches a zone of proximal processes, i.e. cognitive, social and/or physical changes mean that they are ready to acquire new skills
  - coaches can act as facilitators of this process

- according to the ecological psychologists, the child possess actualized and non-actualized genetic potential
  - actualized genetic potential is the amount of potential being used by the child
  - non-actualized genetic potential represents the resources not being used
  - actualized plus non-actualized genetic potential represents the child's full capacity

- ecological psychologists believe in domain-specificity

Social development

- according to Piaget, in the preoperational thought phase children move from being egocentric to becoming aware that they must interact with others
  - their concern remains their own enjoyment not the group's

- in the concrete operations phase, there is little change but they can play in larger groups
  - attention span is short

- in the formal operations stage, the need for affiliation increases
  - adolescents enjoy competition and cooperation

- according to Piaget, moral development follows similar patterns to cognitive development
  - in the preoperational thought and concrete operations phases, rules are set by adults and cannot be altered
  - in the formal operations phase, rules are mutually agreed upon and can be changed

- according to Kohlberg, in the conventional morality phase children will follow the rules

- in the postconventional morality phase, the child follows underlying principles of equality and social equilibrium

Practical implications

- cognitive development affects the complexity of the display with which children can deal perceptually and with regard to decision making

- optimal periods of learning refer to the time when the child is cognitively, socially, emotionally and physically ready to learn a skill.

12

Physiological and Motor Development

Learning objectives

At the end of this chapter, you should

- know the stages of development used by motor developmentalists
- understand the main physiological changes that take place during late childhood and adolescence
- understand the main physiological and motor effects of ageing
- understand selected theories of motor development
- understand the implications of development for the coach.

In this chapter, we examine the physiological and motor development of children from 6 years onwards and also the ageing adult. Motor developmentalists divide the stages of development into *prenatal* (conception to birth), *infancy* (birth to 2 years), *childhood* (2 years to puberty), *adolescence* (puberty to 20 years), *young adulthood* (20 to 40 years), *middle adulthood* (40 to 60 years) and *older adulthood* (60+ years). Childhood is often sub-divided into the *toddler period* (2 to 3 years), *early childhood* (3 to 5 years), *middle childhood* (5 to 7 years) and

Coaching Science   Terry McMorris and Tudor Hale
© 2006 John Wiley & Sons, Ltd

later childhood (7 years to puberty). There are some variations on this, however, and some authors include the toddler period in early childhood.

These stages are also useful when discussing physiological development. Although we concentrate on 6+ years, the reader is reminded than the majority of motor development takes place before 6 years. The key times for physiological development are in infancy and during adolescence. The implications of changes during adolescence are very important with regard to physical training. The interaction between physical changes in adolescence and cognitive and emotional development are major issues in the effect of development on sports coaching.

Physiological development

In this section, we examine physiological development during late childhood, adolescence and in older adults. It is difficult, in all of the stages, to differentiate between development and the effects of physical activity. Moreover, the types of test chosen by researchers will also affect results. In the case of children, the experimental evidence has generally been taken from North American children, although we do have more recent research by Neil Armstrong and his colleagues at Exeter University that give some examples of the situation in Britain. Nevertheless, we should be aware that research is limited. Above all, the reader should remember that all ages given are gross generalizations and individuals can differ greatly.

Late childhood

The period of late childhood is one of relatively little change physiologically. Growth is slow. Average gains in height are about 5–7.6 cm (2–3 inches) per year and increases in body mass are also slow, about 1.4–2.7 kg (3–6 lbs) per year. The development tends to follow the *cephalocaudal* (head to toe) and *proximodistal* (centre to periphery) principle put forward by Gesell (1945). This means that development follows a head to toe and centre to periphery timetable. It also results in large muscles being considerably more developed than smaller ones. Throughout this period girls tend to be about one year ahead of boys. The increase in height and weight is accompanied by slow increases in muscular strength and endurance, speed and agility. However, flexibility tends to show slight decreases after the age of 10 years. Girls are more flexible than boys.

$V_{O_2 max}$ improves slowly during this period but it is difficult to know to what extent this is due to maturation *per se*. Improvements in the cardiovascular system are very much affected by the lifestyle of the individual. Children taking part in sports are likely to show much greater improvements than those who are not active. Maximum heart rate can reach similar levels to that of adults but it is rare that children can push themselves to achieve this. Resting heart rates are similar to adults throughout this period, 60–80 beats min^{-1}.

Adolescence

Pubescence sees a growth spurt, which lasts about 4.5 years. Girls begin adolescence at about 9 years old and boys about two years later. The peak of the growth spurt occurs about two years after its start. Girls continue to increase in height until they are 16 years old and boys until 18 years. The increase in height can be dramatic, even as much as 15–20 cm (6–8 inches) in a year. Weight increases in boys tend to occur almost simultaneously with height. The increase in boys' weight during adolescence is due mostly to increased height and muscle mass. Increases in girls' weight, however, are due to increases in adipose tissue as well as height and muscle mass. Indeed, muscle mass in girls increases less than in boys. Girls' increases in weight lag a little behind their increases in height.

$V_{O_2 max}$ increases for both sexes during this period, although there is a levelling off for girls at about 12 years. Boys have higher $V_{O_2 max}$ values than girls following adolescence; this tends to disappear when we measure oxygen uptake against lean muscle mass. Thus, it is the increase in adipose tissue that is the limiting factor for females. Females also lag behind males in speed, agility, power and muscular endurance, probably due to the fact that male increases in muscle mass are greater than female. However, females remain more flexible. Flexibility can be seriously disrupted during the growth spurt. Bone growth precedes muscle and tendon growth, making it difficult for the individual to have a good range of movement around their joints. As muscles and tendons 'catch up', the problem dissipates.

Ageing

Making generalizations with older adults is more precarious than making generalizations with children and adolescents. I am sure you all know people who are 'fit for their age' and many who are 'unfit for their age'. Cardiovascular and muscular fitness are both supposed to peak around the mid-20s to early 30s. There is then a slow decline up to about 50 years, followed by a fairly rapid decline. This decline accelerates even further at about 70 years. However, a physically active lifestyle can mean that the process is slowed greatly. At the time of writing, the world record for 100 m for 70-year-old men is 13.0 s, for 50-year-olds it is a remarkable 11.2 s, while the record for 40-year-olds is 10.6 s. This gives you some idea of what older people can achieve.

Task 1 At what age do most athletes retire in your sport? Are there many exceptions? What do you think are the main physiological reasons for athletes retiring in your sport?

Motor development

The study of motor development is vital to the coach who is going to work with children or older adults. Motor developmental studies have identified what we can expect people of different stages of cognitive, social and physiological development to be capable of doing. Motor developmentalists tend to provide a litany of skills that can be performed at different ages or, more precisely, a description of how individuals perform basic skills at different stages of development. These lists are found especially in books that draw on information processing theory as the basis of their assumptions of how humans perform. They are, however, also to be found in some texts that draw more heavily on ecological psychology principles (e.g. Haywood and Getchell, 2001). This is despite the fact that the ecological psychologists do not perceive development as progressing in stages. Ecological psychology is more concerned with how the individual develops a movement pattern or skill rather than when a pattern emerges. They emphasize individual differences in when and how skills are developed. Indeed, most of what you will find written in ecological psychology developmental texts is the same as that found in ecological explanations of skill acquisition.

One of the reasons for motor development texts placing so much emphasis on what and how individuals, particularly children, perform at any given age is because there is a wealth of biomechanical research which shows the changes in patterns of movement. If one generalizes, you could say that the changes tend to occur at specific stages of development. Moreover, as with cognitive development, it could be argued than these changes generally occur at certain chronological ages.

There is undoubtedly a great deal of experimental data to show that children of different ages demonstrate different levels of maturity in the way they perform skills. However, there are also some factors that make the decision to definitively proclaim these as motor developmental stages somewhat dubious.

First of all, many children are above or behind the norms for the different skills. More importantly, a child's 'developmental' stage in any particular skill appears to be specific to that skill. It cannot be generalized to other skills. There is often a mismatch even between the different components of a skill. A child might demonstrate a mature pattern in one aspect of a skill but an immature one in another aspect. For example, a child throwing a ball may have a mature arm movement but the leg movements of someone at a much lower stage. This is not as unusual as you might think.

It is impossible to know to what extent the child is performing at a given level because of developmental factors or experience. Therefore, great care must be taken when we examine the literature in this area. However, the literature does give good examples of the development of movement patterns as a skill is acquired. If we examine the descriptions provided, and then watch children in action, it is easy to see at which stage any given child is at that moment in time. As coaches, that is the main factor. Whether our athlete is ahead of or behind his/her contemporaries is not the issue. It is where our athletes are that matters. If we know this then we can help them to further develop their skills, either to 'catch up' to the others or go even further ahead.

Task 2 *Look at a basic motor development text and examine the stages of performing basic skills. When you see children performing these skills, do they appear to follow what is in the textbooks?*

In this section, as with the previous sections in this part of the book, we examine only the stages from 6 years onwards. It should be noted, however, that most motor development takes place in infancy and the toddler period. There are many good texts that cover these periods and it may well be in your interests to examine some of these. This will be especially so if you are coaching children who are 6 years old or less.

Theories of motor development

The motor development literature tends to focus on theories of cognitive and social development, such as Piaget's theory or theories of physiological development such as Gesell's, rather than specific motor development theory. In fact, most so called motor development theories are no more than descriptions of the ages at which research has shown children to be able to perform certain skills. Mostly they provide comment on how each aspect of the skill develops though the different stages. For example, when throwing a ball, children in the early childhood period will not move their feet. As they move into middle childhood, they will step forward but with the foot on the same side of the body as the throwing arm. When they reach late childhood, they will move forward with the other foot (Wild, 1938). In this example, I have only focused on what Wild had to say about the feet. He, in fact, covered the whole body action during the throw. Some theories attempt to provide a rationale for the occurrence of these stages. Gesell claims that they are closely related to the stages of physiological development that he proposed. Kephart (1960) argues that they are closely related to cognitive and perceptual development. Kephart believes that, in order to learn skills, the child must be able to integrate the perceptual information that he/she is receiving from the environment with perception of the movement of his/her own limbs. He claimed that, as perpetual skills developed, so would motor skills.

Gallahue's life span model of motor development

One of the most recent models or theories of motor development is that put forward by David Gallahue (see Gallahue and Ozmun, 1995). Like most other theories, this is a stage theory. The two early stages, the reflexive movement phase and the rudimentary movement phase, are not of interest to us as they occur before children begin learning sports skills. In the *fundamental movement phase*, from 2 to 7 years, children learn to perform 'a variety of stabilizing, locomotor and manipulative movements, first in isolation then in combination with one another. ...They are gaining increased control in the performance of discrete, serial and continuous movements...' (Gallahue and Ozmun, 1995). The ability to combine facets of a movement is an important one and can be seen in the way children improve the quality of their motor output as they develop in this stage.

During the *specialized movement phase* (7–11 years), the individual develops the basic movements of previous phases into specific actions. Up to the age of about 14 years, the child is learning to apply fundamental movements patterns to complex skills. Whether or not this process will continue to be developed in adulthood will depend on the motivation of the person. Gallahue believes that adults will attempt to develop those skills at which they perceive themselves to be good, but not those at which they think they are poor.

Gallahue sees development as being dependent upon heredity and environment. He sees heredity as fixing the level that we can achieve. It is fixed, but the environment is not. It can be engineered to get the most out the 'hereditary pot'. This, of course, is the role of the coach. To Gallahue, lifestyle is part of the environment. In recent years, we have seen many outstanding athletes, all around the world, waste their talent because of poor lifestyles or lifestyles that are not correct for athletes.

Ecological psychology and motor development

It is difficult to differentiate between what the ecological psychologists mean by development and what they mean by learning. The ecological psychologists see both learning and development as coming about by an interaction between the individual and their environment. Therefore, all of the issues we cover in this section are also relevant to ecological theories of learning; and all that we covered in Part II, on ecological theories of learning, is relevant to motor development. According to the ecologists, motor development will take place when the person sets him/herself a goal that requires the acquisition of a new movement pattern. This goal itself will probably depend on some aspect of cognitive or social development, which leads to the desire to learn a new skill. As we saw with cognitive development, when individuals are in this situation they are in what Vygotsky would term a zone of proximal process.

Whatever causes this desire to acquire a new skill is known as a *control parameter*. A control parameter can be almost anything. Significant others, e.g. coaches and parents, often act as control parameters getting the individual to want to learn a more advanced skill. This could be an intrinsic desire to get into a team or it could even be a change in physical attributes. An increase in strength, such as during puberty, may lead the child to want to develop this new found attribute. Just moving from one level of competition to a higher level can also be a control parameter. The person can see that, if he/she is to stay at this new level, he/she must acquire more advanced skills.

Task 3 Can you think of a period in your own life where a coach or parent or friend has acted as a control parameter? Have physical changes, e.g. during puberty, ever acted as control parameters for you?

Once a person has decided that he or she wishes to acquire a new skill, by trial and error he or she attempts to achieve the goal. According to the ecological psychologists, this is possible due to self-organization; i.e., the different muscles, joints and nerves organize themselves in such a way that the person can achieve the goal. The exact way in which this occurs will vary from person to person and even from time to time. The latter is important because no two situations are identical; therefore, the details of the organization will have to change every time the person performs the skill. Physical development plays a key role in this process. For example, an adolescent may have suddenly grown tall and feel that he/she would like to learn to dunk in basketball. If his/her strength has not also developed, he/she may not be able to achieve sufficient height in the jump. Thus, they cannot yet dunk the ball. In this case we say that the strength, or lack of it, is a *rate limiter*. Rate limiters are very evident during the ageing process. As we have seen above, flexibility decreases with age and can have a major effect on how an older person performs a skill, even if he/she maintains their speed and power. Ageing goalkeepers in most sports are good examples of this. Their lessening flexibility affects their agility so that, even if they maintain all their other skills, their lack of agility lets them down.

One of the major differences between the ecological psychologists and other developmentalists is that they do not perceive change as happening in stages. They claim that change is spasmodic. The individual goes through periods of great change and periods of no change. It takes a control parameter to trigger off such a change. This change, however, is not age dependent, *per se*, but periods of time, such as puberty, will act as control parameters. To the ecological psychologists carrying out research into what 11-year-olds can do and 10-year-olds cannot is pointless. What two people can and cannot do is down to the individuals. Similarly, attempting to break a skill down to describe how different age groups perform the skill is a waste of time because each individual performs the skill differently. Moreover, no individual performs it exactly the same way each time. This is totally opposed to the information processing theorists, who claim that we develop motor programs. As we develop and learn, we acquire more and more motor programs, which are permanently stored in our brains.

Development of motor skills

Almost all motor development textbooks spend a great deal of time telling the reader what skills children can perform at different stages and how well they perform them. As I stated earlier, even some books following an ecological psychology approach do this. This is based on empirical evidence and, therefore, has a place in our examination of motor development. We must treat it with some caution, however. The research is almost invariably with North American children or occasionally Europeans. Obviously it is affected by the child's learning experiences as well as development. To Bronfenbrenner, it is measuring actualized potential only. What the child is capable of we really do not know.

By the age of 6 years normal children are *capable* of carrying out basic motor skills, such as walking, running, jumping, catching, skipping, throwing and balancing, at a mature level. I have italicized 'capable' because not all children are at this stage. They would be if they were in an environment that led to them practising these skills. Remember these are skills. They are not innate. They need to be practised. Striking follows a slightly different pattern. At 6 years old the child is capable of striking a static object, in a mature fashion, but has difficulty with a moving object. This is thought to be the result of limitations in psychomotor factors such as eye–hand and foot–eye coordination. We discuss this later.

Performance of these basic skills improves very slowly throughout child-hood, although there are massive inter-individual variations due to opportunities for practice. Boys tend to perform better than girls on all of the skills except balance, where the girls perform the better. Remember that here we are talking about performance not ability. It is very likely that there are social factors affecting the results of research. Boys, perceiving good performance as being a sign of masculinity, may try harder than girls in these tests. Following adolescence, both sexes show improved performance in all tasks. This is probably due to increases in strength, power, speed and perceptual skills. Boys remain better than girls at tasks that require speed and power, and catch up to the girls in balancing skills. Girls' greater flexibility, however, shows in their performance of gymnastic and dance skills, so much so that, in gymnastics, males and females are tested on different skills. Also in dance and ice dance males and females have different roles.

While the basic skills improve during adolescence due to increases in physio-logical factors, striking develops due to improvements in perceptual ability. Most of this improvement appears to occur in the last few years of late child-hood and the early years of adolescence. By 12 years perceptual skills are thought to be at the adult level. These changes appear to occur in line with Piagetian stages. As we saw in the last chapter, visual acuity, figure–ground perception and depth perception have reached maturity by 12 years. There are some large inter-individual differences in visual–motor coordination, however, and it does appear to be greatly affected by the individual's personal experi-ences. This falls in line with cognitivist ideas of perception. In order to develop perceptual skills, we must build up a vast amount of experience, which is held in long-term memory. We can only integrate visual and kinaesthetic informa-tion if we compare what we are perceiving at the present with similar situations held in long-term memory. To the ecological psychologists, however, this is not the case. To them, there is no recourse to memory. They explain the comparative slowness in the development of visual–motor coordination as being due to the person's need to become attuned to the affordances in the environment. This takes time. However, ecological psychologists have yet to explain exactly how this attunement occurs.

Research into the development of motor skills has tended to be carried out with children and very little with the ageing population. Some work has examined balance and shown that it deteriorates with age. This appears to be due to a slowing down of transmission of nerves in the periphery and possibly also in the brain. In general, the performance of all motor skills deteriorates throughout the late stage of adulthood. However, when this begins varies greatly between individuals, dependent on their lifestyles. Performance appears to deteriorate more due to physiological deterioration than anything else. This can be seen by watching 'old timers' sports. The games are slower and there is less power in shots etc. but the techniques are still very evident and the decision making is generally better than when they were younger. I think that deterioration in eyesight and slowing of reaction time must also have an effect, particularly on coincidence anticipation skills.

Task 4 *Younger readers should talk to people who have retired from playing a sport. Ask them which physiological and motor factors led them to retire.*

Practical implications

There are several practical implications for coaches resulting from our knowledge of physical and motor development. As we saw in the last chapter, these cannot be taken in isolation from cognitive and socio-psychological factors. Before examining these issues, we must be aware that the athletes will be greatly affected by what has happened before the coach meets them, regardless of whether they are children or older adults. With children, the years of infanthood and early childhood will provide the basis of their repertoire of skills. If this period has been one rich in experiences, the child will have developed the basic movement skills of walking, running, jumping and balancing. Moreover, their physiological development will be, at least, normal. If, however, the child is from a physically impoverished background, these qualities may not have been developed. This does not mean that the coach cannot help the child make up some of the 'lost ground'. However, it is rare that these 'lost opportunities' can be totally overcome.

There are similar problems with older adults who begin to take an interest in sport late in life. As we saw in Part II, the building up of schemas is important if skills are to be performed well. If the individual has not taken part in a variety of activities throughout their childhood and adult life, they are likely to be behind their peers and unlikely to 'catch them'. We often see this with those talking up golf late in life. If they do not have experience of hitting stationary, or even moving objects, they are at a disadvantage against the performer who has a lifetime of such activities. However, I have seen older adults benefit from taking up sport late in life. I know two long distance runners who started after the age of 40 years and are still competing seriously at 60 years old. The advantage they have is that it is all new to them, both training and competing. Many at this age have lost the desire to continue training in particular. They suffer from what might be termed 'burn-out'. Years of pushing themselves day in day out and week in week out has taken its toll and they are happy to retire. Although many maintain the desire to compete, they may well change to less physically demanding activities such as golf or lawn bowls.

Before leaving the area of basic skills, the coach should be aware that the athlete may lack these. It is doubtful whether an older adult can learn something that they should have acquired as a child. However, those in the late childhood stage, and possibly even adolescence, can be put on 'remedial' work aimed to help them acquire or perfect basic skills that are lacking. If the coach decides to do this he/she must be careful in how he/she goes about it. It is not advisable to say 'You're remedial, you need to learn to run properly'. A little imagination is needed so that the remedial learning is built into the training programme as though it were part of normal training. It can be done as part of the warm-up or cool-down. It can also be included in some obviously more complex training routine so that the learner does not even recognize it as being remedial. My experience as a coach and school teacher suggest to me that this kind of training is probably more necessary than most people imagine.

Mini-games

One of the areas of physical development that has been taken seriously by sports governing bodies is that of size. Technical directors have realized that small children cannot use full-sized equipment. The idea of a 7-year-old trying to wield a full-sized tennis racquet is absurd. While this is commonsense, we sometimes forget that factors such as the weight of the ball are also an issue. As a result, tennis governing bodies have developed the game of mini-tennis, with smaller racquets, lighter balls, smaller nets and smaller courts. These allow the children to develop the skills of the game within their own capabilities.

Conditioned games

Variations of mini-games are conditioned games such as tee-ball. Tee-ball is a version of softball with the ball placed on a tee for the batter to hit rather than being pitched to him/her. It is particularly good with children in the first stages of late childhood, who have little difficulty in hitting static objects but have problems with moving objects, due to the comparatively slow development of perceptual skills. The use of such games, however, leaves the coach with another dilemma, namely when to introduce the moving ball. There is no magical answer and coaches must use their judgment. Obviously it can be introduced gradually. The speed of the pitch can be slowly increased as the players become more proficient.

> *Task 5* *Make a list of five or six mini- and/or conditioned games that you know. How do these aid skill acquisition in children? Try to draw on what you have read in this chapter and also what you read in Part II.*

In cricket, we also see children using tennis balls rather than cricket balls due to the fact that the latter are hard and children, in general, are afraid of them. Again the problem arises with regard to when we introduce the use of the hard ball. If the children have confidence in their own ability, this can be achieved but good equipment is necessary, i.e. batting pads and good quality bats in order to lessen the fear aspect. As a child, I learned to play cricket in the back-streets with a hard ball and no padding. To some this sounds romantic and they recall the days of English cricket at it best. In reality, many children hated it and stopped playing. Many others developed bad habits such as backing away from the line of flight of the ball. Others, like me, ended up in hospital on many occasions.

American football raises a similar issue to that of cricket. It is not possible to move from flag football to full-body contact unless the equipment is available. Similarly, in ice hockey body checking requires the availably of the proper clothing. These sports and rugby also require the individual to have good technique before introducing body contact. Contact is not unduly dangerous if the person has been coached properly. The problems arise due to poor technique. There is one exception to this rule, however.

The exception in question is the problem of inter-individual differences in stages of physical development. The differences in height and weight, particularly around the 11–13-year-old groups, can be huge. As we have seen, children reach adolescence at different ages. It is not unusual to have height differences of 0.3 m (1 foot) and weight differences of 6.4 kg (14 lbs) in the same age group. The Australians and New Zealanders have recognized this in Rugby Union and have competitions based on height and weight rather than age. This is not only better for enjoyment; it is also better for skill development. You are not helping the child who can simply run through the opposition because he/she is bigger, stronger and faster than the others to develop skill. Nor are you helping the child who has skill but lacks power and speed by having them compete against more physically mature athletes. By competing against others of the same physical development they are more likely to develop their skills. Having said all of this, I can give examples of small youngsters who were very skilful and who profited from having to compete against bigger and stronger opponents. Undoubtedly this is an individual matter, and the coach must make a decision based on what he/she observes.

Gender issues

The arguments laid out above lead nicely into a similar issue, i.e. when boys and girls should compete against one another and when not. Pre-puberty, it would seem that the between sexes differences favour the girls, but are not that great. Moreover, there are probably more intra-gender differences than inter-gender differences. Therefore, the idea that boys and girls should compete together appears to be sensible. However, after puberty there are some problems. The larger body mass of the boys and greater muscle power mean that they have a physical advantage, which affects many sports. Sports that require power may be better played separately. However, there are girls whose physical and motor development mean that they would benefit from playing against the boys. I had one group of table tennis players in which the only girl was, by far, the best player. Playing against the physically stronger, but less skilful, boys helped develop her own repertoire of skills. The great American tennis player Christine Evert actually played against men when only a teenager and claimed that this helped her when she came up against the more powerful female players on the professional circuit.

Physical training

The positive effects of physical training, aerobic, anaerobic and muscular strength and endurance, in the post-pubertal child have been known for some time. The infusion of growth hormone, testosterone and other hormones at pubescence mean that, by and large, adult rules concerning training also apply to the adolescent. In boys, massive increases in androgenic steroids mean that resistance training results in large increases in muscle mass and strength. There are some potential problems with overtraining and epiphyseal damage, which we deal with later.

With the pre-pubescent child, however, it was thought for a long time that training was of little use. The lack of growth hormone and testosterone were thought to be particularly major hurdles making training inefficient. However, more recent research, and some more advanced interpretation of previous research, has shown that training can and does aid the pre-pubescent athlete. Improvements in $V_{O_2 \, max}$ have been shown but they are generally less than in adults. Although some improvements of more than 15 per cent $V_{O_2 \, max}$ have been shown, even good training programmes only appear to result in increases of between 10 and 15 per cent. The quality of the programme needs to be at least as great as in adults in intensity, frequency and duration. There is even some evidence to say that intensity needs to be greater than that in adults because children's OBLA occurs at a higher oxygen uptake value than adults.

Research has also shown that anaerobic capacity can be improved, albeit in smaller amounts than with adults. Similarly, muscle strength has been shown to improve. The surprising thing with this is that it is not accompanied by changes in muscle mass. It appears that muscle mass is heavily hormone dependent, but changes in strength performance may be due to neuromuscular adaptation and/or what Rowland (1996) termed 'intrinsic muscle force production', which includes such factors as excitation–contraction coupling. Thus, even weight resistance training can be useful with child athletes.

In the past, and even today, there is much criticism of the use of resistance training with pre-pubescent children and even with adolescents. Much of this is based on problems with epiphyseal damage. The epiphyseus is found between joints and the end of large bones. It is, in effect, an area of growth, sometimes called the growth centre or growth plate. The joint side contributes to the development of the joint surface, while the bone side or physis contributes to the longitudinal growth of the bone. Until growth stops it is cartilaginous in nature and so is lacking the strength of mature bone. The ligaments and tendons controlling the joints are stronger than the epiphyseus and so, if stress is placed on the joint, they tend to cause damage to the epiphyseus. Lifting heavy weights is one way of putting stress on the joints. As a result, many sports governing bodies recommend that only sub-maximal weights should be used. Some go as far as to say that it is better for pre-pubescent children to work against their own body resistance, e.g. doing pull-ups and press-ups rather than using weights. I am loath to take sides in this argument because I believe that a great deal more research is necessary before we can make definitive statements about this. Doctors complain that they are not able to be certain about the merits and de-merits of resistance training because there is insufficient evidence from general practitioners, hospitals and coaches concerning injuries resulting from weight training.

Another problem with epiphyseal injuries occurs due to overtraining. This is particularly a problem with activities that really stress joints. The best reported problem has been 'Little League elbow', i.e. damage to the epiphyseus in the elbow joint due to too much pitching in Little League baseball. The Little League authorities have limited the number of innings that pitchers can play in order to stop this problem. In England, the Football Association have made efforts to limit the amount of competitive football played by adolescent boys to stop overuse injuries. A major problem with epiphyseal damage is that it is notoriously difficult to diagnose. It can easily be missed. Coaches need to be aware of asking children to do too much. They need also to listen to the children. If someone complains of aches and pains you must not say 'Oh, it's only growing pains, it will go soon'. When a child complains the coach should watch the child carefully and never be afraid to err on the side of caution.

This last point brings me to a key issue with regard to physical training in children, both pre- and post-puberty. Coaches need to decide what their priorities are. How important is aerobic capacity, anaerobic fitness, power and so on for the child athlete? That is, how important is it compared to other factors such as technique and skill? We must ask ourselves whether time spent on fitness would be better spent on developing skill. As we will see in the next part of this book, we can, in fact, work on both at the same time. We need also to be very aware of the motivation of our athletes. Many game players do not like physical training and much prefer learning skills. Are we in danger of boring them with physical training? Having to do the physical work will come soon enough in adulthood; it may be better to develop skills during childhood and leave the fitness to later. If, however, we are coaching track and field athletes or swimmers then physical work is essential. These athletes, however, have generally chosen these activities because they are good at them and enjoy doing the training.

Key points

- motor developmental theorists divide childhood (2 years to puberty) into the toddler period (2 to 3 years), early childhood (3 to 5 years), middle childhood (5 to 7 years) and late childhood (7 years to puberty)

- adolescence is thought to last from puberty to 20 years

- adulthood is divided into young adulthood (20 to 40 years), middle adulthood (40 to 60 years) and older adulthood (60+ years)

- late childhood is a period of little physiological growth
  - development follows the cephalocaudal (head to toe) and proximodistal (centre to periphery) principle
  - girls develop about one year faster than boys

- during pubescence there is a growth spurt
  - girls begin puberty about two years earlier than boys
  - height, weight and muscle mass increase dramatically
  - $V_{O_2 \, max}$ increases
  - males become stronger than females
  - females remain more flexible than males

- individuals differ greatly in the timing of the onset of the ageing process
  - an active lifestyle slows the advance of old age

- lifestyle greatly affects motor development
  - lots of opportunities for activity in infancy and childhood aid motor development

- performance of specific basic skills, such as running, jumping and throwing, tend to follow set stages

- Gallahue and Ozmun identified stages of motor development
  - in the fundamental movement phase (2–7 years), the child can learn basic motor movements (e.g. gymnastic skills, swimming strokes)
  - in the specialized movement phase (7–11 years), these basic skills can be developed into complex skills (e.g. striking a ball with a bat can be developed into cricket, baseball or hockey skills)

◆ after 14 years, these skills can be refined and reach very high levels if the person continues to practise

● according to Vygotsky, children develop during periods of proximal processes, i.e. the child sets him/herself a goal, which requires the acquisition of a new movement

● factors that cause a child to enter a zone of proximal processes are called control parameters
  ◆ control parameters can be coaches or parents; an increase in strength or power; a change in the environment, such as meeting new friends

● by the age of 6 years most children are capable of carrying out basic motor skills
  ◆ at 6 years, children can strike static objects but have difficulty with moving objects

● at 12 years of age, perceptual skills are thought to be at adult level

● mini-games and conditioned games overcome some of the physiological and perceptual factors than limit performance in children

● pre-puberty, there are no reasons why boys and girls should not compete against one another
  ◆ post-puberty, boys' extra strength can cause problems in some activities

● care needs to be taken with physical training pre-puberty but it can be beneficial
  ◆ damage to the epiphyseus is a major problem
  ◆ overtraining is a problem for children.

V

Integrated Factors

Introduction

In this part of the book, we examine two major areas of coaching, namely the planning of annual programmes and integrating physiological, mental, technique/skill and tactical practice. I have included the planning of annual programmes under the title 'Integrated Factors' because it is, in essence, integrated. The athlete competes as a whole. Even if they wanted to, athletes could not separate the physical and mental aspects of their performance. Poor technique has a physiological cost. Lack of physical fitness affects the performance of skill. Anxiety can disrupt decision making and technique and so on. So athletes must train in an integrated manner. They must prepare for competition physiologically, technically and mentally. Moreover, their annual planning needs to take into account all factors that will affect their performance.

In developing the integrated warm-ups and practices outlined in Chapters 14 and 15, I have drawn heavily on the work of the late George Wardle. George was one of the first ever Football Association coaches. He worked for many years as youth team coach at Middlesborough FC. George developed a vast array of integrated practices, many of which are now in common use in football. Most have been adapted for use in other sports. I have not only stolen ideas from George. Throughout my coaching career, I have copied ideas from many coaches from a wide variety of sports. I hope that you can alter the different drills and practices, given as examples in the following chapters, to suit your own sports. I am grateful to the coaches who have provided the examples used below.

13

Developing Annual Programmes

Learning objectives

At the end of this chapter, you should

- understand the principles involved in developing an annual programme
- be able to devise an annual programme
- know how to divide your programme into phases, sub-phases and cycles.

In this chapter, we examine the nature of annual programmes and, in particular, how we go about organizing them. A history of warfare from the Ancient Greeks to the modern day shows the necessity of planning. However, the Greeks were aware that planning should not just happen immediately before the event but be an ongoing process. Coaches need to know what they intend to do throughout the coming year. Admittedly there will have to be flexibility in their planning and changes will almost certainly need to be made. However, the basic plan should be set. In most sports this will be an annual programme. However, athletes may set biannual programmes. For example, someone looking to compete in a major championship in two years time will set a programme covering that length of time. Many Olympic athletes set quadrennial programmes. One of the most successful quadrennial programmes was that used by the 1992 Olympic pursuit

Coaching Science   Terry McMorris and Tudor Hale
© 2006 John Wiley & Sons, Ltd

cycle gold medal winner Chris Boardman. At that time, I had the pleasure of sharing an office with Boardman's coach, Pete Keen. I was able to see Pete and Chris develop their programme in minute detail. Nothing was left to chance; even rest days were accounted for.

The annual programme is closely linked to goal setting (see Chapter 3). Just as goal setting is broken down into long- and short-term goals, so an annual programme is broken down into *phases*. Tudor Bompa (1999), who is generally regarded as the leading authority on annual programmes, divides the programme into three phases, the *preparatory, competitive* and *transition*. The titles for the preparatory and competitive are self-explanatory, while the transition phase represents the period between the end of one annual programme and the beginning of the next. Some authors (e.g. Galvin and Ledger, 2003) call this the *recovery* phase, as it is a recovery from competition. Bompa breaks the phases into sub-phases. The preparatory phase is divided into the *general preparation* and *specific preparation phases*. He divides the competitive phase into the *pre-competitive* and *competitive*. Some coaches see the pre-competitive sub-phase as being part of the specific preparation phase.

These sub-phases are then further broken down by Bompa into the *macro-* and *micro-cycles*. Galvin claims that there are three cycles, the macro-, *meso-* and micro-cycles. This can be confusing, but some of it is semantics. Galvin's macro-cycles are very similar to Bompa's sub-phases and his meso-cycles are similar to Bompa's macro-cycles. Regardless of the terms used, all theorists agree that programmes need to be broken down into phases or cycles, a process they call *periodization*. The annual programme itself will be closely linked to the long-term goals of the athletes and/or team, while the macro-cycle (following Bompa's approach) will reflect the short-term goals. The micro-cycle depicts the methods to be used to achieve the short-term goals. (Throughout the rest of this chapter, we will use Bompa's notion of what constitutes macro- and micro-cycles.)

Figure 13.1 shows some of the factors that the coach must take into account when determining the cycles. From the task demand point of view, the coach should use some of the methods of task analysis that we examined in Chapters 6 and 7. The coaching manuals of sport governing bodies are geared very well to this, as are most coaching award courses. Therefore, I do not perceive this as causing any difficulty. However, someone studying biomechanics, physiology and psychology may wish to analyse at a deeper level. Whether or not this level of analysis should be shared with the athletes will depend on their level of understanding. However, analysis of the athletes' strengths and weaknesses must be shared with them.

In order to analyse the athletes' fitness, the coach can take advantage of physiological testing. If there is the money available, sophisticated laboratory

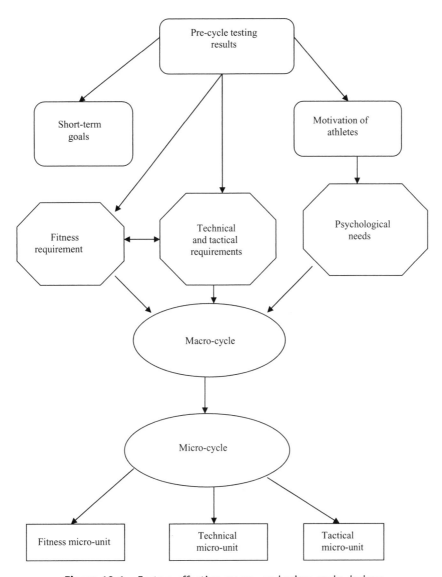

Figure 13.1   Factors affecting macro- and micro-cycle designs

based tests can be used. However, in most cases the coach will have to use field based tests, such as the bleep test. Testing is not only a very useful tool, in that it provides empirical data, but it also has a motivational effect. Most athletes like to know their level of fitness. Moreover, being naturally competitive they will compete against team-mates. If the information is used correctly, the coach can set goals and organize the cycles so that the athletes have targets to work towards in the coming weeks. Technical aspects can also be examined in the same way, although there are few really good, valid and reliable tests of technique in most sports. Psychological aspects are less easy to determine empirically and the coach may need to work on these through simply observing the athletes in practice and talking to them. However, as I stated in Part I, this may be best left to a sports psychologist.

> **Task 1** *Draw up a list of physiological and skill tests that you might want to use with a group of athletes in your own sport. Try to include some laboratory tests and some tests that can be undertaken by anyone with only a limited amount of equipment. Why have you chosen these particular tests? Try to draw on the theoretical aspects of physiology and skill acquisition that you have covered in this book when giving your answer.*

Once the baseline is known, the coach and athletes can begin working on the cycles. How much input the athletes have will depend on the leadership style of the coach and on the knowledge level of the athletes. At the very least, the athletes should know why these particular cycles have been chosen. I have seen coaches with a sound knowledge of how to periodize coaching fail to explain the periods to the athletes. The result in one case was close to catastrophic. Only the intervention of a sports psychologist stopped an athlete revolt. Once the reasoning behind the periodization was explained to the athletes, they were happy and had a successful season.

Macro-cycles

Macro-cycles can vary from 2 to 6 weeks and the annual programme will consist of between 3 and 20 macro-cycles. Each macro-cycle has a *specific* object. For example, pre-season the objective of a macro-cycle might be to work on strength training or aerobic training. A tennis player may spend one macro-cycle working on serves and the next on ground strokes. The main factor, however, is that the macro-cycles should be coordinated with one another and fit into the annual plan. They should work together to serve the aims of the annual programme. Their timing in terms of length and when they occur needs to follow the principles of training and practice that Tudor Hale covered in Part III.

The first one or two macro-cycles should form the general preparation sub-phase. As far as fitness is concerned, this is the time when an aerobic base is developed. The length of time this will take will depend on the information we receive from our pre-testing. It will also depend on how important an aerobic base is to the particular activity. As we saw in Part III, an aerobic base is vital in almost every sport but obviously is more important in say basketball or American football than in the shot putt. Muscular endurance also needs to be developed. In this phase the physical work will be low in intensity but high in duration and frequency. Strength also needs to be developed in this period, but here intensity should be high and duration short, i.e. heavy weights but with only one to three repetitions. Strength is the antecedent to power. Power is necessary for speed to be developed. Another area that can be worked at is flexibility, which is necessary for good agility.

From a technical/tactical point of view, most coaching manuals recommend that the macro-cycles, in this period, be concerned with technique. It is actually an excellent time to integrate the technical with the physical. The athlete can improve technique and at the same time be developing an aerobic base (see Chapter 15 for how this can be done). I would argue that tactical practice can also begin in this phase. As with technique, it can be done as part of the aerobic training.

Goal setting should begin in earnest at this time. Athletes are normally looking forward to the next season. They want to do well. Coaches should sit down with their athletes and work out what the goals are to be. In setting the goals, the coach and athletes should take into account the annual programme. They should decide how the goals of each macro-cycle will serve the goals of the programme. They can build in reappraisal times for the goals. These could be linked to testing or performance results. As well as goal setting, the preparatory phase allows the coach, or a sports psychologist, to work with the athletes on developing their mental skills. Remember that such things as imagery and mental rehearsal are skills. They need to be practised. It is a good time for the coach to bring in a sports psychologist and gives the psychologist time to work with the athletes in preparation for the demands of competition.

The third and fourth macro-cycles will form the specific preparatory period. In these macro-cycles everything becomes more specific. General components are phased out. Fitness work becomes greater in intensity, though frequency or duration may be lessened. Sports teams will play practice games among themselves and against other teams. Track and field athletes will take part in practice-type competitions. Tactical work in team games will become very important. The athletes will be ready to undertake anaerobic training. Strength training will give way to power work and flexibility work will be replaced by agility training.

The final macro-cycle of the preparation phase is *tapering*. If the physical aspects of training have been carried out correctly, some fatigue will be experienced by the athlete. It is pointless letting the athletes enter the competition phase tired. Therefore, a tapering period of between 10 and 21 days should occur. In this period training will be 100 per cent in intensity but the duration or frequency will be seriously cut down. How much they are cut back will depend on the initial fitness level of the athletes and the amount of training they have undertaken. If this period is correctly assessed, the athletes will be ready and raring to go come competition time.

Another set of macro-cycles makes up the *competition* phase. The nature of the macro-cycles in this phase will be greatly affected by the type of competition in which the athletes take part. There is a massive difference between the make-up of this phase for a track athlete compared with that of a team game player, who competes every week and sometimes two or three times a week. For the team game player, physical work in this phase will be maintenance. On the other hand, a track athlete may build in several macro-cycles, which are aimed at peaking for specific competitions. Thus one cycle might include intense work, followed by a tapering period and then a major competition. The next cycle will then be a short recovery one. This will be followed by another cycle of intense work, then tapering leading to a second major competition. This could happen several times in a competition phase. Figure 13.2 shows this in diagrammatic form. For all types of athlete, the coach can alter intensity, duration or frequency of training in order to achieve the aims of the macro-cycles. Goals may need to be re-assessed as a result of competition results.

Task 2 *How might the cycles in the competition phase differ between a track athlete competing intermittently and a team game player competing once or twice a week? Give an example of each.*

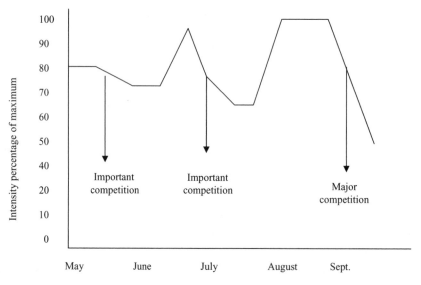

Figure 13.2 Diagrammatic representation of intensity of training in the competition phase for a track athlete

The final set of macro-cycles constitutes the *recovery* period. Athletes must rest. They must rest physically and mentally. So time has to be taken to give them a break. A complete break of some kind is recommended, but the coach must take into account the effects of detraining. It is not unusual to see team game athletes return to training overweight and having suffered massive detraining effects. At least one, probably two or three, macro-cycles in this phase should include some attempt to lessen the detraining effect. An aerobic base should be maintained as much as possible. One way this can be done is through cross-training. Athletes can work at activities that they enjoy but which help them maintain some form of aerobic fitness. While it may be more beneficial, in a purely physiological sense, to have the athletes continue training specifically, psychologically the change is beneficial. Also, some team coaches like to take their players away as a group at this time in order to try to develop social cohesion. As we have seen, social cohesion may not, in fact, be very important (see Chapter 4), but such activities can act as a motivator for the players. They feel that the club and coach value them. This can be positive in itself.

This is also the time for the coach and athletes to sit down and appraise the season or annual programme. Were the goals achieved and if not, why not? They must begin to work on next year's goals. In this period it is more important for the coach to appraise than the athlete, especially team game coaches who may need to decide whom they will retain in the team and whom they will try to bring in – new signings or draft choices. To the athletes, the beginning of the next annual programme may be a better time to appraise, before they begin goal setting for the next season.

Micro-cycles

Micro-cycles make up the macro-cycles. They last about seven days. These cycles determine the intensity, duration and frequency of physical training. They decide what technical and tactical aspects will be worked on; also whether mental practice is necessary. The micro-cycles themselves can be broken done into *micro-training units*, so a typical training session might consist of several micro-training units. The athletes may work on their technique (one unit), then tactics (another unit) and finally fitness (a third unit). This is, in fact, a typical training session for most team game players.

One aspect of micro-cycles that is often forgotten is that a cycle can include breaks from practice. In fact, a whole micro-cycle may consist of rest. Rest is very important both physically and mentally. Another factor with micro-cycles is that they might include some from of mini-tapering. This is particularly to be recommended in team games. Light training sessions one or two days before a game are more sensible than heavy ones. The player must be 'fresh' physically and mentally for the game. The other aspect of micro-cycles often forgotten is that they should include regular periods of testing fitness, assessing technical and tactical performance and ascertaining the psychological well-being of the athlete. Goals will need to be reappraised from time to time depending on the outcome of the tests and appraisals.

Task 3 Design a micro-cycle, including micro-training units, for your own sport. Using what you have learned so far, justify this design.

Summary

In planning each year or a period of time up to a major event, e.g. the Olympics, the coach should use periodization. Training and practice sessions should be divided into macro- and micro-cycles. The macro-cycle should be based around the short-term goals of the athletes and/or team. Macro-cycles should have specific aims. In the preparation phase the macro-cycles can be broadly divided into general and specific preparation cycles, and a tapering cycle. The latter will occur just prior to the beginning of competition. In turn, the macro-cycles should be broken down into micro-cycles, which are basically the weekly training and practice programmes.

Figure 13.3 is an example of an annual programme for a ladies hockey team playing at senior level. The programme is based on one kindly provided for me by my colleague at Chichester, Paul Robinson, who is coach to Chichester Ladies hockey team. (In case anyone disagrees with this programme, I must accept all of the blame as I have adapted Paul's programme. The actual programme is much more detailed – as it should be – but for the sake of brevity I have shortened it.) Macro-cycle one is the general preparation phase. Although we use the word 'general', Paul actually includes mostly hockey specific work in the micro-cycles. This has the effect of aiding motivation and does not waste valuable training and practice time. His team are amateur and time is a premium. Therefore, Paul integrates physical training and practice as much as possible. The second macro-cycle is more specific than the first and the micro-cycles become more intense in nature, although, towards the end of this macro-cycle, the duration of the physical element in the micro-cycles is decreased ready for the beginning of the season. This is, of course, tapering.

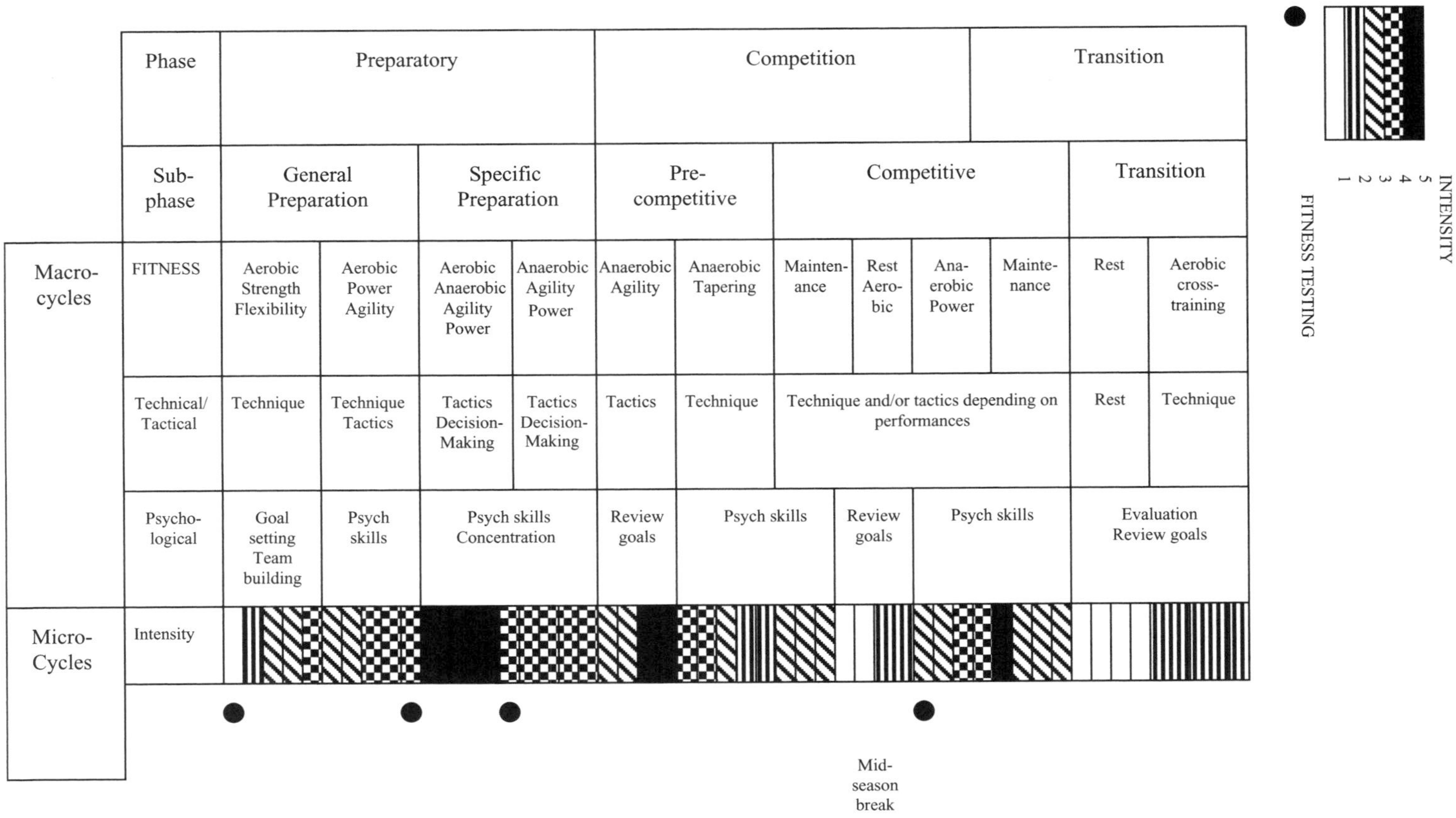

Macro-cycles	Preparatory				Competition						Transition	
Phase	Preparatory				Competition						Transition	
Sub-phase	General Preparation		Specific Preparation		Pre-competitive		Competitive				Transition	
FITNESS	Aerobic Strength Flexibility	Aerobic Power Agility	Aerobic Anaerobic Agility Power	Anaerobic Agility Power	Anaerobic Agility	Anaerobic Tapering	Mainten-ance	Rest Aero-bic	Ana-erobic Power	Mainte-nance	Rest	Aerobic cross-training
Technical/ Tactical	Technique	Technique Tactics	Tactics Decision-Making	Tactics Decision-Making	Tactics	Technique	Technique and/or tactics depending on performances				Rest	Technique
Psychological	Goal setting Team building	Psych skills	Psych skills Concentration		Review goals	Psych skills	Psych skills	Review goals	Psych skills		Evaluation Review goals	
Intensity												

Mid-season break

Figure 13.3 Annual programme based on one for a ladies hockey team

As hockey in England has a winter break around Christmas, Paul begins a new macro-cycle then. The first micro-cycle, of this period, consists of a time for recovery from the first part of the competition phase; this lasts about three weeks. There will be very little, if any, detraining effect; therefore, the ladies are ready to start intense training in the second micro-cycle. Throughout the competition phase, in both macro-cycles two and three, tactics are appraised and changed whenever necessary. Macro-cycle four begins post-season or in the recovery period. Paul makes good use of cross-training in this time.

Task 4 Draw up an annual programme for a sport of your choice. Decide on the level of competition, amount of time available for practice and age of the athletes before beginning your design.

Key points

- annual programmes should be broken down into phases
  - ◆ Bompa divides programmes into three phases, preparatory, competition and transition
  - ◆ Galvin calls the transition phase the recovery phase

- Bompa divides the preparatory phase into the general and specific preparation sub-phases and the competition phases into pre-competitive and competitive

- Bompa breaks the sub-phases into macro- and micro-cycles

- Galvin divides the sub-phases into the macro-, meso- and micro-cycles

- testing athletes' fitness and skill levels should be part of the programme

- assessing the athletes' psychological state should be part of the programme

- macro-cycles should have a specific objective

- macro-cycles should be coordinated

- an aerobic base and strength should be built up in the general preparation phase

- technique should be developed in the general preparation phase

- goal seating should be undertaken in the general preparation phase

- in the specific preparation phase, fitness work becomes more intense
  - tactics are worked on
  - strength training gives way to power training
  - the final sub-phase of the specific preparation phase should be one of tapering

- the content of the competition phase varies greatly from sport to sport

- in the recovery phase, athletes must be given a time to rest
  - appraisal of the season should take place
  - training should be maintenance
  - cross-training is useful motivationally

- micro-cycles can be broken down into micro-training units (sub-divisions of the practice session)

- micro-cycles should include breaks from training and practice

- coaches may wish to use biannual or quadrennial programmes.

14

Integrated Warm-Up

Learning objectives

At the end of this chapter, you should

- understand the nature of warm-up
- be able to devise an integrated (physiological, technical and psychological) warm-up
- know how to use warm-up to help overcome anxiety.

In Chapter 3, we examined preparation for competition purely from a psychological perspective. However, the athlete does not only perform psychologically. Athletes need to be physically ready to act. This obviously requires physiological preparation. Similarly, prevention of injury is also necessary, so joints and muscles must be readied for the rigours of competition. In this chapter, we examine how these different aspects of preparation can be worked on simultaneously during integrated preparation.

Warm-up

A story often told, true or not I do not know, is that the famous Victorian athlete C. B. Fry 'warmed up' for his world record long jump by having a glass

Coaching Science   Terry McMorris and Tudor Hale
© 2006 John Wiley & Sons, Ltd

of wine and talking to friends. Certainly until very recently warm-up has been a somewhat haphazard affair. Athletes in the highly physical sports such as track and field, swimming and cycling have been well ahead of others in their preparation for events. Warm-up has normally revolved around two major issues – to guard against injury and improve motor control. In fact, the latter is, in itself, a major factor in avoiding injury. Track and field athletes have been aware for many years that, in order to get the best from their bodies, they need to raise core temperature by at least 2 °C. They also make sure that they stretch well so that joints are not likely to cause tears in muscles and themselves be displaced.

More recently, track and field athletes have become aware of the need to incorporate, in their warm-up, some form of mental preparation. Even the highly physical sports involve having the correct mental approach as well as the physical. This is more true the higher the level of competition, where individual differences in ability are not very great. Due to the fact that most track and field athletes, cyclists and swimmers take a long time over the physical aspects of their warm-ups, they have time to carry out the mental preparation at the same time as they undertake the physical. In team games, the tendency has been to listen to an 'inspirational' team talk and do the physical warm-up separately. The skill aspects were worked at even separately from the physical, while tactical warm-up was never even thought about. At last, this is changing and not before time.

I am not suggesting that we do away with the team talk; I think that it has great value (see Chapter 3), but we must be aware that when players perform they do so as whole beings. Their physical, mental, and psychological functions do not perform in a multi-disciplinary way but in an integrated fashion. Moreover, tactics are not performed in isolation of skill and both, in turn, are not carried out without physical activity. Therefore, it is sensible to use integrated warm-ups.

Developing integrated warm-up is more complex than using a multi-disciplinary approach. The first stage is, as with annual programmes, to examine the nature of the activity in detail. Once we know what the athletes need to do in performance, we have to work out the best way to get them into the correct physical and mental states to perform at their best. During warm-up there has to be a slow progression from gentle to vigorous exercise. You could say that the beginning of the warm-up should be a warm-up for the next stage and so on. To many athletes, arriving at the event includes a lot of socializing. There are team-mates, spectators and opponents to talk to. Sometimes these are people they have not seen for some time. All of this can be off-putting. Moreover, in top class sport there may be the media to deal with and autograph hunters and so on. Often athletes have to sort out tickets for friends and relatives. It is best if these jobs can be taken from them as much as possible, but not all social activity can be done away with. The beginning of the warm-up can act as a definitive breaking point for such activity. It is like the performance routines we talked about in Chapter 5, e.g. carrying out a set routine before serving in tennis or taking a penalty kick in rugby.

The warm-up must have a definite starting point. I have seen many professional football matches in England where different players join the warm-up at different stages. More often than not they also leave it at various points. The coach should have a starting point. This can be very simple and could be a slow jog even. However, the key point at this time is that the coach is, in effect, saying to his/her athletes 'Ladies and gentlemen, the competition starts *now*'. In order to ensure that this is the case, the athletes must be put almost immediately into situations in which they have to think as well as act. This is particularly important in team games, where tactics and teamwork are involved. It is probably best not to have too many demands on cognition at this stage but having to think will start the athletes' focusing more on the event. Whether or not Aunt Agnes has got her seat in the stand can no longer be a priority.

Many athletes involved in highly physical activities like to 'tune into their own bodies' at this stage. They enjoy the gradual build-up in intensity of the physical aspects of the task. Feeling themselves perform powerfully has many psychological effects. First of all, it is the correct psychological or activity set for such an athlete. Second, it acts as a motivator and an aid to self-confidence. Team game players are generally less interested in the physical feelings. They are more concerned with skills and tactics. So at this stage, simple skill practices can be included. These may be technique practices or drills, at first, with the emphasis on concentrating on the very basic (see Figure 11.1(a) for an example). However, such activities do not require much in the way of cognition. Therefore, soon the coach must include some decision making in the drills (see Figure 14.1). In the drill shown in Figure 14.1, the players have to pass and run across the same space; therefore, they must be aware of one another. This forces them to make decisions about *when* to pass the ball, not only *how* to pass it, as in Figure 11.1. Thus the player begins to get into the correct activity set.

Task 1 *Draw up some integrated warm-ups like those shown in Figures 11.1 and 14.1 for a team games sport. Try to devise your own rather than copying some you have seen previously.*

If the intensity of the activity is increased at this time, the athlete will be ready to undertake some dynamic stretching. Dynamic stretching cannot be

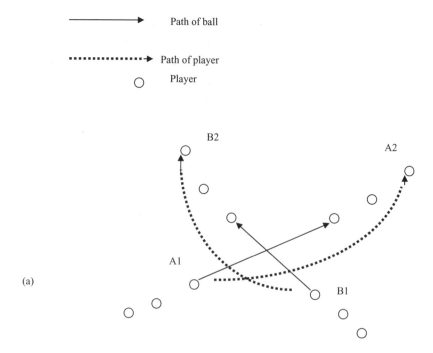

(a)

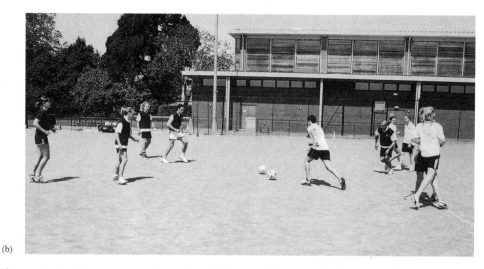

(b)

Figure 14.1   (a) A more complex passing drill shown diagrammatically. (b) A photograph of the same drill. By having to pass the ball across the central space and cross it themselves, the players need to be aware of where they are running, where the players from the other group are running and whether or not there is a clear pathway through which to pass the ball. This develops perceptual and decision-making skills

Table 14.1   Outline of warm-up used for soccer

1. Passing drill as in Figure 11.1
2. Passing drill as in 14.1 above but distances to be covered increased
3. Passing drill as in Figure 14.1 but with large distances to be covered
4. Passing drill as in 3 above but with fewer players per group, thus forcing players to run at
   ¾ pace
5. Passing drill as in Figure 11.1 but players sprint after turning
6. 3 v 1 game, one touch
7. Attack v defence phase of play

undertaken until muscles are warm and blood flow has increased. Following the dynamic stretching, the athlete can return to greater intensity of running. As they have undergone the stretching, the chances of muscle and joint damage with hard activity is greatly lessened, so they can do some sprinting. In team games, I would suggest that some sort of game is played at this stage. It can be a small sided game or a phase (attack versus defence) practice. In Table 14.1, I have outlined a warm-up used by myself for my football teams.

Task 2 What kinds of stretch would you use for your sport? Using what you have read in Part III, justify your choice.

In deciding on the length and intensity of the warm-up, the coach must take into account several factors (see Figure 14.2). As we have seen, the first of these is the nature of the activity itself. We also need to know a great deal about the athletes. Their fitness levels will affect what they can do. There is no point in having an elaborate warm-up if it places too much strain on the athletes, with the result being that they fatigue before the end of the competition. We also need to understand something about their motivation and personalities. Most track and field athletes like a long elaborate warm-up. While warming up, they are doing what they really enjoy – acting physically. Team game players, on the other hand, often see warm-ups as a necessary evil. It may be best with these athletes to keep the warm-up fairly short. Some team game players hate warming up and these people can be a problem. Injury prevention is a necessary factor in warm-up. Many game players think that stretching is the 'be all and end all' of this aspect of warm-up, but increasing blood flow and core temperature is more important. While massage can have an effect here, I would suggest that you try to explain to these people the necessity for the physical aspect of warm-up. Similarly, mental rehearsal can be used to help athletes into the correct activity set, but a mixture of the physical and mental appears to be far more beneficial. One of the reasons for this is that physical plus mental

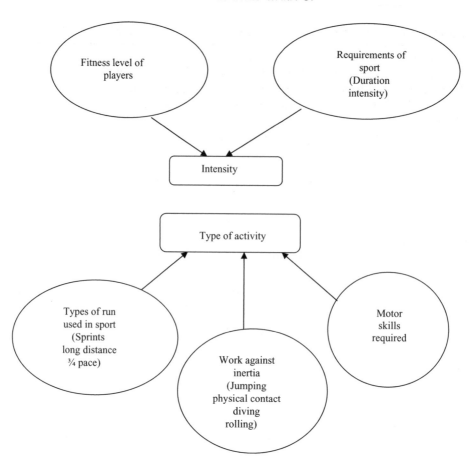

Figure 14.2   Factors to be considered when devising a warm-up

warm-up ensures that the two key aspects of arousal – the cognitive and the physiological – are dealt with. As I have just said, mental rehearsal gets the athlete into the correct way of thinking about the task – tactically and technically – while the physical increases concentrations of hormones and neurotransmitters in both the PNS and CNS.

Studies with animals have shown that exercise increases the concentrations of the neurotransmitters noradrenaline, dopamine and serotonin in the CNS. Studies with humans show some indirect evidence of this. With humans, it is not possible to use the same research techniques as with animals. Well, not without ending up in jail. Nevertheless, we know that noradrenaline, dopamine and serotonin regulate arousal and that moderate concentrations are ideal for optimal levels of performance. One of the main problems, however, in inducing increases in CNS concentrations of these neurotransmitters is the fact that research has shown that it may be necessary to work at a fairly high intensity of exercise to induce such changes. My own research (e.g. McMorris *et al.*, 1999) and that of Jan Chmura (e.g. Chmura, Nazar and Kaciuba-Uścilko, 1994) in Poland has found that we need to exercise above OBLA. This is because the neurotransmitters act in the same way as lactate and at these intensities they also show a dramatic increase in concentrations. The problem is that working at this intensity could have repercussions later in a game or competition, with fatigue setting in.

> **Task 3** *Show how you would develop a warm-up to increase physiological intensity while also increasing the technical and psychological demands.*

In an ideal world, the coach would warm up the athletes and the game or competition would begin immediately. However, in top level competition, this is not the case. There are pre-game ceremonies and conventions. Think of the poor track athlete who has warmed up to perfection only to have to wait while announcements are made, the television camera thrust into her face and so on, or the situation that international rugby and football teams regularly face, with the playing of national anthems and introduction of the teams to dignitaries. So what can the coach do in these circumstances? Mental rehearsal can be continued. Athletes can learn to remain focused. Physically, they can attempt to be as active as possible. Any chance to start running should be taken. Their muscles will not have cooled down too much and the effect of stretching should remain for some time. Wearing tracksuits will help maintain some warmth. However, noradrenaline, dopamine and serotonin dissipate quickly. Mental rehearsal should help maintain the activity set and the beginning of the action should see a return of optimal levels of these neurotransmitters fairly quickly.

Warm-up and anxiety

Carrying out the warm-up in the actual playing arena can be very useful as an aid to deal with any anxiety that may be due to performing in front of a large audience. The *actual* size of the audience is not the issue here; it is all comparative. To top class athletes a crowd of 100 000+ is not unusual, but to amateurs much smaller numbers can cause anxiety. I have seen schoolboys 'freeze' in front of crowds of less than 100. This is not surprising, as they are used to playing in front of only a handful of people. By getting out in front of the crowd to do the warm-up, they get an actual taste of what it is like. The initial fear can be dissipated to some extent. This is particularly important in away fixtures. Research has shown repeatedly that there is a home advantage. The crowd bias is thought to be a factor but only one factor. The unfamiliarity of the venue to the away team is another factor. By warming up in that environment there can be some familiarization. Admittedly this is not going to solve all problems. Simply warming up in front of a hostile crowd does not stop their hostility.

The problem of playing in front of crowds is part of the phenomenon of *social facilitation*. The original research into social facilitation was concerned with performing while in the presence of others. This was shown to have a positive effect on performance. Social facilitation research was further developed to examine the effect of a crowd or audience. It was found that, in line with drive theory, performance improved if the task was well learned, but deteriorated, or was not affected, if the task was not well learned. Research into home advantage, however, has questioned this interpretation. The home advantage occurs even with top class athletes, to whom habit strength is very high. It would appear that it is not merely an arousal issue but that other factors are having an effect. Certainly whether the audience is passive or active has an effect. It would appear that vociferous, antagonistic audiences can disrupt performance. However, some athletes are able to use crowd hostility to aid their performance. Whether or not an athlete can do this, merely becoming familiar with the presence of the crowd should be beneficial.

Substitutes warming up

One of the major problems facing substitutes, in many games, is having to enter a game when everyone else is in 'full flow'. Time and time again we see the poor substitute looking lost. Often the game appears to be 'going on around them'. In some situations there is not time or space to have a proper warm-up. So what we can we do? We know that imagery and mental rehearsal can aid preparation for performance. As imagery is best carried out in quiet and with some form of relaxation it is difficult for this to happen if the athlete is sat on the bench. I have seen some substitutes disappear into the changing rooms when they know that they are going to come into play. This is fine if there is time. In most situations, there is not. However, mental rehearsal does not need the same environmental controls. Substitutes can mentally rehearse while doing their stretches and/or aerobic activities. As we saw in Chapter 3, Sir Alex Ferguson, manager of Manchester United, claimed that Ole Gunnar Solksjaër was excellent as a substitute because he constantly followed the game and became mentally immersed in it. This allowed him to enter the action and be successful immediately.

Substitution can have extra problems in a game such as ice hockey, where players work in shifts, or American football, where there are offensive and defensive players and special teams. Not only do the players need to warm up; they need to warm down after their shift. This can be almost impossible to do in ice hockey. The player leaves the ice and immediately sits down, thus not helping lactate to dissipate. It may be beneficial for ice hockey players to stand and do some minor physical work on the spot rather than sit down. It is interesting that American footballers rarely sit on the bench; they are nearly always walking about.

Summary

Integrated physical–skill–psychological warm-up has many advantages. Pragmatically, it saves time. More importantly, it helps the athlete to control what Kahneman identified as the two major aspects of arousal – the cognitive and the physiological. The link between the physical and mental components of arousal have been known for some time, indeed since the beginning of the 20th century (Yerkes and Dodson, 1908). If carried out properly, an integrated warm-up can ensure that the athletes not only increase arousal but also develop the correct activity set. This can have a major impact on the beginning phases of team games. An integrated warm-up can also help the athlete control the negative problems of anxiety, although this will only work in conjunction with other methods.

Key points

- warm-up helps guard against injury
  - stretching should be included in the warm-up

- warm-up improves motor control
  - core temperature should be raised by 2 °C

- warm-up should include some form of mental preparation

- warm-ups should be task-specific
  - physical intensity should increase gradually

- ♦ skills and tactics can be integrated with the physical aspects
- ♦ duration, intensity and types of activity depend on the nature of the sport and fitness levels of the athletes

- warm-up should be at an intensity slightly above the lactate threshold in order to increase arousal

- warm-up can be used as an aid to combating anxiety

- substitutes may need to use mental preparation before entering the action.

15

Integrating Practice and Training

Learning objectives

At the end of this chapter, you should

- be able to develop integrated (physiological, technical and tactical) drills and practices
- design a skills/fitness circuit
- design a pressure training session.

One of the biggest problems facing coaches of amateur and part-time professional athletes and teams, in particular the latter, is finding the time to practise basic skills. Although time is less of a problem for coaches of full-time athletes, repetition of basic skills can be boring to most team game players. Game players are also notoriously indifferent to physical training, particularly training aimed at building up an aerobic base. By combining skill practice and physical training, the coach can overcome many of these problems. Many basketball players hate doing repeated sprints up and down the court, but give them a ball and have them practice lay-ups and they will run all day. Similarly, the idea of running for 10 km for rugby forwards is a nightmare. However, they will willingly cover 10 km in practice sessions involving a ball and/or scrum machine.

Coaching Science   Terry McMorris and Tudor Hale
© 2006 John Wiley & Sons, Ltd

By combining skill practice and physical training the coach can use the skill practice as 'sugar to the pill' of physical training. The training can also help to break the monotony of continuous practice of skills. It could be argued that the running or other exercise can aid the practice in the same way, as practising different skills results in a contextual interference effect. It is important that the coach has a definite aim for each session and that this is pointed out to the athletes unambiguously. The aim can be to use the skill as the 'sugar', or the skill can be the more important factor in the session, or there may be equal emphasis on both skill and technique. Moreover, coaches need to keep the aim in mind themselves. I have seen coaches forget what the aim is. If the main aim is fitness then the coach cannot be stopping the players and giving feedback on the performance of the skill. However, if the skill is the primary aim then poor performance cannot be ignored.

Skill–fitness practices

The drills that we covered in Chapter 14 can also be used as skill–fitness practices. If the coach wishes to work at the skill primarily then simply increasing the time spent on the drills should be useful, although, given that most athletes easily get bored with repetitive practice, it will be best to use several drills. The coach should be ready to change as soon as he/she sees signs of boredom setting in. The coach should also take into account variability of practice and change the nature of the drill for that reason   alone.

If the emphasis is on the physical, the coach must alter the duration and/or intensity of the drills. If the aim is aerobic training, the coach should decide how much running the athletes need to do. If we take the drills in Figures 11.1 and 14.1 as examples, the coach can work out how far the athletes will run in completing one time through the drill. They can then work out how long the athletes will need to work in order to complete the desired amount of running. The coach will also be able to decide if, and when, they will need a break and how long the break should be. Figure 15.1 shows how the addition of cones to the drill shown in 11.1 can be used to increase the distances to be run, so that the athlete has more time running at a moderate pace. Moreover, if the numbers in each row are lessened, the athlete will have to run more quickly if they are to get back into position to receive the ball when it is their turn. The latter is another way in which intensity can be increased. Fewer players in each group means that the ground must be covered more quickly. The coach must also have spare balls ready if the practice is aimed primarily at fitness, because it will break down and unplanned breaks will occur while someone goes to get the ball. Unscrupulous payers will deliberately make mistakes to get a break.

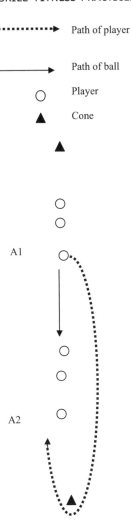

Figure 15.1 A diagrammatic version of how to develop the drill shown in Figure 11.1 in order to increase the distance run by the players

> *Task 1* *What are the typical distances and intensities of run in your sport? How much work against inertia is there required? Try to devise at least three drills that athletes could use for training.*

Skill and fitness does not only mean running while performing skills. Other aspects of fitness can be included, e.g. local muscular power and endurance. You have probably all, at some time, used skill circuits. These are ways of getting players to practice skills and they take into account the contextual interference effect. They can also be used to get lazy athletes to do fitness exercises. Figures 15.2(a)–(c) show a football player undertaking an agility/jumping

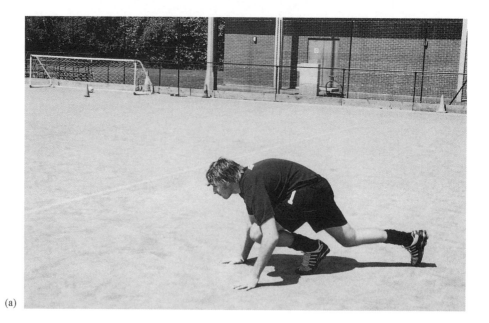

(a)

(b)

Figure 15.2 (a)–(c) A soccer player working on agility and jumping without a ball. (d) The addition of a ball in the final jump stage can increase enjoyment and add a skill aspect

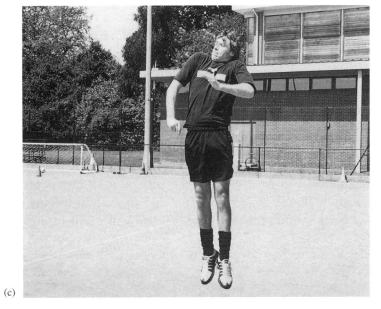

(c)

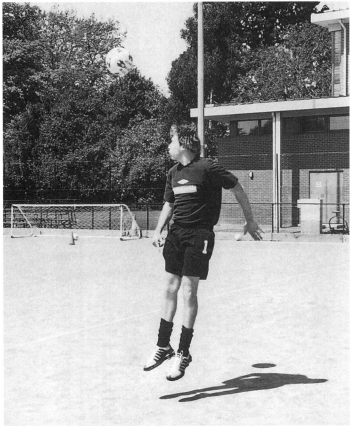

(d)

Figure 15.2 (*Continued*)

task. Figure 15.2(d) shows that if, in the jump phase, we have him head a ball, he can practise heading and make the exercise more enjoyable. Thus motivation is increased and understanding of the game is improved. Figure 15.3 shows how a ball can be used during sit-ups to achieve the same effect. These activities can also be included in drills. Figure 15.4(a) shows the football players having to jump and head the ball as an extension to the drill shown in Figure 11.1(a). We can even add some competition to these sessions. Figure 15.4(b) is the same drill as in 15.4(a) but this time the two players compete for the ball.

If we look again at the basketball skills circuit shown in Figure 6.3 we can see how these practices can be used with the emphasis on fitness rather than the skill. Obviously both will be stressed. It is easy to see that forcing the player to do the skills quickly and repeatedly for 30–40 s will result in the development

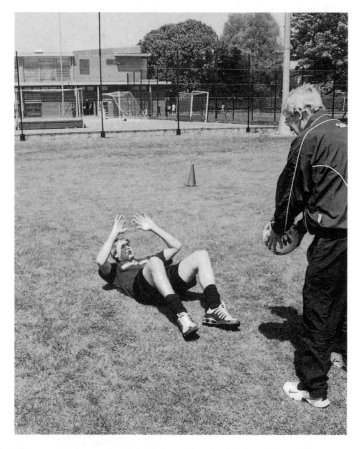

Figure 15.3   Sit-ups can be made more interesting by having the goalkeeper catch the ball. Exactly the same exercise can be used with basketball players. Soccer outfield players can be made to head the ball back to the coach

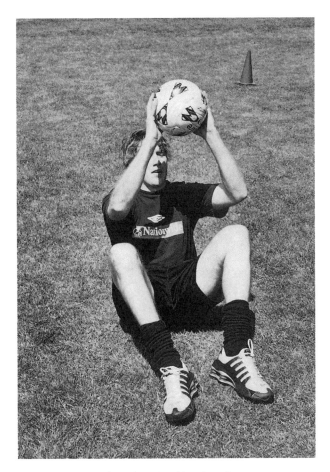

Figure 15.3 *(Continued)*

of muscular endurance and work on the energy systems. In order to add a physical component to the shooting practice shown in 6.3(b) the player would need to run from one shooting position to another as quickly as possible.

Task 2 Devise a skills/fitness circuit for your own sport.

Fitness work, however, does not only have to be in drills or circuits; fitness can be included in most practices. The great Internationale Milan football coach of the 1960s, Helenio Herrera, used to have his players practice in a full game for only one hour. However, in that time they never stopped. If a ball went out of play another was immediately put into play. Moreover, he expected everyone to work harder and faster than they would in a full 90 min game. This can also be done in any skills practices. However, it must be pointed out to the players that the emphasis has moved to fitness.

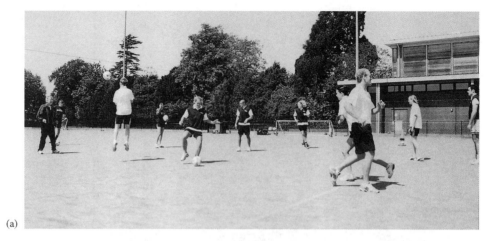

(a)

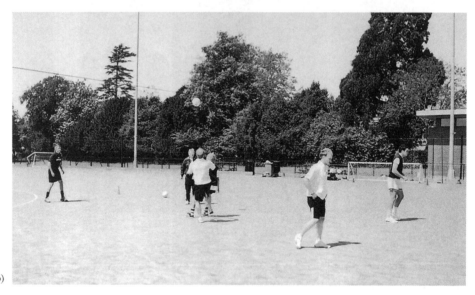

(b)

Figure 15.4   (a) The same drill as in Figure 11.1 except that, when the passer reaches the back of the line, he must jump and head a ball fed to him by the coach. (b) is similar except that the passers coming from the near and far groups compete for *one* ball fed by the coach

One of the major effects of using skill and training combined is that athletes actually practice and train in sport-specific contexts. Hockey players have to run with the stick in hand, while rugby players run while carrying the ball. The biomechanics of these techniques is different to running without the stick or ball. Yet we often see hockey and rugby players undertaking training that does not take into account what they have to do in a game. Of course, this applies to other sports. How many cricketers practice running carrying a bat and wearing pads? The principle of specificity of practice applies both to skill acquisition and physical training.

Skill–perceptual training

The skill drills outlined above can be used to practice both technical skills and perceptual skills. While the latter is far better coached and practiced in real game situations, for coaches with limited time and facilities it may be useful to use integrated skill–perceptual practice. I do not believe that this can be done if the athletes have not previously been introduced to the skill in real sport-specific situations. However, some generic factors can be practised. In Chapter 14, I showed a drill (see Figure 14.1) that forces the players to 'get their heads up' and look round at where the others players are positioned. From an ecological psychology perspective, they have to search for affordances to pass the ball. These affordances disappear if someone is in the way. To the information processing theorists they are improving their selective attention and building up a long-term memory store with regard to the timing of the pass. They also get into the habit of searching the environment. However, psychologists are a little divided as to whether this will transfer into the real game.

As we saw in Chapter 7, transfer of training refers to the effect that practice on one task has on the learning or performance of another task. The kind of transfer that we are talking about is intra-class transfer. Intra-class transfer is when there is transfer between variations of the same task. However, transfer does not always occur. In Figure 14.1 the player is trying to decide when to pass (timing) and pass accurately (accuracy). This is the same as happens in the game, therefore there would be some transfer. Admittedly there are differences between the two tasks, but the timing and accuracy of the pass are the same. According to Holding (1976), positive transfer will occur when a new but similar stimulus requires the use of a well learned response. In our drill in Figure 14.1 the response, passing the ball, is the same as in a game, but the stimulus is slightly different. That is, in the drill the ball has to be passed to someone who is not being marked by opponents and who is standing still. The stimulus, however, is sufficiently similar to what happens in a game for transfer to occur.

To the ecological psychologists, moving from drills to the game should be simple. All you are doing is changing the task constraints. As long as the athlete knows that he/she must search for affordances that are somewhat different in the actual game, there will be no problem. However, the players will have had to have been introduced to sport-specific situations prior to undertaking the drill if they are to know which affordances to search for in the game. This is not dissimilar to the claim of the information processing theorist Bryant J. Cratty (1967), who argued that transfer will only occur *if the athletes are informed as to how what they are practising will transfer to the game.* This last point also has major implications with regard to motivation. If the athletes understand the nature of the drill, they are more likely to work at it with enthusiasm.

Performing skills when fatigued

Just by observing individuals trying to perform skills when they are fatigued, we know that it is not easy. However, how often do performers practise their skills when they are in a state of fatigue? Fatigue results in a breakdown of neurotransmitters, an increase in lactate concentrations and glycogen depletion in the body. It also affects cognitive performance. Fatigue causes increases in the neurotransmitters noradrenaline, dopamine and serotonin in the CNS. In most texts, it is stated that these increases result in overarousal and a deterioration in perceptual and decision-making performance. However, research findings do not fully support this. Most of the research examining this has used tasks such as reaction time tests or decision-making tests that do not require the athlete to do anything physical. The little research that has examined the effect on tasks requiring both a motor and a cognitive response, as skill does, do show a negative effect of fatiguing exercise.

Allen Wade (1967) suggested that coaches should occasionally have their players carry out a heavy training session and follow it with skill practice. He believed that, in this way, the athletes would get used to performing while fatigued and that this would lessen the debilitative effect. Despite this, it is something one rarely sees and there is no actual research to support Wade's argument. However, commonsense suggests that it is correct. I have carried out a lot of research into the effect of exercise on cognition and my research suggests strongly that, as we become familiar with the stressor, i.e. the fatigue, we become less negatively affected by it. It is not in the scope of a text like this to go into the psychophysiology of exercise other than to say that it is possible that, when the individual is familiar with feeling fatigued, the CNS produces less noradrenaline, dopamine and serotonin and hence we do not become overaroused.

Perhaps most importantly of all, however, are the biomechanical changes that occur. When we are fatigued our range of movements changes. The recruitment of motor units becomes different. Therefore, we have to alter the nature of the movement: not a great deal, but we do alter it. Watch someone performing a skill when fresh and when fatigued. You can actually see the differences even with the naked eye. According to schema theory, we have altered the response parameters. To the ecological psychologists, our organismic constraints have changed and so our self-organization must change. If we practise while fatigued, the athlete becomes used to performing in this way. The 'new' movement patterns become more established and the deterioration in performance is less. Note that I am not saying that we can eliminate the debilitating effect of fatigue, but we may be able to limit it.

As well as championing the use of practising kills while fatigued, Wade was a great supporter of *pressure training*. Figure 15.5 shows the use of pressure training. The players are working on their defensive skills. They work non-stop for a set amount of time. It is rare that they can manage more than 60–90 s. They must repeatedly perform the task as quickly and efficiently as possible. Although players get better as they use this method of training, the skill still eventually breaks down due to fatigue.

Task 3 *Devise two or three pressure training sessions for your own sport.*

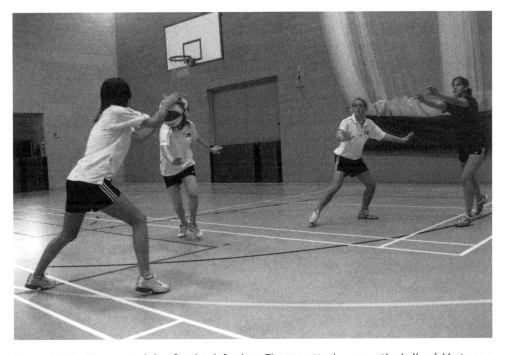

Figure 15.5 Pressure training for the defenders. The two attackers pass the ball quickly to one another repeatedly and the two defenders have to quickly change position. This lasts for 1 min. The intensity of the drill can be increased by speeding up the passing

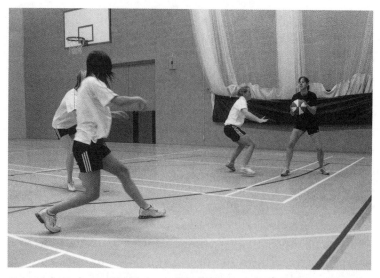

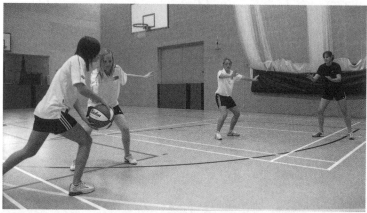

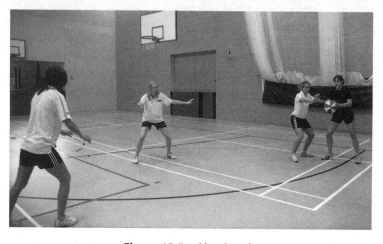

Figure 15.5   (*Continued*)

Practising skills under stress

As we saw in Chapter 3, a moderate amount of stress can be beneficial to performance, but above that it is normally negative. Under stress, the same psychophysiological effects are experienced by the CNS as outlined in the previous section, but with the addition of increases in cortisol. Moreover, even peripherally there can be problems. Stress can lead to antagonist muscles contracting, with the result that movements become less well coordinated. However, athletes must perform when under stress. Practising skills, or even playing practice games, under stress is very useful. However, inducing stress, other than physical stress, is notoriously difficult.

Large crowds can be a source of stress, particularly for those not used to this situation. Teams and individual athletes can practise with crowd noises being transmitted over public address systems. This acts as a form of inoculation. It is not the same as will be found in the real game but at least it provides some exposure to what the athlete will have to experience. Players can carry out drills with fines being imposed if they make an error in order to increase stress. Of course, one must be careful with this. I suggest that it is used once and no fines are actually collected. 'Punishments' in the form of doing extra physical training are also possible. I do not like this because it suggests that physical training is negative. However, other minor but irritating punishments can be used, e.g. cleaning out the changing rooms, cleaning footwear. Another method is to let the public into training sessions. If there are players who are easily put off by negative comments from spectators, the coach can instigate this by getting accomplices in the crowd to start barracking the player. It is probably best if this is only used following discussion with a sports psychologist. This method of anxiety control, called *implosion*, does work if carried out under control. One must be careful not to go too far and negatively affect the athlete. It will only work if the athlete is being unrealistically self-conscious and temperamental.

Rehabilitation and tactical practice

I am not aware of any coaches who attempt to have injured athletes practise an aspect of skilful performance during periods of rehabilitation. One area that is open to practice during rehabilitation is the tactical and/or decision-making aspect of skill. The Canadian ice hockey coach, Charles Thiffault, put forward this idea as far back as the 1970s (Thiffault, 1978). Thiffault suggested that while doing their rehabilitation training the players could use tachistoscopic presentations of game situations to aid their decision making. Thiffault developed a series of slides of typical ice hockey game situations and showed them to the players using a slide projector fitted with a tachistoscopic timing device (hand timing could be used). He could show the slides for anything from 0.5 s upwards. The injured player had to say whether the player with the puck should skate, shoot or pass. They were told to answer as quickly and accurately as possible. Thiffault claimed that this method was successful in improving skilful decision making. Moreover, it made the rehabilitation training more pleasant for the athlete. Working on a cycle ergometer while having to make decisions is better than simply looking at the wall or the physiotherapist (the latter will, of course, depend on the physiotherapist).

Since Thiffault's work using tachistoscopes, technology has developed. The Belgians Werner Helsen and Jan Pauwels (1988) developed videos of game situations and froze the action at the point when the decision was to be made. This is more realistic than the tachistoscope. Moreover, more options were added for the player, e.g. dribble. Paul Ward and Mark Williams (2003) provided empirical evidence for the use of video training in improving football goalkeepers' ability to save penalty kicks. Williams has developed many videos covering a variety of perceptual skills. I have further developed Thiffault's original decision-making work to include decisions to be made for a player not in possession of the ball, e.g. a defender or a team-mate of the player in possession (McMorris and Graydon, 1996). It is therefore possible to actually work on skills, or rather the cognitive and perceptual aspects of skills, with players who are undertaking rehabilitation training.

Task 3 *What kinds of tachistoscopic and/or video test might you use in your sport?*

Summary

Practising skills and undertaking physical training at the same time can save time and improve motivation for physical training. The skill takes the athletes' minds off the physical stress of training. Not only is undertaking physical work while running or doing some other form of exercise less boring, but also the physical activity can result in a contextual interference effect. The most common skill–fitness types of practice are drills, but fitness and skill can be worked on simultaneously in game situations.

Practising skills while undertaking fatiguing exercise, in drills or using pressure training, is another use of integrated practice. This kind of practice can result in the negative effects of the fatigue becoming somewhat lessened. It would appear that familiarity with the physical stress results in less of a psychophysiological reaction in the CNS. A final use of integrated practice is with athletes rehabilitating from injury. Although this was put forward by Thiffault in the 1970s, it is rarely used but has great potential.

Key points

- duration and intensity of the drills and practices depend on the requirements of the sport
    - the types of activity should be sport specific: this may mean hockey players running while carrying sticks; American footballers wearing all their equipment
    - intensity can be altered by lengthening the distances to be covered
    - intensity can be altered by changing the number of players in each group

- skill circuits can be combined with physical circuits

- decision making can be incorporated into drills
    - for this to transfer to the real activity, athletes need to be informed as to how it will transfer

- athletes should practise performing skills while fatigued
    - pressure training can do this
    - occasionally athletes should undertake heavy physical exercise before beginning skill and/or tactical practice

- occasionally practice should take place in front of an audience
    - this helps athletes perform when under the pressure of being assessed by spectators

- tachistoscopic and video tests of perceptual tasks can be undertaken by athletes when training in order to rehabilitate from injury.

References

Adams, J. (1976). Player analysis: is it worth it? *Soccer Insight*, 2, 20–21.

Albrecht, P. R. and Feltz, D. L. (1987). Generality and specificity of attention related to competitive anxiety and sport performance. *Journal of Sport Psychology*, 9, 231–248.

Allard, F., Graham, S. and Paarsalu, M. E. (1980). Perception in sport: basketball. *Journal of Sport Psychology*, 2, 14–21.

Allard, F. and Starkes, J. M. (1980). Perception in sport: volleyball. *Journal of Sport Psychology*, 2, 22–33.

Anderson, J. R. (1982). Acquisition of cognitive skill. *Psychological Review*, 89, 369–406.

Åstrand, P.-O. and Rodahl. K. (1986). *Textbook of work physiology*, 3rd ed. McGraw-Hill: Singapore.

Bandura, A. (1977). Self-efficacy: Toward a unifying theory of behavioral change. *Psychological Review*, 84, 191–215.

Barrow, J. C. (1977). The variables of leadership: a review and conceptual framework. *Academy of Management Review*, 2, 231–251.

Battig, J. W. (1979). The flexibility of human memory. In L. S. Cermak and F. L. M. Craik (Eds.), *Levels of processing in human memory* (pp. 23–44). Erlbaum: Hillsdale, NJ.

Bompa, T. O. (1999). *Periodization: theory and methodology of training*, 4th ed. Human Kinetics: Champaign, IL.

Bredermeier, B. J. and Shields, D. L. (1986). Game reasoning and interactional morality. *Journal of Genetic Psychology*, 147, 257–275.

Bronfenbrenner, U. (1989). Ecological systems theory. In R. Vasta (Ed.), *Six theories of child development: Revised formulations and current issues* (pp. 185–246). JAI Press: Greenwich, CT.

Bronfenbrenner, U. and Ceci, S. J. (1994). Nature–nurture reconceptualized in developmental perspective: A bioecological model. *Psychological Review*, 101, 568–586.

Burke, V. and Collins, D. (1996). Physical challenge and development of conflict management skills. In J. Annett and H. Steinberg (Eds.), *How teams work in sport and exercise psychology* (pp. 49–56). British Psychological Society: Leicester.

Butler, R. J. and Hardy, L. (1992). The performance profile: theory and application. *The Sport Psychologist*, 6, 253–264.

Carr, G. (2004). *Sport mechanics for coaches*, 2nd ed. Human Kinetics: Champaign, IL.

Carron, A. V. (1984). Cohesion in sports teams. In J. M. Silva and R. S. Weinberg (Eds.), *Psychological Foundations of Sport* (pp. 340–351). Human Kinetics: Champaign, IL.

Chelladurai, P. and Saleh, S. D. (1978). Preferred leadership in sport. *Canadian Journal of Applied Sport Sciences*, 2, 9–14.

Chmura, J., Nazar, K. and Kaciuba-Uścilko, H. (1994). Choice reaction time during graded exercise in relation to blood lactate and plasma catecholamines thresholds. *International Journal of Sports Medicine*, 15, 172–176.

Cratty, B. J. (1967). *Movement behavior and motor learning*, 1st Ed. Lea and Febiger: Philadelphia, PA.

Duda, J. L. (1989). Relationship between task and ego orientation and the perceived purpose of sport among high school athletes. *Journal of Sport and Exercise Psychology*, 11, 318–335.

Easterbrook, J. A. (1959) The effect of emotion on cue utilization and the organization of behavior. *Psychological Review*, 66, 183–201.

Ekblom, B., Åstrand, P-O., Saltin, B. and Wallstrom, B. (1968). Effect of training on circulatory response to exercise. *Journal of Applied Physiology*, 24, 518–528.

Ekblom, B. and Hermansen, L. (1968). Cardiac output in athletes. *Journal of Applied Physiology*, 25, 619–625.

Ericsson, K. A., Krampe, R. T. and Teschrömer, C. (1993). The role of deliberate practice in the acquisition of expert performance. *Psychological Review*, 100, 363–406.

Eysenck, M. W. and Calvo, M. G. (1992). Anxiety and performance: the processing efficiency theory. *Cognition and Emotion*, 6, 409–434.

Fiedler, F. E. (1967). *A theory of leadership effectiveness*. McGraw-Hill: New York.

Fitts, P. M. and Posner. M. I. (1967). *Human performance*. Brooks/Cole: Belmont, CA.

Gallahue, D. L. and Ozmun, J. C. (1995). *Understanding motor development*. Brown and Benchmark: Madison, WI.

Galvin, B. and Ledger, P. (2003). *A guide to planning programmes*. SportsCoachUK: London.

Gesell, A. (1945). *The embryology of behavior*. Harper: New York.

Gibson, J. J. (1979). *The ecological approach to visual perception*. Houghton Mifflin: Boston, MA.

Gill, D. L. (1993). Competitiveness and competitive orientation in sport. In R. N. Singer, M. Murphey and L. K. Tennant (Eds.), *Handbook of research on sports psychology* (pp. 314–327). Macmillan: New York.

Gruber, J. J. and Gray, G. R. (1981). Factor patterns of variables influencing cohesiveness at various levels of basketball competition. *Research Quarterly for Exercise and Sport*, 52, 19–30.

Hale, B. D. (1982). The effects of internal and external imagery on muscular and ocular concomitants. *Journal of Sport Psychology, 4,* 379–387.

Hale, T. (2003). *Exercise physiology – A thematic approach*. Wiley: Chichester.

Hanin, Y. L. (1989). Interpersonal and intragroup anxiety. Conceptual and methodological issues. In D. Hackfort and C. D. Spielberger (Eds.), *Anxiety in sports: An international perspective* (pp. 19–28). Hemisphere: Washington, DC.

Hardy, L. and Parfitt, G. (1991). A catastrophe model of anxiety and performance, *British Journal of Psychology*, 82, 163–178.

Hay, J. G. (1993). *The biomechanics of sports techniques*, 4th ed. Prentice-Hall: Englewood Cliffs, NJ.

Haywood, K. M. and Getchell. (2001). *Life span motor development*, 3rd ed. Human Kinetics: Champaign, IL.

Helsen, W. and Pauwels, J. M. (1988). The use of a simulator and training of tactical skills in soccer. In T. Reilly, A. Less, K. Davids and W. J. Murphy (Eds.), *Science and football* (pp. 493–497). Spon: London.

Helsen, W. F., Starkes, J. L. and Hodges, N. J. (1998). Team sports and the theory of deliberate practice. *Journal of Sport and Exercise Psychology*, 20, 12–34.

Holding, D. (1976). An approximate transfer surface. *Journal of Motor Behavior*, 8, 1–9.

Horne, T. and Carron, A. V. (1985). Compatibility in coach–athlete relationships. *Journal of Sports Psychology*, 7, 137–149.

House, R. J. (1971). Path goal theory of leader effectiveness. *Administrative Science Quarterly*, 16, 321–339.

Hughes, M. and Franks, I. M. (1994). Dynamic patterns of movement of squash players of different standards in winning and losing rallies. *Ergonomics*, 37, 23–29.

Hull, C. L. (1943). *Principles of behavior*. Appleton–Century–Crofts: New York.

Humphreys, M. S. and Revelle, W. (1984). Personality, motivation and performance: a theory of the relationship between individual differences and information processing. *Psychological Review*, 91, 153–184.

Jones, G. and Swain, A. (1995). Predispositions to experience debilitative and facilitative anxiety in elite and nonelite performers. *The Sport Psychologist*, 9, 201–211.

Jones, G., Swain, A. and Hardy, L. (1993). Intensity and direction dimensions of competitive state anxiety and relationships with performance. *Journal of Sport Sciences*, 11, 525–532.

Jowett, S. and Ntoumanis, N. (2004). The Coach–Athlete Relationship Questionnaire (CART-Q) development and initial validation. *Scandinavian Journal of Medicine and Science in Sports*, 14, 245–257.

Judd, C. H. (1908). The relation of special training to general intelligence. *Educational Review*, 36, 28–42.

Kahneman, D. (1973). *Attention and effort*. Prentice-Hall: Englewood Cliffs, NJ.

Keele, S. W. (1968). Movement control in skilled motor performance. *Psychological Bulletin*, 70, 387–403.

Kephart, N. C. (1960). *The slow learner in the classroom*. Merrill: Columbus, OH.

Kerr, R. (1982). *Psychomotor learning*. Saunders: Philadelphia, PA.

Knudson, D. V. and Morrison, C. S. (1997). *Qualitative analysis of human movement*. Human Kinetics: Champaign, IL.

Kohlberg, L. (1976). Moral stages and moralization: the cognitive developmental approach. In T. Lickona (Ed.), *Moral development and behavior: theory, research and social issues* (pp. 31–53). Holt, Rinehart and Winston: New York.

Lee, T. D. and Magill, R. A. (1983). The locus of contextual interference in motor skill acquisition. *Journal of Experimental Psychology: Learning, Memory and Cognition*, 9, 730–746.

Lees, A. (2002). Technique analysis in sports: a critical review. *Journal of Sports Sciences*, 20, 813–828.

Lyle, J. (1999). Coaches' decision making. In N. Cross and J. Lyle (Eds.), *The coaching process: Principles and practice for sport* (pp. 210–232). Butterworth Heinemann: Oxford.

Magill, R. A. (1993). *Motor learning: Concepts and applications.* Brown and Benchmark: Madison, WI.

Martens, R. (1975). *Social psychology and physical activity.* Harper and Row: New York

Martens, R. (1977). *Sport competition anxiety test.* Human Kinetics: Champaign, IL.

Martens, R. (1982). *Sport competition anxiety test.* Human Kinetics: Champaign, IL.

Martens, R. (1987). *Coaches guide to sport psychology.* Human Kinetics: Champaign, IL.

Martens, R. and Peterson, J. A. (1971). Group cohesiveness as a determinant of success and member satisfaction in team performance. *International Review of Sports Sociology*, 6, 49–61.

Martens, R., Vealey, R. S. and Burton, D. (1990). *Competitive anxiety in sport.* Human Kinetics: Champaign, IL.

Masters, R. S. W. (2000). Theoretical aspects of implicit learning in sport. *International Journal of Sport Psychology*, 31, 530–541.

McClelland, D. C., Atkinson, J. W., Clark, R. W. and Lowell, E. L. (1953). *The achievement motive.* Appleton–Century–Crofts: New York.

McMorris, T. (1999). Cognitive development and the acquisition of decision-making skills. *International Journal of Sport Psychology*, 30, 151–172.

McMorris, T. (2004). *Acquisition and performance of sports skills.* Wiley: Chichester.

McMorris, T. and Graydon, J. (1996). The effect of exercise on soccer decision-making tasks of differing complexities. *Journal of Human Movement Studies*, 30, 177–193.

McMorris, T., MacGillivary, W. W., Sproule, J. and Lomax, J. (2006). Cognitive development and performance of 11, 13 and 15 year olds on a soccer-specific test of decision making. *International Journal of Sport and Exercise Psychology*, 4, in press.

McMorris, T., Myers, S., MacGillivary, W. W., Sexsmith, J. R., Fallowfield, J. and Graydon, J. (1999). Exercise, plasma catecholamine concentrations and decision-making performance of college soccer players on a soccer specific test. *Journal of Sports Science*, 17, 667–676.

Mosston, M. and Ashworth, S. (1994). *Teaching physical education*, 4th ed. Macmillan: New York.

Nacson, J. and Schmidt, R. A. (1971). The activity-set hypothesis for warm-up decrement. *Journal of Motor Behavior*, 3, 1–15.

Newell, K. M. (1986). Constraints on the development of coordination. In M. G. Wade and H. T. A. Whiting (Eds.), *Motor development in children: Aspects of coordination and control* (pp. 341–360). Nijhoff: Dordrecht.

Nicholls, J. G. (1978). Development of concepts of effort and ability, perception of academic attainment, and understanding that difficult tasks require more ability. *Child Development*, 49, 800–814.

Nicholls, J. G. (1984). Achievement motivation: conceptions of ability, subjective experience, task choice, and performance. *Psychological Review*, 91, 328–346.

Nideffer, R. M. (1976). Test of Attentional and Interpersonal Style. *Journal of Personality and Social Psychology*, 34, 394–404.

Osgood, C. E. (1949). The similarity paradox in motor learning. *Psychological Review*, 56, 132–143.

Pascual-Leone, J. (1970). A mathematical model for the transitional rule in Piaget's developmental stages. *Acta Psychologica*, 32, 301–345.

Piaget, J. (1952). *The origins of intelligence in children*. International Universities Press: New York.

Piaget, J. (1969). *The psychology of the child*. Basic: New York.

Reilly, T. and Thomas, V. (1976). A motion analysis of work rate in different positional roles in professional football match play. *Journal of Human Movement Studies*, 2, 87–97.

Roberts G. C. (1993). Motivation in sport: Understanding and enhancing the motivation and achievement of children. In R. N. Singer, M. Murphey and L. K. Tennant (Eds.), *Handbook of research on sports psychology* (pp. 405–420). MacMillan: New York.

Roth, D., Slone, M. and Dar, R. (2000). Which way cognitive development? An evaluation of the Piagetian and the domain-specific research programs. *Theory and Psychology*, 10, 353–373.

Rowland, T. W. (1996). *Children's exercise physiology*. Human Kinetics: Champaign, IL.

Schmidt, R. A. (1975). A schema theory of discrete motor skill learning. *Psychological Review*, 82, 225–260.

Schutz, W. C. (1966). *The interpersonal underworld*. Science and Behavior: Palo Alto, CA.

Schwartz, G. E., Davidson, R. J. and Coleman, D. J. (1978). Patterning of cognitive and somatic processes in the self-regulation of anxiety: Effects of meditation vs. exercise. *Psychosomatic Medicine*, 40, 321–328.

Shea, J. B. and Morgan, R. L. (1979). Contextual interference effects on the acquisition, retention and transfer of a motor skill. *Journal of Experimental Psychology: Human Learning and Memory*, 5, 179–187.

Singer, R. N. (1968). *Motor control and human performance*, 1st ed. Macmillan: London.

Smith, R. E., Smoll, F. L. and Schutz, R. W. (1990). Measurement correlates of sport specific cognitive and somatic trait anxiety: The Sport Anxiety Scale. *Anxiety Research*, 2, 263–280.

Smodlaka, V. N. (1978). Cardiovascular aspects of soccer, *Physician and Sports-medicine*, 6, 66–70.

Spence, K. W. (1958). A theory of emotionally based drive and its relation to performance in simple learning situations. *American Psychologist*, 13, 131–141.

Spielberger, C. D. (1971). Trait–state anxiety and motor behaviour. *Journal of Motor Behavior*, 3, 265–279.

Stadulis, R. E., Eidson, T. A. and McCracken, M. J. (1994). A children's form of the competitive State Anxiety Inventory (CSAI-2). *Journal of Sport and Exercise Psychology*, *16*, S109.

Thiffault, C. (1978). Tachistoscopic training: an aid to improve hockey players' visual perception of tactical situations. Paper presented at the CIAU Hockey Seminar, Moncton, NB.

Thorndike, E. L. (1927). The law of effect. *American Journal of Psychology*, *29*, 212–222.

Tortora, G. J. and Graboswki, S. R. (2003). *Principles of anatomy and physiology*, 10th ed. Wiley: New York.

Tuckman, B. W. (1965). Developmental sequences in small groups. *Psychological Bulletin*, *63*, 384–399.

Turvey, M. T. (1992). Ecological foundations of cognition: invariants of perception and action. In H. Pick, P. Van Den, and D. Knill (Eds.), *Cognition: Conceptual and methodological issues* (pp. 85–117). American Psychological Association: Washington, DC.

van Geert, P. (1993). A dynamics systems model of cognitive growth: Competition and support under limited resource conditions. In E. Thelen and L. Smith (Eds.), *A dynamic systems approach to development: Applications* (pp. 265–331). MIT Press: Cambridge, MA.

Vealey, R. S. (1986). Conceptualization of sport-confidence and competitive orientation – preliminary investigation and instrument development. *Journal of Sport Psychology*, *8*, 221–246.

Vygotsky, L. S. (1978). *Mind in society*. Harvard University Press: Cambridge, MA.

Wade, A. (1967). *The Football Association guide to training and coaching*. Heinemann: London.

Ward, P. and Williams, A. M. (2003). Perceptual and cognitive skill development in soccer: The multidimensional nature of expert performance. *Journal of Sport and Exercise Psychology*, *25*, 93–111.

Welford, A. T. (1968). *Fundamentals of skill*. Methuen: London.

Widmeyer, W. N., Brawley, L. R. and Carron, A. V. (1990). *The measurement of cohesion in sport teams: The Group Environment Questionnaire*. Sports Dynamics: London, ON.

Wild, M. (1938). The behavior patterns of throwing and some observations concerning its course of development in children. *Research Quarterly for Exercise and Sport*, *9*, 20–24.

Yerkes, R. M. and Dodson, J. D. (1908). The relation of strength of stimulus to rapidity of habit formation. *Journal of Comparative Neurology and Psychology*, *18*, 459–482.

Yukelson, D., Weinberg, R. and Jackson, A. (1984). A multidimensional group cohesion instrument for intercollegiate basketball teams. *Journal of Sport Psychology*, *6*, 103–117.

Index

Coaching Science   Terry McMorris and Tudor Hale
© 2006 John Wiley & Sons, Ltd